Dose-Exposure-Response Modeling

This thoroughly revised and updated new edition reflects the progress that has been made in dose-exposure-response (DER) modeling. As the title suggests, the new edition covers more topics on dose and dose adjustment. A large part of the book has been rewritten, including an updated Bayesian analysis and modeling chapter with new materials on approximate Bayesian modeling with misspecified models, Bayesian bootstrap for the "cut-the-feedback" approach, and meta-regression with Stan codes for implementation. Two new chapters in this edition include one on causal DER modeling, with an introduction to the concept of causal DER relationship, approaches such as the generalized propensity score and instrumental/control function approaches for adjustment for observed and unobserved confounders, and Bayesian causal DER modeling. Another new chapter is dedicated to learning DER relationships with the concept and methods of machine learning, including applications to adaptive dose finding trials by bandits, contextual bandits, and Thompson sampling with Bayesian bootstrap, adaptive control for tracking using a dynamic model with an application for individual warfarin dosing. The new appendix contains non-standard materials used in the book.

Applied statisticians and modelers can find details on how to implement new approaches, while researchers can find topics for or applications of their work. In addition, students can see how complicated methodology and models are applied to practical situations.

Key Features:

- Provides SAS, R, and Stan codes that will enable readers to test the approaches in their own scenarios.
- Gives a systematic treatment of concepts and methodology.
- Helps with understanding concepts and evaluating the performance of new methods, particularly those in Chapters 7, 8, and 9.
- Includes a large amount of R codes for methods introduced in the new materials in chapters on Bayesian analyses, causal inference, and dose-adjustment.
- Includes a simulation to show how some complex methods such as generalized propensity score adjustment and adaptive dose adjustment can be implemented with simple codes.

Jixian Wang is a statistical methodologist in Bristol Myers Squibb, Switzerland. He has worked on drug development for over 20 years and was an academic researcher before joining the pharmaceutical industry. His research interests include statistical methodology and its applications to real problems in pharmaceuticals, including exposure-safety, PKPD modeling, treatment/dose selection, health economics, benefit-risk, and health technology assessments, and optimal trial design with 60+ publications on peer-reviewed journals.

Chapman & Hall/CRC Biostatistics Series
Series Editors: Mark Chang, *Boston University, USA*

Development of Gene Therapies
Strategic, Scientific, Regulatory, and Access Considerations
Edited by Avery McIntosh and Oleksandr Sverdlov

Bayesian Precision Medicine
Peter F. Thall

Statistical Methods for Dynamic Disease Screening and Spatio-Temporal Disease Surveillance
Peihua Qiu

Causal Inference in Pharmaceutical Statistics
Yixin Fang

Applied Microbiome Statistics
Correlation, Association, Interaction and Composition
Yinglin Xia and Jun Sun

Association Models in Epidemiology
Study Design, Modeling Strategies, and Analytic Methods
Hongjie Liu

Likelihood Methods in Survival Analysis
with R Examples
Jun Ma, Malcolm Hudson, and Annabel Webb

Biostatistics for Bioassay
Ann Yellowlees and Matthew Stephenson

Power and Sample Size in R
Catherine M. Crespi

R for Health Technology Assessment
Gianluca Baio, Howard Thom, and Petros Pechlivanoglou

Advanced Statistical Analytics for Health Data Science with SAS and R
Ding-Geng Chen and Jeffrey Wilson

Group Sequential and Adaptive Methods for Clinical Trials
Christopher Jennison and Bruce W. Turnbull

Machine Learning for Microbiome Statistics
Yinglin Xia and Jun Sun

Exposure-Response: Methods and Practical Implementation
Jixian Wang

For more information about this series, please visit: www.routledge.com/Chapman--Hall-CRC-Biostatistics-Series/book-series/CHBIOSTATIS

Dose-Exposure-Response Modeling

Methods and Practical Implementation

Second Edition

Jixian Wang

CRC Press
Taylor & Francis Group
Boca Raton London New York

CRC Press is an imprint of the
Taylor & Francis Group, an **informa** business
A CHAPMAN & HALL BOOK

Designed Cover Image: Jixian Wang

Second edition published 2026
by CRC Press
2385 NW Executive Center Drive, Suite 320, Boca Raton, FL 33431

and by CRC Press
4 Park Square, Milton Park, Abingdon, Oxon, OX14 4RN

CRC Press is an imprint of Taylor & Francis Group, LLC

[First edition published by CRC Press 2015]

ISBN: 978-1-032-59625-9 (hbk)
ISBN: 978-1-032-59962-5 (pbk)
ISBN: 978-1-003-45700-8 (ebk)

DOI: 10.1201/9781003457008

Typeset in Nimbus Roman font
by KnowledgeWorks Global Ltd.

Publisher's Note: This book has been prepared from camera-ready copy provided by the author.

Contents

Symbol Description

$\text{argmin}_x g(x)$	x that minimizes $g(x)$
$\text{argmax}_x g(x)$	x that maximizes $g(x)$
$\min_x g(x)$	the minimum of $g(x)$
$\max_x g(x)$	the maximum of $g(x)$
$a \in A$	a is an element of A
$\|\mathbf{A}\|$ or $det(\mathbf{A})$	Determinant of $\mathbf{A}$
$P(A)$	Probability of occurrence of A
$E(y\|x)$	Expectation of y conditional on x.
$E_x(f(x))$	Expectation of $f(x)$ over x.
$E^g(X)$	Geometric mean of X : $\exp(E(\log(X)))$
$\hat{\beta}$	Estimate of β
$X \perp Y\|Z$	X and Y are independent given Z
$\int_x f(x)dG(x)$	Expectation of $f(x)$ over $x \sim G(x)$, where the distribution $G(x)$ is specified explicitly.
$g(x) \propto f(x)$	$g(x) = Kf(x)$ where K is not a function of x.
$y \sim F(.)$	y follows distribution $F(.)$.
$y\|x \sim F(.)$	y follows distribution $F(.)$ conditional on x.
$Y_i \to Y$	Y_i converges to Y (all types).
$\mathbf{X}^T$	Transpose of matrix $\mathbf{X}$.
$\mathbf{I}$	An identity matrix of a conformable dimension (if not specified).
$Bin(p)$	Bernoulli distribution with parameter p
$\text{logit}(p)$	$\log(p/(1-p))$
$\text{expit}(l)$	$1/(1+\exp(-l))$
$a \leftarrow a+b$	Update the value of a with $a+b$
$\chi^2_k(h)$	The χ^2 distribution with k degrees of freedom and non-central parameter h (may be omitted if $h = 0$.)
$\frac{dy(x)}{dx}$, or $\dot{y}(x)$	The derivative of $y(x)$ with respect to x.
$\frac{\partial f(\mathbf{x})}{\partial \mathbf{x}}$, or $\nabla_{\mathbf{x}} f(\mathbf{x})$	Partial derivatives of $f(\mathbf{x})$ with respect to $\mathbf{x}$.
$\frac{\partial^2 f(\mathbf{x})}{\partial \mathbf{x} \partial \mathbf{x}^T}$, or $\nabla^2_{\mathbf{x}} f(\mathbf{x})$	2nd order partial derivatives of $f(\mathbf{x})$ with respect to $\mathbf{x}$.
$N(\mu, \sigma^2)$	Normal distribution with mean μ and variance σ^2.
$N(\boldsymbol{\mu}, \boldsymbol{\Sigma})$	Multi-variate normal distribution with mean $\boldsymbol{\mu}$ and variance-covariance matrix $\boldsymbol{\Sigma}$.
$\phi(x)$, $\Phi(x)$	Density and distribution functions of standard normal distribution.

$U(a, b)$	The uniform distribution within the range (a, b).
$IG(a, b)$	The inverse gamma distribution with parameters a and b

.

Preface

Exposure-response modeling is a very general topic, since both the exposure and the response are general concepts covering different scenarios in a number of areas of research and applications. Typical areas where exposure-response modeling is widely used are pharmacological modeling and simulation (or pharmacometrics), toxicology and epidemiology. In pharmacometrics the exposure often refers to drug concentration in human body and the responses are good (intended) reactions or bad (unintended) reactions to the treatment. In toxicology, the exposure could be a drug, a chemical or other material or conditions that may be harmful and response may vary dramatically since a toxicology study could be in-vitro (using cells or tissues) or in-vivo (using animals). The exposure in an epidemiological study could be the strength of drug exposure measured by drug dose and duration, exposure to harmful conditions such as radiation (which can also be measured by its dose and duration) and the response could be any measure for the health outcome of a population. Comparing with the other two areas, in an epidemiology study, the investigator has much less control (if any) to the exposure and her data comes from observation, in contrast to a study in the other areas where the investigator can design and conduct a study to control other factors so that the exposure-response relationship is easier to determine.

In recent years, there has been considerable activity in the applications of, and methodological research for, exposure-response modeling in several areas including the aforementioned ones. Diversity of the aspects in different areas means that different approaches have to be used and developed. However, there are still considerable common elements that makes exposure-response modeling a systematic approaches with a uniform framework for researches and applications. For example, it has been a well-known fact that even in a clinical trial confounding factors exist when a pharmacokinetic-pharmacodynamic (PKPD) modeling, a typical example for exposure-response modeling, is used to determine the exposure-response relationship. There has been a significant development in approaches coping with confounding bias and causal effect estimation econometrics and statistics, which has found applications in epidemiology, but rarely in pharmacology modeling.

Another reason calling for a uniform framework is that in a number of areas ER modeling has been extended considerably leading to similar scenarios or applications of similar approaches. For example, traditional PKPD modeling uses concentration as a measure of exposure, while a new approach known as K-dynamic modeling uses drug dose, yet still capture the dynamic of exposure-response relationship. In the same time, researchers in epidemiology and drug safety developed approaches to consider the dynamic of drug exposure change and risk of adverse events (AE), using a similar approach. Apparently neither side knew the development of the other.

The book reflects the author's experiences in ER modeling in a number of areas including experimental toxicity, clinical epidemiology and drug safety, outcome studies (studies to evaluated treatment effects in the target population), clinical trial statistics and pharmacological modeling and simulation, particularly experiences on using approaches available in different softwares, some are rather basic but a large number of them are newly developed and advanced, to solve problems of different natures, but with considerable similarity in statistics and modeling aspects.

There have been several books concerning the same or similar topics. For PKPD modeling, Bonate (2006) is an excellent book written for modelers in this area. In addition, there are a number of books, although not purely for PKPD (or exposure-response) modeling but cover topics in PKPD modeling, such as. In statistics two books on the main tool of PKPD modeling: nonlinear mixed models (NLMM) are Davidian and Giltinan [2017] and Pinheiro and Bates [2000]. The book is different from existing ones in the following aspects. The current book tries to bridge gaps between difference research areas to allow borrowing well developed approaches from each other. This is an application book, but it does not stop at using simple models and approaches. It goes much further to recently developments in a number of areas and describes implementation and methodologies and interpretation of fitted models and statistical inference based on them. Although the focus is on recent developments, no assumption on intensive knowledge on ER modeling is needed to read the book and implement the methods. There are models given in general forms with matrix notations. This may not be necessary when a model is explicitly specified (as in NONMEM), but is useful to understand the concept of some advanced approaches, particularly when using software with model specified in general forms such as R and SAS. The contents are arranged to allow the reader to skip these formulae yet still be able to implement the approaches.

I would like to thank my colleagues at Bristol Myers Squibb, in particular Ram Tiwari and Inna Perevozskaya, and Lara Spieker and the publication team of Taylor & Francis for their help in many ways. The new edition also benefits from suggestions and discussion of relevant topics from external colleagues in the pharmaceutical industry, in particular, Zhiwei Zhang, Tomas Dumortier, and others in Causal Inference in Pharmacometrics working group. Finally, my big thank you goes to my wife Sharon for her support in the last one and a half years.

Preface to the second edition

It has been ten years since the first edition of the book. Much progress has been made in dose-exposure-response (DER) modeling during this period, although the basic methods still apply to areas such as population PK and PK-PD modeling. The second edition aims to reflect some new development while still keeping the basic method and implementation parts. One major change is, as suggested in the new book title, that dose-exposure and dose-response modeling is considered explicitly, while the first edition mainly focuses on exposure-response modeling. The rationale for this change reflects the important role of dose, particularly dose adjustment in both dose-response and exposure-response relationship, in recent developments in areas such as adaptive clinical trial design and optimal individualized dosing.

About one third of the contents of this edition are new materials. In Chapter 7, newly added are Bayesian approaches with misspecified models and priors, the use of a loss function to replace the likelihood function, and Bayesian bootstrap approaches for approximate Bayesian inference. In addition, Causal Bayesian approaches can be found in Chapter 8 and Bayesian bootstrap for Thompson sampling is used in reinforcement learning in Chapter 9.

We have seen substantial development in causal inference in the last ten years, although mainly for binary and categorical treatments. The modeling and inference of the causal DER relationship have also attracted research work in pharmacometrics [Rogers et al., 2023]. Hence, a new chapter 8 is dedicated to this topic. Starting from basic concept causal inference, the chapter covers the basic and recent development of key causal inference methods for continuous treatments such as generalized propensity scores, instrumental variables, and control functions and their use for causal inference for exposure-response and dose-response relationships.

The last chapter covers a wide range of topics on dose optimization and adjustment with DER modeling, with a focus on the use of machine learning approaches. Key topics include optimal design for dose-finding trials with and without DER models by Thompson sampling for reinforcement learning, individualized dose adjustment with dynamic DR models with a combination of machine learning and automatic control approaches. A new example extensively used in this chapter is the Warfarin dosing dataset, which includes individual patient dosing and response data with response-dependent dose adjustment. This chapter also gives a new view on some well-known topics such as the dose-titration paradox and retrospective fitting dose-response models for dose-escalation trials.

The new appendices also reflect the changes above, with some rather standard materials removed and new materials such as approximate Bayesian methods and dynamic dose-response models and their connection to some causal inference models.

The new edition includes a large amount of R codes for methods introduced in the new materials in chapters on Bayesian analyses, causal inference, and dose-adjustment. Some of them include simulation to show how some complex methods such as generalized propensity score adjustment and adaptive dose-adjustment can be implemented with simple codes, some are to illustrate concepts of the methods and their applications. Some lengthy codes can be found in the online appendix.

Due to the space limit, many original references for methods cannot be all cited. Instead, only one or two textbooks or recent review papers are cited to provide the reader with an entry point to relevant literature. Apologies for the omission of these references.

I would like to thank my colleagues at Bristol Myers Squibb, in particular Ram Tiwari and Inna Perevozskaya, for their help in many ways. The new edition also benefits from suggestions and discussion of relevant topics from external colleagues in the pharmaceutical industry, in particular, Zhiwei Zhang, Tomas Dumortier and others in Causal Inference in Pharmacometrics working group. Finally, my big thank you goes to my wife Sharon for her support in the last one and a half years.

It took more than one and a half years to write this edition. Despite the time spent on this effort, I am sure there are still many typos and other errors in this edition. I sincerely welcome corrections/suggestions and criticisms from the readers.

Jixian (Jason) Wang
Cortaillod, Switzerland

1

Introduction

1.1 Multi-faceted dose-exposure-response relationships

Dose-exposure-response (DER) relationships refer to a collection or combination of different types of relationships between dose, exposures, and their responses, including dose-exposure (DE), exposure-response (ER), and dose-response (DR) relationships. They can be modeled separately or jointly. The DR relationship can be modeled directly or by combining the DE and ER models; the latter is a common practice of population pharmacokinetics (PK) and pharmacokinetics-pharmacodynamics (PKPD) modeling [Bonate, 2006] for dose selection, taking both exposure and response data into account. This book is concerned with modeling quantitative DE, ER, and DR relationships of drugs or chemicals, with an emphasis on their application in the pharmaceutical environment, especially in drug development and pharmacoepidemiology. However, the approaches described in this book are readily applicable to a wider range of topics such as environmetric modeling and areas in biostatistics where the source of exposure is not drugs or chemicals.

In many biostatistics-related areas, DER relationships carry important information about how dose and exposure influence outcomes of interest. For example, in pharmacology, dose refers to the drug dose given to a patient. Exposure is the drug concentration of the dose which induces the response of the patient. Often exposure cannot be directly controlled, but we may indirectly control it by changing the dose, e.g., in a randomized concentration controlled (RCC) trial [Holford et al., 1993a,b; Wang, 2014] in which patients are randomized into a number of concentration ranges and the concentration in an individual patient is controlled by dose titration to achieve the target range. Environmental exposures could be air or water pollution, radiation, or exposure to risk factors in an industry environment, where often we have no control over them but may be partially controlled by environmental policies. In pharmacoepidemiology the dose can be referred to the prescribed dose, and exposure is the dose actually taken by the patient.

By DER relationships, we mean causal relationships rather than correlations. For example, the causal DR relationship describes how the response changes as a consequence of a dose change. The causal DR relationship can

DOI: 10.1201/9781003457008-1

be easily modeled if the dose is randomized, e.g., in a randomized dose finding trial, but it may be difficult to model or estimate if individual doses depend on factors affecting the response (known as confounding factors). This problem is more common in ER modeling, as exposure is not randomized directly and is often subject to the impact of confounding factors.

1.2 Practical scenarios in ER modeling

We will use several real and hypothetical examples to illustrate practical aspects of DER modeling, as well as a practical background for methodological development. These examples can only cover a small fraction of all aspects of DER modeling in practice, but they may represent some typical scenarios. Therefore, it is important to identify the similarities and differences between approaches and between models applied to seemingly different practical scenarios so that appropriate approaches can be selected and adapted. This point will be emphasized from time to time in this book, wherever appropriate. The following are four examples of different types from the area of pharmaceutics.

1.2.1 Moxifloxacin exposure and QT prolongation

The QT interval in electrocardiography (ECG) is an important measure for the time from heart de-polarization to re-polarization. QT interval prolongation (QT prolongation hereafter) is often used as a measure to assess the cardiac safety of new non-cardiovascular drugs. Since the interval depends on the heart rate (or equivalently the RR interval, i.e., the interval between two consecutive R-waves in the same ECG), the QT interval should be corrected by heart rate to eliminate the impact of the RR difference among people with very different heart rates. A commonly used corrected QT interval is $QTcF = QT/RR^{1/3}$, known as the Fridericia correction. QT prolongation is believed to suggest an increased risk of cardiac arrest and sudden death. A 10 millisecond (ms) prolongation in QTcF has been used by drug regulators as a threshold to indicate increased cardiac risk. Another approach called categorical analysis calculates frequencies of QTc higher than certain thresholds (e.g., 30 ms and 60 ms). A thorough QT (TQT) study, which includes a placebo, a positive control, and two doses of a test drug, all with baseline QT measurements, is used to show that a drug has no QT effect, normally does not need complex ER modeling. However, modeling approaches can be very useful in situations where the TQT study fails to demonstrate no QT effects at the current doses.

Moxifloxacin is known to have a stable QT prolongation effect and is safe to use as a positive control in TQT trials. We use the moxifloxacin data in a TQT trial as an example to show (i) potential uses of modeling approaches, (ii) the need for advanced modeling techniques, and (iii) some potential problems leading to further development of models and model fitting techniques. We will revisit this example in later chapters, when a model or a method can be applied to it. The dataset consists of ECG and moxifloxacin concentration data from a crossover design in which a total of 61 subjects received a single dose of placebo, moxifloxacin, or the test drug in each period, and the concentration and ECG measures were taken at several time points. The ECG parameters were corrected by subtracting the baseline value and the (post-baseline – baseline) difference in the placebo period measured at the same time (known as the $\Delta\Delta$ parameters). Figure 1.1 plots $\Delta\Delta QTcF$s vs the corresponding concentrations at all time points. There appears to be a linear trend of increasing QTcF along with an increase in exposure. However, since the data contain multiple ECG measures from individual patients, we cannot simply use a least squares (LS) method to fit a linear regression model. A correct approach is to use an appropriate repeated measurements model as described in Chapter 3. One may be tempted to use a very intuitive approach: first fit the slopes for individual subjects, then analyze the slopes by taking the mean and standard deviation (SD) of them. This approach is, in fact, one type of two-stage approach for fitting a repeated measurement model. Figure 1.2 shows the distribution of individual LS slope estimates together with estimates based on a linear mixed model, assuming the slope for each subject follows a normal distribution. One interesting point is that the individual estimates are highly variable and the distribution shows heavy tails, particularly at the right-hand side. It seems that the mixed model estimates are shrunken toward the center. Details of linear mixed models can be found in Chapter 3.

Apart from the obvious need to deal with repeated measures, other characteristics in this dataset are also worth exploring. First, the concentration-QT relationship may not be linear. Although the trend in Figure 1.1 appears linear, it is not sufficient to conclude that the use of a linear repeated measurement model is sufficient. Second, the relationship may not be instantaneous, as the drug effect can accumulate and cause a delay (known as hysteresis) of the response to exposure.

All three features are important when modeling approaches are used to help further develop a drug that shows some QT prolongation. For example, if a tested dose showed unacceptable prolongation of QT, it would be useful to find the maximum dose that has an acceptable QT effect and test if it also delivers satisfactory efficacy. A valid ER relationship allows calibrating that dose by taking model fitting uncertainty and inter- and intra-subject variabilities into account. Another approach to reducing QT effects may be to change the drug formulation to reduce the peak concentration while maintaining a comparable overall exposure. Two key factors to be considered here are exposure accumulation and correct estimation of the upper percentiles of subjects with very long prolongation, e.g., defined for category analysis. If exposure accumulates over time, the effect of cutting peak concentration on reducing QT prolongation may be much lower than estimated

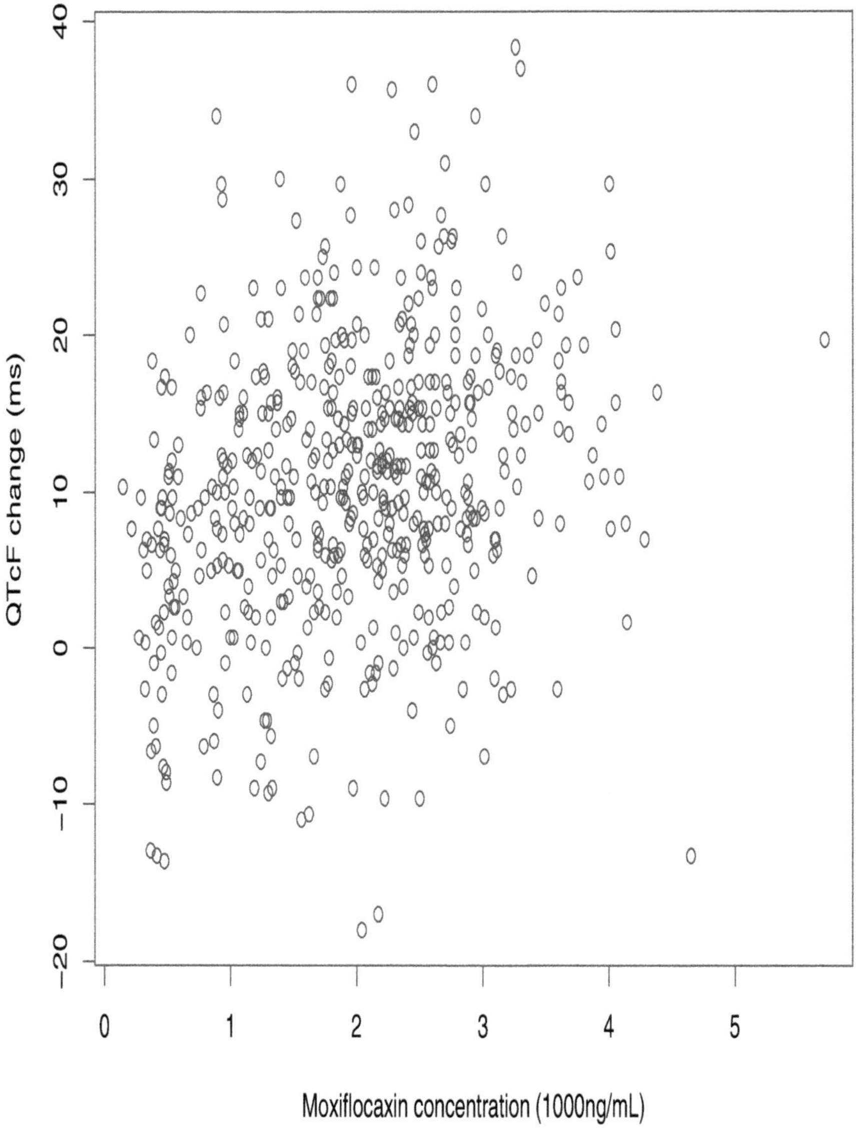

Figure 1.1
Pooled $\Delta\Delta QTcF$s vs. moxifloxacin concentrations from 61 subjects measured at multiple time points.

from a model assuming an instantaneous exposure effect. The appropriate assessment of the effect requires developing a dynamic model that describes the temporal relationship between the PK time profile and the QT time profile. This type of model and related analytical methods will be described in Chapter 6.

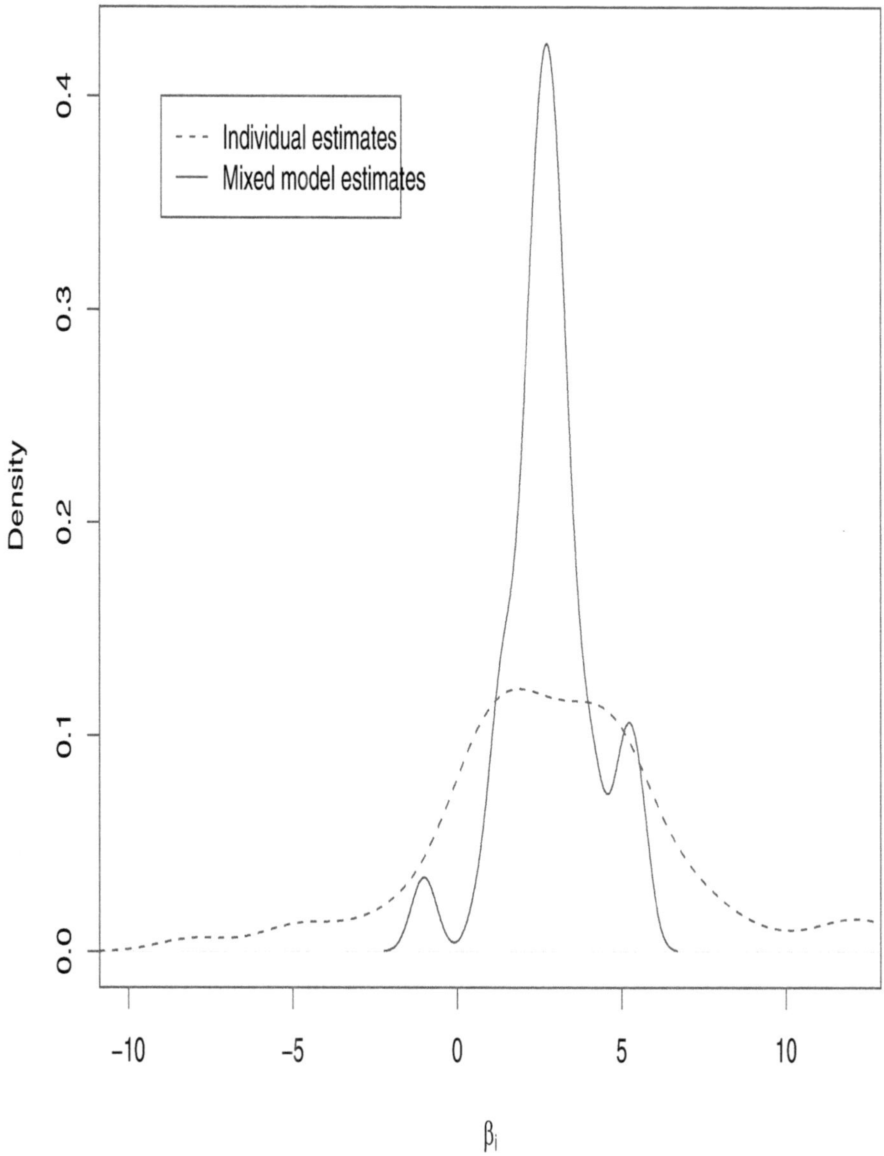

Figure 1.2
Individual parameter estimates by linear least squares and linear mixed model estimates for the slope of $\Delta\Delta QTcF$ and moxifloxacin concentration (1000 ng/mL).

1.2.2 Theophylline and peak expiratory flow rate

This example comes from a study to find the optimal concentration of theophylline for the management of acute airways obstruction. This is an early study using a RCC design [Holford et al., 1993a,b]. In the study, 174 patients were randomized to a target concentration of 10 or 20 mg/L. Theophylline concentrations from individual patients were controlled with dose adjustment. From each patient, the concentration and peak expiratory flow rate (PEFR) were measured multiple times at the same time. The dataset includes PEFR and concentration together with patient characteristics. However, the randomization and dosing data were lost due to a power outage (Halford, private communication). Therefore, we cannot fit a population PK (popPK) model to the data, hence some non- and semi-parametric approaches were used, including those in Holford et al. [1993a,b]. An attempt was made by the author of this book to recover the dosing information from the figures in the references above. PK and PEFR measurements are plotted in Figure 1.3 together with recovered randomization information. A small number of measurements cannot be identified and are marked as "+" in the plots. A scatter plot of theophylline concentration against PEFR, pooling all the repeated measures, is presented in Figure 1.4. An interesting finding when comparing the graphs is that although it seems that there is a trend of increasing PEFR with increased concentration, there is no significant difference between the two groups, while the observed exposure levels are quite different between them (Figure 1.3). We will revisit this issue in later chapters.

1.2.3 Argatroban and activated partial thromboplastin time

Argatroban is an anticoagulant for multiple indications including prophylaxis or treatment of thrombosis in some patients. It is administered intravenously, and plasma concentrations of the drug reach a steady state in a few hours after infusion. Its anticoagulant effect was measured by the activated partial thromboplastin time (APTT), a measure of the speed of blood clotting, and it was expected that increasing exposure would increase the APTT values. The dataset in Davidian and Giltinan [2017] contains 219 measures from 37 argatroban patients administered as a 4-hour infusion, with repeated concentration measures taken up to 6 hours after the start of the infusion. Figure 1.6 shows individual APPT time profiles for these patients.

APTT values were not all measured at the same time as the PK samples were measured. So, to investigate the ER relationship, we need to predict the concentration at the time when each APTT is measured. This can be done using a nonlinear mixed model [Davidian and Giltinan, 2017] to fit the PK data and using the fitted model to predict the APTT at a given time. The APTT values and predicted argatroban concentrations show a strong linear trend, as shown in Figure 1.6. However, appropriate modeling approaches are needed to deal with potential repeated measures, nonlinearity, and hysteresis to quantify the relationship between exposure and APTT.

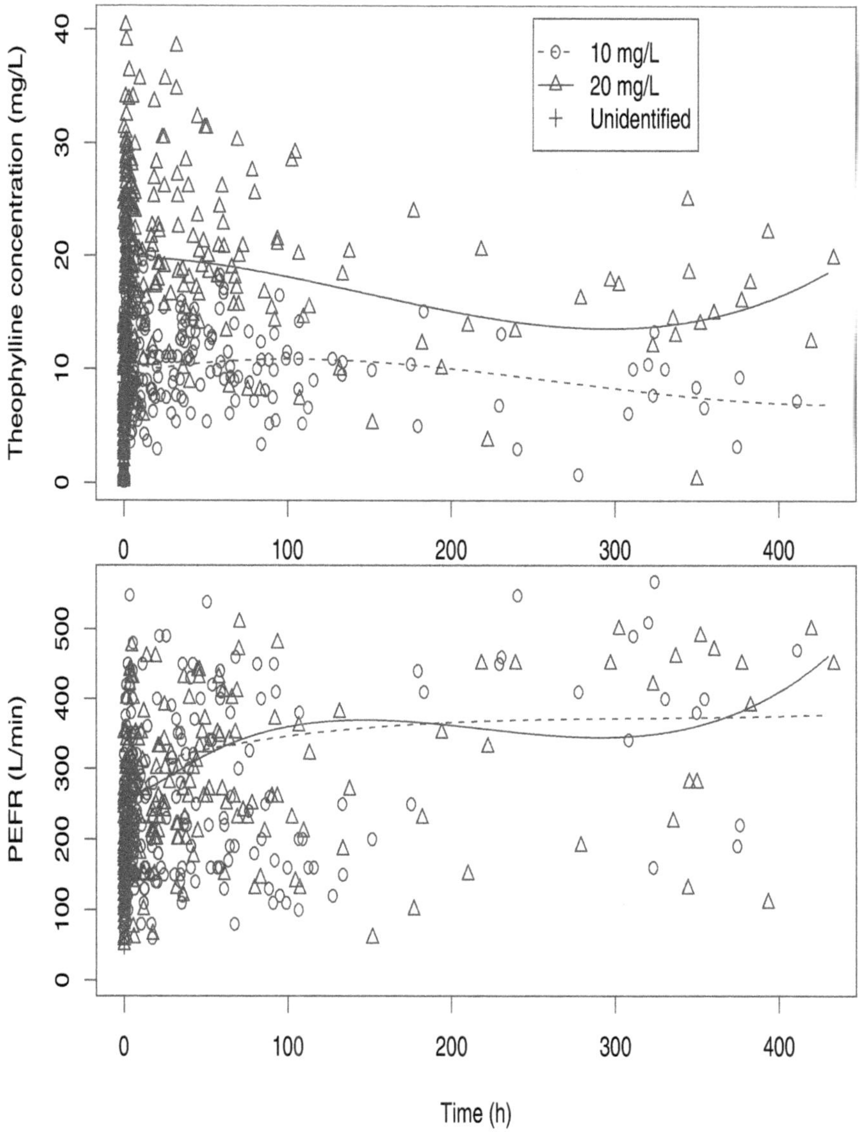

Figure 1.3
Theophylline and PFER time profiles with non-parametric curves fitted by spline functions via linear mixed models for both dose groups.

1.2.4 Response-dependent warfarin dose adjustment

Warfarin is commonly used as an anticoagulant to prevent blood clots in patients post-myocardial infarction (MI) to reduce the risk of further cardiovascular events. For these patients, the dose should be adjusted to keep the

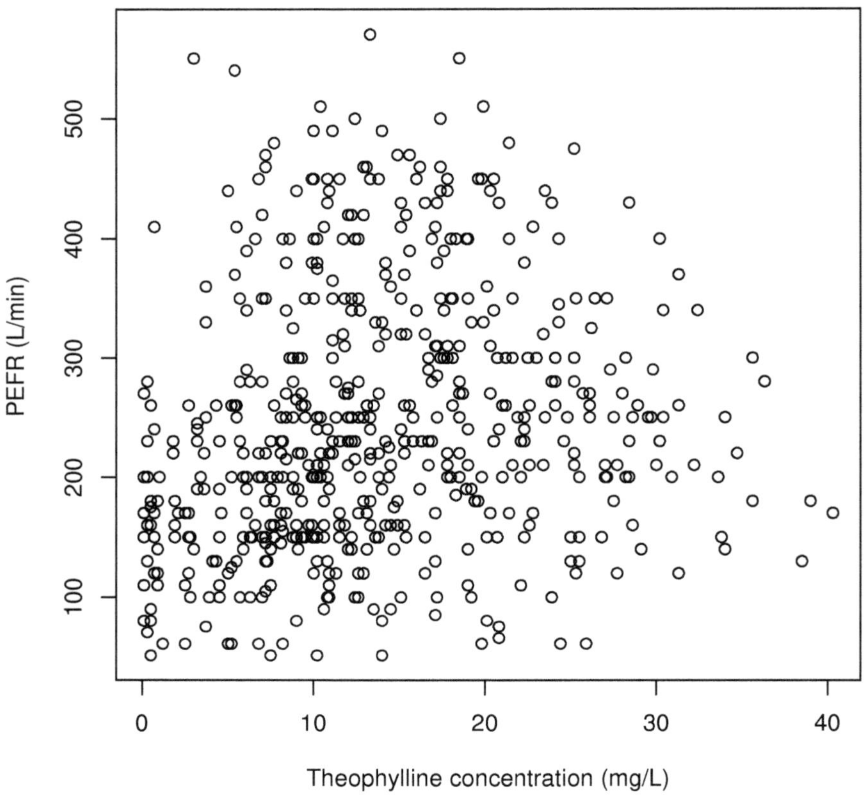

Figure 1.4
Theophylline concentrations and PEFR values pooling all the repeated measures.

international normalized ratio (INR) in the range of 2 to 3. The dose to achieve this goal varies among patients; therefore, after the initial dose, response-dependent adjustment is often needed. We use the dataset in Avery et al. [2020] to illustrate special issues in modeling data with response-dependent dose adjustment and approaches to deal with them. The DR relationship is dynamic, since the effect of a dose adjustment is delayed and can only be seen over time. Figure 1.7 shows the INR and previous warfarin dose (mg) of patient 3 (which is randomly selected and represents typical patients in the dataset) at all visits, together with the target INR range. The initial dose increase appeared to be a reaction of lower INR than 2, then the dose reduction in visits in the middle was to correct the INR higher than 3. Finally, the dose increased again to respond to the low INR. From this subject, we may expect an obvious DR relationship between warfarin dose and INR at the population level. Interestingly, when we look at the marginal DR relationship in Chapter 8 without dealing with response-dependent dose adjustment, we find none. This issue is known in pharmacometrics as the dose-titration paradox.

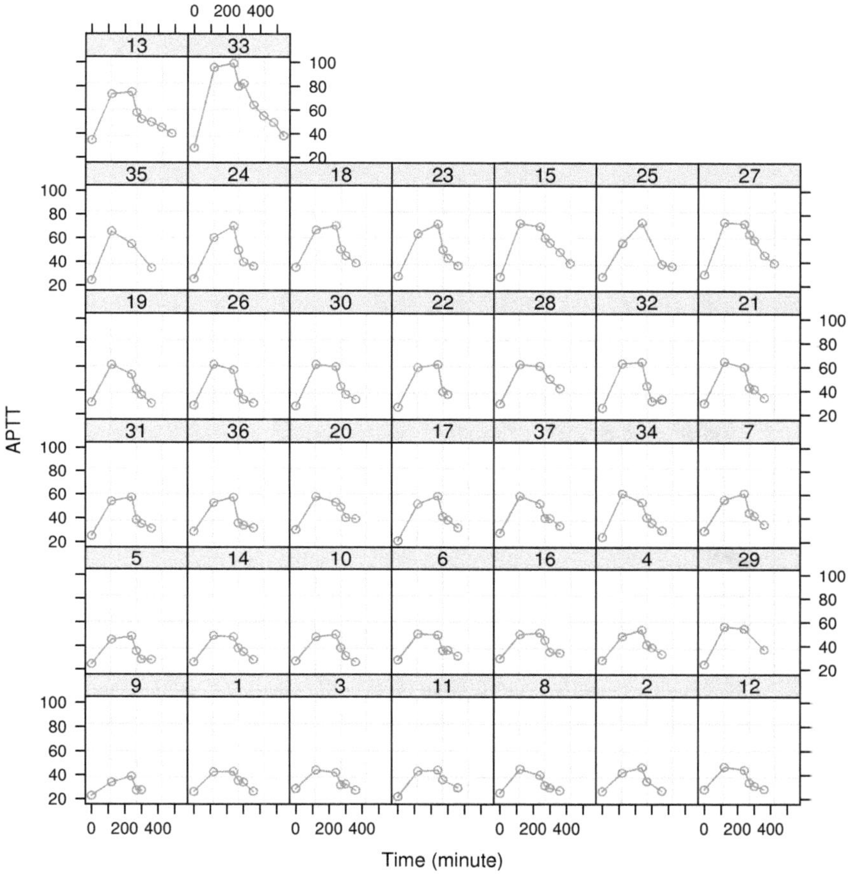

Figure 1.5
Individual argatroban concentration time profiles of 37 patients after a 4-hour infusion.

We will show how this problem is related to the causal DR relationship and under what conditions the underline causal DR relationship can be identified in Chapter 8.

1.3 Models and modeling in dose-exposure-response analysis

There are many different types of DER models, which we will classify into empirical and mechanistic models. Pharmacometrics is the main area in which

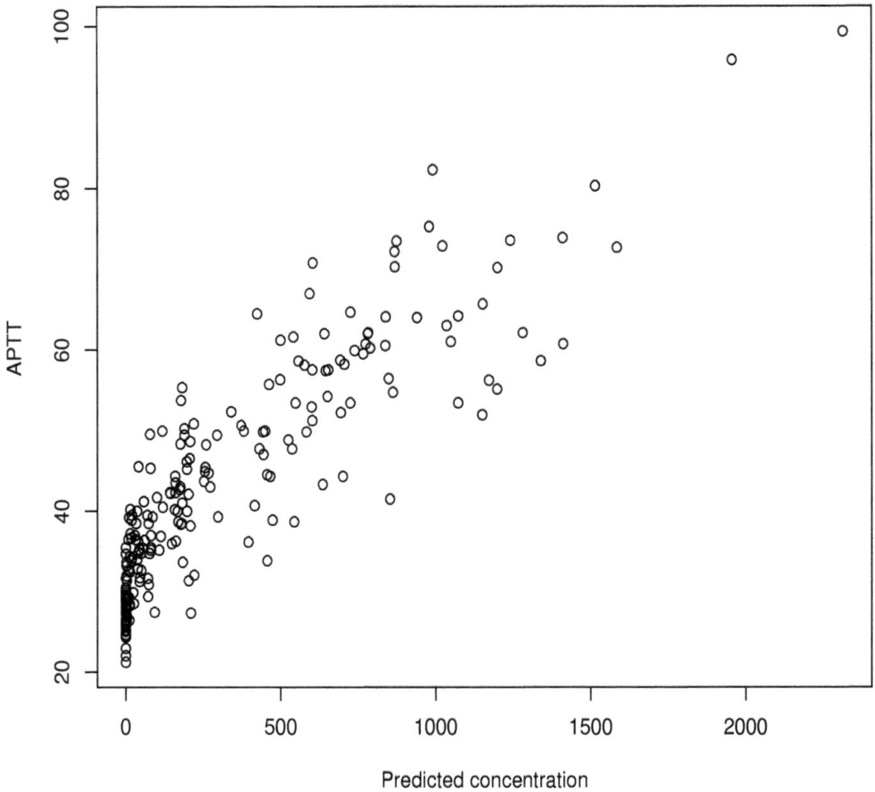

Figure 1.6
Observed APPT and predicted argatroban concentration by a nonlinear mixed model.

mechanism models are widely used for DER relationships. For DE modeling, PK modeling has a long history of describing the PK characteristics of drugs and fitting dose-concentration data [Bonate, 2006]. Compartmental models, derived from physical models of drug disposition have been well developed. Similarly, PKPD modeling is an approach for ER relationship. Recently, mechanistic models for ER relationships have also been developed. Empirical models describe the data in a quantitative manner, taking potential factors affecting the exposure and ER relationship into account.

In contrast, for fitting dose and response data without exposure, DR models are often empirical models, since the mechanism may be either unknown, or too complex to be identified without exposure data. DE, DR and ER models of both types may be written in the following abstract form

```
Exposure=h(Dose, factors,DE parameters)+Error
Response=g*(Dose, factors,DR parameters)+Error
Response=g(Exposure, factors,ER parameters)+Error
```

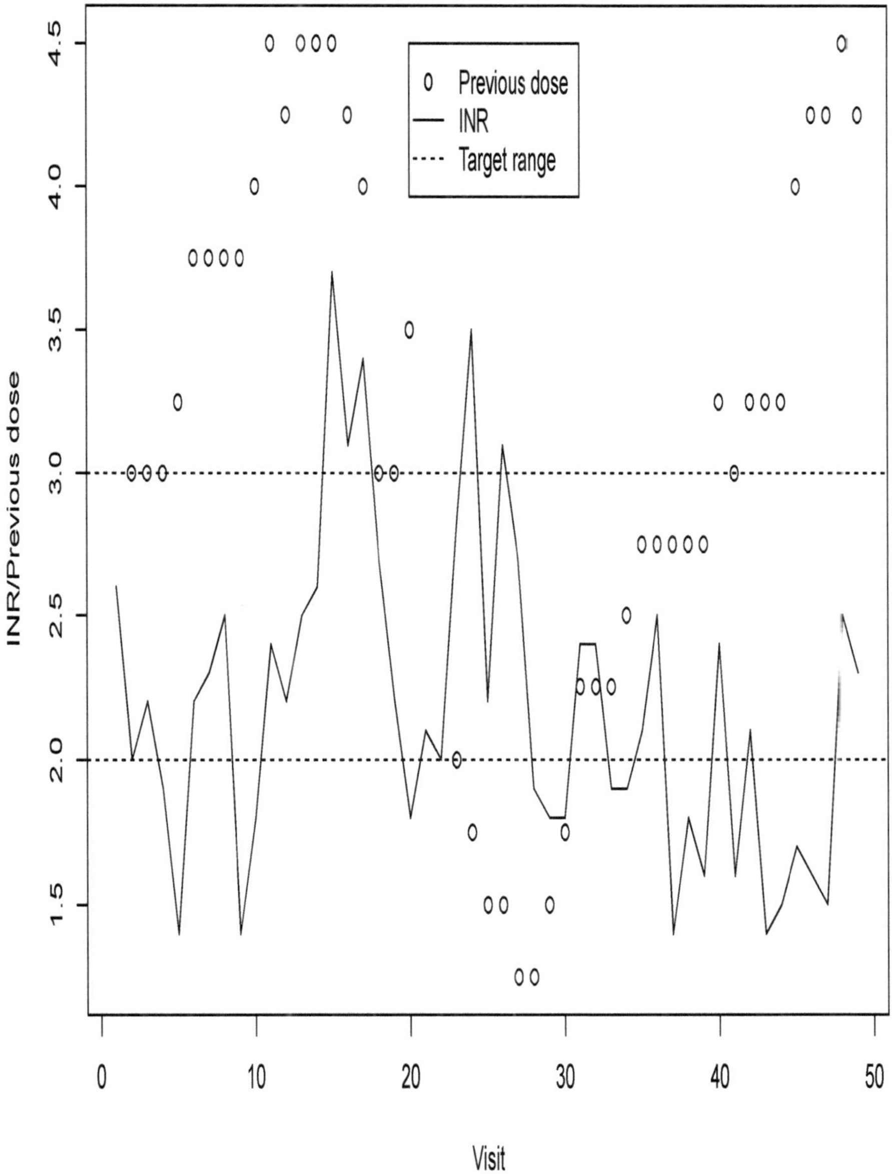

Figure 1.7
INR and previous warfarin dose (mg) of patient 3 over all visits, with target INR range.

where g, $g*$ and h describe the DE, DR and ER relationships. The tasks of modeling include fitting the two models to estimate the parameters, assessing the models as well as quantifying the error terms, and variability and uncertainty in the fitted model and estimated parameters. The models can be used to determine the exposure level corresponding to the desired response level, and how to achieve the exposure by adjusting the dose (or in other ways to control the exposure). The DE and ER model can also be combined to predict the response at a given dose. The importance of quantifying variability and uncertainty may be less obvious than estimating the parameters, but it is an important aspect of statistical modeling and provides important information for model-based decision making, e.g., dose determination.

A mechanistic model has obvious advantages over an empirical model since it may support empirical evidence with a quantified pharmacological relationship. It may also indicate further investigation in specific directions. In contrast, empirical models are more flexible and can often be as good as mechanistic models for prediction. An empirical model may also be used for an alternative or a sensitivity analysis to validate or confirm a mechanistic model-based analysis.

The ER relationship can also be analyzed without using a model. For example, the mean responses of each dose in a dose-finding trial can be used to show the DR relationship; but a model-based approach is more efficient for using the data, and can quantify the whole relationship including the parts in between assigned dose levels. These model-independent analyses also have their advantages, but are beyond the scope of this book.

1.4 Model-based decision making model-informed drug development

Drug development is a long, complex, and expensive process that involves making difficult decisions at many stages in different scenarios. Decision analysis (DA) has been introduced in several stages of drug development and is playing an increasing role. Due to the complexity of drug exposure and its outcome, modeling is a key part of decision analysis. A typical area where modeling has played a key role is to find the right dose to maximize drug effects while maintaining an acceptable safety profile. Typically, both the safety and efficacy responses increase with increasing exposure levels. The drug developer hopes that there is an exposure range in which efficacy is satisfactory and toxicity is at an acceptable level, and that appropriate doses can be determined so that the exposure in most patients is in that range. Therefore, selecting a suitable dose involves a proper balance of safety and efficacy. DER modeling provides key information for making such a decision.

Often a critical question at a certain stage is whether a trial is needed to obtain further information about safety and efficacy, given that the trial is expensive and takes a long time to run. The information may be used to find a more accurate dose or to determine the efficacy and safety profile of an existing dose. Decision analysis calculates the value of information (VoI) to assess whether the benefit of running such a study is worth the costs (both money and the possible delay in the development process). Decision analysis offers tools to evaluate the benefit and compare it with the costs. For this, ER models are needed to provide information about efficacy and safety at a given or a range of doses. On a larger scale than the decision on a single trial, the whole drug development process that involves a large number of trials can be considered as a complex process, and decision makers make multiple decisions step by step, taking up-to-date information into account.

Decision analysis is increasingly used to optimize individual treatment for personalized medicine. For example, if a drug has highly variable exposure between patients, therapeutic dose monitoring, which monitor the exposure periodically and adjust the dose if necessary, may be needed to ensure that individual patients are at the right exposure level. Taking the measure has a considerable cost and incontinence for the patient. How long do we have to measure before stop? In fact, the question should be when collecting further information does not justify the costs and inconvenience. The recent development of dynamic treatment regimes also brings decision analysis to the frontline of the development of optimal treatment regimes that maximize the benefit of drugs for individual patients through response-dependent adaptation.

Most of these decision-making problems require making optimal decisions sequentially. The decision process itself needs a complex model to evaluate. The decision tree is a common tool to solve some simple problems. For complex problems, a dynamic programming approach is needed. For both, ER models have to be integrated into this decision model.

DER modeling plays a key role in model-informed drug development (MIDD), which is defined as "the strategic use of computational modeling and simulation (M&S) methods that integrate nonclinical and clinical data, prior information, and knowledge (e.g., drug and disease characteristics) to generate evidence" [International Council for Harmonisation, 2023]. MIDD has been promoted by drug regulators worldwide. MIDD uses several types of models, DER models are a key part of them.

DER modeling has played an important role in drug development as well as in drug regulation. Modeling approaches are now frequently used to support the submission of a new drug application (NDA). The Food and Drug Administration (FDA) published a guidance on the analysis of exposure-response relationships [Food and Drug Administration, 2023], in which exposure may refer to dose or PK concentration. The guidance suggests that determining the exposure-response relationship can play a role in drug development to

- support the Drug Discovery and Development Processes,
- support a Determination of Safety and Efficacy,
- support New Target Populations and Adjustment of dosages and dosing regimens.

The importance of PKPD (ER) relationship, compared with the DR relationship was recognized: "... concentration-response relationships in the same individual over time are especially informative because they are not potentially confounded by doses selection/titration phenomena and inter-individual PK variability".

The guidance considered confounding bias in exposure-response analysis an important issue. It states that if one simply uses the observed drug concentration in a PKPD analysis "...potential confounding of the concentration-response relationship can occur and an observed concentration-response relationship may not be credible evidence of an exposure-response relationship". The RCC design, which uses individual dose adjustment to achieve exposure levels randomly assigned to patients, was recommended.

The guidance also gives some details on specific situations when PK/PD modeling may provide important information: "Where effectiveness is immediate and is readily measured repeatedly ..., it is possible to relate clinical response to blood concentrations over time, which can provide critical information for choosing a dose and dosing interval." The guidance suggests that the modeling strategy be described clearly and include a statement of the problem, assumptions used, model selection and validation, and for a PK/PD analysis for a submission, this information should also be presented in the exposure-response study report. Since the publication of the guidance, there have been several recent developments on DER modeling for drug development, including developments in confounding bias and causal effect estimation, modeling temporal ER relationships, and Bayesian DER modeling. The reader can find details of these in later chapters.

1.5 Examples and modeling software

As this is a book about applied statistics, a large number of numerical examples are included. Some of them are illustrations of real examples, such as the PK-QT and PK-PEFR trial data, and the warfarin dose-adjustment datasets. Simulated datasets are also used to create practical scenarios to assess the performance of procedures or simply to demonstrate some specific properties of them. Using real data is the best way to demonstrate the implementation of an approach in practice, but a simulation has the advantage of focusing on the key issues and knowing the correct answers to specific questions (e.g., the true values of parameters). The selection of numerical examples is a compromise between using real examples only and, at the other extreme, using simulated data only.

For all simulated data and examples, the codes for simulation and analysis are available such that the reader can not only reproduce the results, but also explore further in the direction the reader is interested.

In the last 20 years, we have seen a dramatic increase in computing power. Its impact on modeling is the rapid development of software that can fit very complex models. Most applied statistics texts now include a substantial amount of their content dedicated to using software to solve specific problems and implementing approaches. This book is not an exception, since modern exposure-response modeling is heavily dependent on the use of software. We will mainly use three software: SAS [SAS Institute Inc., 2011], R [R Core Team, 2013] and Stan [Stan Development Team, 2023] (for Bayesian analysis) but will not use them to repeat the same task. NONMEM [Bauer, 2010] has been very popular for modeling and simulation, but is less user-friendly than the others. Finally, Stan with its R-interface, Rstan and a PKPD modeling library Torsten make the implementation of Bayesian methods for Bayesian DER analyses very easy.

Compared with the previous edition, this edition added many implementations with R and Stan. Short codes are included in the text, sometimes together with a screenshot of results, and long and complex ones can be found in the online appendix.

Although there is no space for a detailed comparison between R, SAS and NONMEM, a few words may help to make a selection if the reader has a choice, particularly among SAS/R and NONMEM. SAS and R are universal software that provides a large number of statistical tools. NONMEM was developed for modeling and simulation using population PK and PKPD models. The core part is a nonlinear mixed model fitting algorithm, very similar to that of SAS proc NLMIXED, and the other parts allow easily implementation, e.g., of a standard compartmental PK model. There are R-packages such as lme4 with similar functions for fitting nonlinear mixed models, but with less flexibility than proc NLMIXED. Since NONMEM lacks other facilities, such as graphic functions, a partner software is needed, and the common selection is R. For those without access to commercial software (SAS and NONMEM among the three), R alone is sufficient in most cases.

2

Basic exposure and exposure-response models

This chapter introduces simple models for modeling DE and ER relationships. It serves as the basis for more complex models for repeated or longitudinal measurement data. Some modeling tools such as transformation are also introduced here.

2.1 Models based on pharmacological mechanisms

2.1.1 Example of a PKPD model

Some ER models such as PKPD models are derived from drug pharmacological mechanisms, although often based on some simplified assumptions. Csajka and Verotta [2006] give an excellent review of this type of PKPD model. A typical example of such a model is derived from the drug receptor occupancy theory. According to this theory, the drug must bind to its receptor to form a drug-receptor complex to produce its effects. Often, there are only a limited number of receptors. There are two processes that occur simultaneously: free receptors and drug molecules bind to form the complex, and the complex disassociates back to free receptors and drug molecules. Let $R_c(t)$ be the amount of the complex and $C(t)$ be the drug concentration at time t. We assume that the change of $R_c(t)$ follows

$$\frac{dR_c(t)}{dt} = K_{on}(R_{max} - R_c(t))C(t) - K_{off}R_c(t) \tag{2.1}$$

where K_{on} and K_{off} are, respectively, the rates of forming the complex and disassociating back to free drug molecules and receptors and R_{max} is the total amount of receptors. This is a dynamic model and $R_c(t)$ is a function of time. But if $C(t) = C$ is constant, at the steady state (i.e., when association-disassociation reaches equilibrium so that $dR_c(t)/dt \approx 0, t > t_s$, with a reasonably large t_s), we can solve $R_c = R_c(t_s)$ easily and get

$$R_c = \frac{R_{max}C}{K_d + C}, \tag{2.2}$$

DOI: 10.1201/9781003457008-2

where $K_d = K_{off}/K_{on}$. When the response Y in proportional to R_c, this theory leads to an Emax model

$$Y = \frac{E_{max}C}{K_d + C}, \tag{2.3}$$

where E_{max} is the maximum effect when all R_{max} receptors have become R_c, when the drug concentration tends to infinity. K_d is also known as the concentration that gives the effect of $E_{max}/2$ and is also known as EC_{50}, and the model is known as the E_{max} model. In the following, we often write this model as $Y = E_{max}/(K_d/C + 1)$ to shorten formulas, which should read as (2.3), in particular, $Y = 0$ when $C = 0$. The basic form has a number of variants. The reader is referred to Csajka and Verotta [2006] or a specialized text [Bonate, 2006] for more details. Emax model is the most commonly used PKPD model. This model may also be used for the dose-response relationship by replacing C with the dose of a drug with linear PK, that is, the concentration is proportional to dose D: $C = KD$. In this case, $EC_{50} = K_d/K$ is the dose level that gives $E_{max}/2$ effect.

There is a rich literature on PKPD models and mostly these models are dynamic and used to describe temporal ER relationships. Some typical models will be introduced in Chapter 6.

2.1.2 Compartmental models for PK modeling

Compartmental models are commonly used for drug concentrations, and sometimes for general exposures. A compartmental model describes drug absorption, disposition and elimination in and out of different body compartments (although some are hypothetical) [Gibaldi and Perrier, 1982]. For example, the following are differential equations for an open one-compartment model with first-order absorption.

$$\begin{aligned} \frac{dA_1(t)}{dt} &= -K_a A_1(t) \\ \frac{dA_2(t)}{dt} &= K_a A_1(t) - K_e A_2(t) \end{aligned} \tag{2.4}$$

where $A_1(t)$ and $A_2(t)$ are, respectively, the amount of drug at the absorption site and in the blood circulation (the central compartment) at time t, and K_a and K_e are the absorption and elimination rates, respectively. The solution of this system depends on the state at $t = 0$ (initial values). For a bolus injection of dose D, the amount to be absorbed is $F \times D$ where F is bioavailability, which we set at 1 without loss of generality. Therefore, the initial values are

$$\begin{aligned} A_1(0) &= D \\ A_2(0) &= 0. \end{aligned}$$

Solving the ODEs (2.4) gives the analytical form

$$A_1(t) = DF\exp(-K_a t) \tag{2.5}$$

$$A_2(t) = \frac{DK_aF}{(K_a - K_e)}(\exp(-K_e t) - \exp(-K_a t)), \tag{2.6}$$

which can be converted to drug concentration in the central compartment as $C(t) = A_2(t)/V$, where V is the volume of distribution, an important PK parameter. K_e is often parameterized as $K_e = Cl/V$ in terms of drug clearance Cl.

If the drug of dose D is given by a bolus injection that immediately delivers the drug to the central compartment, the model is simplified to

$$C(t) = \frac{DF}{V}\exp(-K_e t). \tag{2.7}$$

This model may also be considered as an approximation to model (2.6) when the absorption is very fast. This can be verified by letting $K_a \to \infty$ in model (2.6). This model may be generalized to allow parameters depending on covariates. For example, V often depends on weight or body surface area. Some PK parameters such as the area-under-curve defined as $AUC = \int_0^\infty C(t)dt$ and the maximum concentration $C_{max} = \max_t(C(t))$ are important exposure measures that can be derived from the models. In the last example, we have $AUC = DF/(VK_e)$ and $C_{max} = DF/V$

2.2 Statistical models

The models introduced in the last section describe theoretical situations, while there are almost always random variations in drug exposure and response data. Statistical models can take into account random variations in response, exposure, and model parameters, but we will introduce them by steps. Here, we introduce a random error term in the observed exposure and response in the DE and ER models, respectively, Variations in model parameters will be introduced in the next chapter, and measurement errors in the exposure in DER models will be introduced in Chapter 4.

A statistical model may be based on a mechanistic or empirical model. An empirical ER model, e.g., describes the relationship between exposures and responses but is not derived from the biological or medical mechanism between them. Drug exposure and its relationship with dose and other factors may also be modeled using an empirical model. Sometimes, a mechanistic model may take a simple form. For example, taking a log-transformation of model (2.7) we obtain

$$\log(C(t)) = \log(D) + \log(F) - \log(V) - K_e t. \tag{2.8}$$

Therefore, a simple linear empirical model for log-concentration may also have a mechanistic interpretation. One such model includes log-dose and other factors such as age and weight as covariates, known as the power model, and is frequently used as an empirical alternative to the compartmental model.

In this book, we focus on cardinal (rather than ordinal) dose and exposure measures. Obviously, drug concentration is a cardinal measure. For the DE and DR relationships, there are often only a few dose levels available or observed. Although technically the dose can be considered as an ordinal categorical variable, we will treat it as a cardinal measure, since this way allows, e.g., model-based calibration or prediction at any dose level based on a fitted model. Therefore, we mostly consider DER models with a cardinal measure of dose or exposure, although covariates of other types may be included.

The DR and ER models for a particular analysis depend mainly on the type of response. When the response is a continuous variable, the following regression models are the main candidates. Let Y_i be the response, C_i be the exposure (which may not always be drug concentration), and $\mathbf{X}_i$ be a set of covariates of subject i. A simple linear ER model is

$$Y_i = \beta_c C_i + \mathbf{X}_i^T \boldsymbol{\beta}_x + \varepsilon_i \tag{2.9}$$

where ε_i is a random variable with zero mean. A DR model may take the same form, with C_i replaced by dose. Here, the key parameter is β_c as it measures how Y_i changes with C_i. To fit the model, the simple least squares (LS) procedure is often sufficient, based on the key assumption that C_i and ε_i are independent. This assumption obviously holds when C_is are randomized dose levels. If C_i is observed, the assumption depends on whether the adjustment for $\mathbf{X}_i$ is sufficient. This issue will be left for Chapter 8. Replacing C_i with doses will lead to a DR model and the same model-fitting approach applies under the assumption that dose and ϵ_i are independent.

As typical ER models such as PKPD models are nonlinear; one example is the E_{max} model (2.3). In general, a nonlinear model with an additive random error can be written as

$$Y_i = g(C_i, \mathbf{X}_i, \boldsymbol{\beta}) + \varepsilon_i. \tag{2.10}$$

where $g(.)$ is a known function. Note that here we classify a model as nonlinear when the relationship between Y_i and the model parameters, not that between Y_i and C_i, is nonlinear, since it is this nonlinearity that has a substantial impact on the statistical inference and model fitting. For example, a model $Y_i = \beta_0 + \beta_c \log(C_i) + \varepsilon_i$ is considered a linear model and statistical inference and model fitting approaches apply. One special form of model (2.10) is

$$Y_i = g(\boldsymbol{\beta}_c, C_i) + \mathbf{X}_i^T \boldsymbol{\beta}_x + \varepsilon_i. \tag{2.11}$$

in which the part $\mathbf{X}_i^T \boldsymbol{\beta}_x$ is linear. This model is often referred to as a partial linear model, and the partial linear structure, specifically the linearity between

Y_i and $\boldsymbol{\beta}_x$, may be used to facilitate model fitting and statistical inference based on the model.

Often, the variance of ε_i in (2.10) may not be constant, a situation called variance heterogeneity. $\text{var}(\varepsilon_i)$ may be a function of the mean of Y_i, e.g., $\text{var}(\varepsilon_i) = \sigma_0^2 + ag^b(C_i, \mathbf{X}_i, \boldsymbol{\beta})$, where σ_0^2 is the constant component, and a and b are parameters determining how $\text{var}(\varepsilon_i)$ changes with $g(C_i, \mathbf{X}_i, \boldsymbol{\beta})$. This occurs when Y_i is a non-negative measure such as a biomarker measure and its variation or measurement error may increase with its mean.

In model (2.10) the error term is additive to $g(C_i, \mathbf{X}_i, \boldsymbol{\beta})$. Sometimes a model with multiplicative error term

$$Y_i = g(C_i, \mathbf{X}_i, \boldsymbol{\beta})\varepsilon_i. \tag{2.12}$$

may be more appropriate. This model is particularly useful when the value range of Y_i is positive, e.g., the level of a biomarker, or within a range, e.g., the percentage reduction in tumor size from baseline size. In this case, one may assume that $\log(\varepsilon_i) \sim N(0, \sigma^2)$, therefore Y_i is always positive as long as $g(C_i, \mathbf{X}_i, \boldsymbol{\beta}) > 0$. In contrast, the additive model with $E(\varepsilon_i) = 0$ cannot guarantee this property. The PK model (2.7) is also a multiplicative model.

Both (2.9) and (2.12) assume that Y_i is continuous, hence they cannot describe some types of response measures such as the status of dead or alive or the number of epileptic events within a day. A class of models known as generalized linear models (GLM) provides tools to model these types of response [McCullagh, 2019]. A GLM assumes that the distribution of Y_i belongs to the exponential family, and the mean of the response $E(Y_i)$ is linked to a linear structure with a link function $g(.)$ in the form

$$g(E(Y_i)) = \mathbf{X}_i^T\boldsymbol{\beta}_x + \beta_c C_i \tag{2.13}$$

or equivalently $E(Y_i) = g^{-1}(\mathbf{X}_i^T\boldsymbol{\beta}_x + \beta_c C_i)$. This model preserves the linear structure in model (2.9), but allows for nonlinearity in the link function. The linear part $\mathbf{X}_i^T\boldsymbol{\beta}_x + \beta_c C_i$ is known as the linear predictor. GLMs can be used to model a range of outcome types such as continuous variables with a positive distribution, binary, count, and categorical variables, since the exponential family contains a wide range of distributions.

Two commonly used GLMs are Poisson and logistic regression models [McCullagh, 2019]. The former is used for count data, e.g., $Y_i \sim \text{Poisson}(\lambda_i)$ may be the count of AE events on patient i with the log-link function

$$\log(\lambda_i) = \mathbf{X}_i^T\boldsymbol{\beta}_x + \beta_c C_i, \tag{2.14}$$

where the right hand side is the linear predictor and β_c is log-risk ratio (log-RR) for a 1 unit increase in C_i. The logistic regression models binary responses (e.g., $Y_i = 1$ if the patient had an AE and $Y_i = 0$ otherwise), then Y_i may follow the logistic model

$$\text{logit}(P(Y_i = 1)) = \mathbf{X}_i^T\boldsymbol{\beta}_x + \beta_c C_i \tag{2.15}$$

where $\text{logit}(p) = \log(p/(1-p))$ and β_c is log-odds ratio (log-OR) for a 1 unit increase in C_i. A GLM model can be fitted using the maximum likelihood estimation (MLE) (Section 10.2.1) to obtain $\hat{\boldsymbol{\beta}}_x$ and $\hat{\beta}_c$ as well as their variance-covariance matrix.

Now we apply the logistic regression model to the QT prolongation data in the example in Chapter 1. Since the mean PK concentration had the maximum around 2 hours, we explore the relationship between the concentration and the probability that QTcF prolongations would be longer than 20 ms around 2 hours. Using the 20-ms instead of the 30-ms threshold used by drug regulators is due to the very small number of patients with QTcF 30-ms in this dataset. Since QTcF was also measured during the placebo period, we can treat these measures as taken at 0 concentration. Fitting the logistic model to the data for the placebo and moxifloxacin periods, we obtain logOR = 0.468 (SE = 0.215) for an increase in concentration of 1000ng/ml, which shows a significant increase in the risk of prolongation of 20 ms at the level 5%. However, when the model is fitted to moxifloxacin data only, the log-OR becomes -0.104 (SE = 0.557), indicating that there is no ER relationship. In fact, this situation is not uncommon in exposure-response modeling when control (i.e., no exposure) data are available, since fitting the same model with and without control data may lead to completely different results. The difference often suggests that the dose-response relationship in the whole exposure range is complex and may need a more complex model. A simple model is likely to be misspecified in some exposure ranges. Using such a model may give very misleading predictions in these ranges.

Several special situations need careful consideration when using a GLM model. For example, if Y_i is the number of asthma attacks of patient i within a week, a Poisson regression model can be used to model Y_i since it is a count of events. However, Y_i may have a higher variance than $E(Y_i) = \lambda_i$: the variance of Y_i if it is Poisson distributed. This situation is known as over-dispersion, often caused by correlation between the events in the same patient. One way to accommodate over-dispersion is to assume that λ_i is a random variable following a gamma distribution. This leads to a negative binomial distribution for Y_i with $\text{var}(Y_i) = \lambda_i + \phi\lambda_i^2$ where ϕ is an over-dispersion parameter which can be estimated from the data [Cameron and Trivedi, 2013].

Over-dispersion may also be found in the distribution of the number of failures (or responders) Y_i among n_i subjects. In toxicology experiments, the responses of animals in the same litter are often correlated. Therefore, the number of deaths Y_i may not follow a binomial distribution and $\text{var}(Y_i) \neq n_i p_i(1-p_i)$, where p_i is the probability of an event. The effect leading to this correlation is known as the litter effect, but it can be found in other areas under similar situations. A common model to take into account positive correlation is to assume that p_i follows a beta distribution. The resulting distribution for Y_i is the beta-binomial distribution with $\text{var}(Y_i) = n_i p_i(1-p_i)(1+(n_i-1)\phi)$ where ϕ is the over-dispersion parameter.

Over-dispersion may not always occur even when p_i is a random variable. For the beta-binomial distribution, when $n_i = 1$, ϕ has no effect and the variance is $\text{var}(Y_i) = p_i(1 - p_i)$. Hence, there is no over-dispersion in a binary response variable. Intuitively, in an animal toxicology experiment, if there is only one animal in a litter, then there is no over-dispersion due to variation between animals. It is easy to verify that if $Y_i \sim Bin(p_i)$ and $p_i \sim F(p)$ where $F(p)$ is any distribution within (0,1), the marginal distribution Y_i is always binary.

Although one may use a MLE approach with an appropriate distribution such as negative- or beta-binomials for fitting over-dispersed data, in practice, an empirical approach is often sufficient and more convenient. The approach uses a robust estimate, rather than its parametric form (e.g., $\text{var}(Y_i) = n_i p_i(1 - p_i)$ for the binomial distribution) to estimate $\text{var}(Y_i)$, then uses the estimate to calculate the SEs of $\hat{\boldsymbol{\beta}}$ so that the Wald test-based statistical inference is valid under over-dispersion. In SAS proc GENMOD, [SAS Institute Inc., 2011] the option "PSCALE" in the "model" statement asks to estimate ϕ by the Pearson χ^2 statistic based on the empirical variance estimate $\sum_{i=1}^{n}(Y_i - E(Y_i))^2/(n - q)$ where q is the number of parameters in the model. Another option "DSCALE" uses the deviance to calculate ϕ. Often the resulting difference in $\text{var}(\hat{\boldsymbol{\beta}})$ by using the two options is small. Although ϕ is introduced by a mixture of distributions that only allows for over-dispersion, the robust approach also works for under-dispersion, i.e., when $\text{var}(Y_i) < \lambda_i$ in the count model example. In this case, it is often worthwhile to consider if under-dispersion is likely before deciding if one of the options should be used. NONMEM is a likelihood based software, so there is no readily used option to deal with over-dispersion. One may use either a full likelihood approach with the likelihood function for the beta-binomial or negative binomial distribution, or the so called quasi-likelihood approach. See Chapter 3.

Sometimes, extra variations occur at a particular value. The most common scenario can be found in data with more zero counts than it should be if a Poisson, or even a negative binomial distribution is assumed. This scenario is known as zero-inflation and has often been seen in biomedical outcomes, e.g., in the counts of asthma or epilepsy attacks, or adverse events under drug exposure. To describe this type of data, zero-inflated Poisson (ZIP) [Cameron and Trivedi, 2013] is introduced as follows. A ZIP distribution is denoted as $ZIP(\lambda_i, \rho_i)$ and defined as

$$P(Y_i = y) = \begin{cases} \rho_i + (1 - \rho_i)\exp(\lambda_i) & y = 0 \\ (1 - \rho_i)tPoisson(y, \lambda_i) & y > 0 \end{cases} \tag{2.16}$$

where $tPoisson(y, \lambda_i)$ is the truncated Poisson distribution (conditional on $y > 0$) and ρ_i is the probability of $Y_i = 0$. Therefore, we have $E(Y_i) = (1 - \rho_i)\lambda_i$. As both λ_i and ρ_i may depend on exposure and covariates, they can be fitted in separate models. These models are also known as two-part models.

Similarly, a zero-inflated NB (ZINB) distribution can be defined $Y_i \sim ZINB(\lambda_i, \phi, \rho_i)$ and has the chance $1 - \rho_i$ to follow the NB distribution and the chance ρ_i to always be 0. Zero-inflated models have been widely used for medical decision making, in which some outcomes such as the number of hospital visits are often zero-inflated. A DER model may help assess the impact of dosing and dose adjustment on costs due to, e.g., adverse events leading to hospitalization.

To link the two distributions to exposure and covariates, one may use a GLM structure for both λ_i and ρ_i:

$$\begin{aligned} \text{logit}(\rho_i) &= \mathbf{X}_i^T \boldsymbol{\beta}_a + C_i \gamma_a \\ \log(\lambda_i) &= \mathbf{X}_i^T \boldsymbol{\beta}_b + C_i \gamma_b \end{aligned} \tag{2.17}$$

where each model may only include part of the covariates in $\mathbf{X}_i$. The likelihood function of ZIP can be written based on its distribution (2.16), and can be maximized numerically to obtain estimates for the parameters in both parts. Fitting some standard zero-inflated models is easy with software such as SAS proc GENMOD [SAS Institute Inc., 2011]. Alternatively, proc NLMIXED can fit a wide range of models consisting of two parts with a regression model for each.

A similar issue may also occur when the outcome is a continuous variable. An example is the duration of hospital stay for a population of patients. The duration may be modeled by a log-normal or a gamma distribution, but for those without any hospitalization, the duration is zero. A similar approach can be applied. But since a positive continuous distribution does not contain zero value, it has no contribution to zero count, as we have seen $(1 - \rho_i)\exp(\lambda_i)$ in the ZIP distribution (2.16). Hence, the models for the probability of having zero value and the non-zero values can be fitted separately.

The logistic model can be extended to model ordered categorical responses. Examples may include clinical outcomes such as a three-level category of responding to treatment, stable disease and disease progression. One may model such an outcome with a general polynomial distribution $Poly(p_1, ..., p_k)$ with $p_k = P(Y = k)$ being the probability of outcome y in the kth category, and $\sum_{j=1}^{k} p_k = 1$. Although each p_k can be linked to exposure and covariates, to exploit the order of categories, a model can be used to represent a trend between, e.g., exposure and the level of outcome. For example, a higher exposure may increase the odds of being in a higher category, which is the basic assumption of proportional odds model with

$$log(P(Y_i > k)/P(Y_i \leq k)) = \beta_c C_i + \mathbf{X}_i^T \boldsymbol{\beta}_k \tag{2.18}$$

where β_c is the common log-OR for a 1 unit increase in C_i for all ks, but different $\boldsymbol{\beta}_k$ are needed, as $\mathbf{X}_i$ includes the intercept, which typically changes with k. An alternative is to use a reference category, e.g., level 1 so that the model assumes

$$log(P(Y_i = k)/P(Y_i = 1)) = \beta_c C_i + \mathbf{X}_i^T \boldsymbol{\beta}_k. \tag{2.19}$$

Both models include the logistic model a special case when the category has two levels. Fitting such a model is straightforward with current software for GLMs such as proc GENMOD.

2.3 Transformations

Transformation is a very useful approach in modeling to transform dose, exposure and/or response variables as well as parameters. We will leave transformation of parameters (also known as re-parameterizations) to a later part where we treat parameters as random variables. The log-transformation is the most commonly used transformation and plays a central role in DER modeling. Sometimes, a transformation should be applied to both the variable and the model for it. This is known as the transform-on-both sides (TBS) approach [Carroll and Ruppert, 2017]. One reason for using a transformation from a statistical aspect is to make the distribution of the response easy to handle with a simple model. Transformation can also convert a multiplicative model to an additive one, and the latter is often much easier to fit. Some transformations are proposed from purely statistical aspects, particularly those depending on extra-parameters, such as the Box-Cox transformation are used less frequently than the log-transformation in DER modeling. Here we will mainly focus on the latter.

Consider the theophylline concentration data. Since there are no dosing history data, we modeled the concentration data before any dose adjustment was made. Let C_i be the concentration of patient i at 0.01h. We fitted a linear model for log-transformed C_i and covariates:

$$\log(C_i) = \mathbf{X}_i^T \gamma + e_i, \tag{2.20}$$

where $e_i \sim N(0, \sigma_e^2)$. Note that this model might be considered as an approximation to model (2.7). The data were fitted by the linear regression function lm(.) in R. After fitting models with different combinations of covariates in $\mathbf{X}_i$, we found that only age is related to C_i (denoted THEO in the output) and the fitted model is

```
lm(formula = log(THEO) ~ log(AGE), data = short[short$TIME ==0.01, ])

Coefficients:
             Estimate Std. Error t value Pr(>|t|)
(Intercept)   -0.8623     0.9418  -0.916   0.3618
log(AGE)       0.5699     0.2655   2.147   0.0339
```

The other factors included in the dataset may have been sufficiently adjusted when planning the initial dose. Transforming back to the original scale, we get the geometric mean of C_i as

$$\exp(\mathbf{X}_i^T \hat{\gamma}) = \exp(-0.862)\text{AGE}^{0.570} \tag{2.21}$$

which is in the form of the power model. The key feature is that the contributions of the factors are multiplicative to each other. Note that $\exp(\mathbf{X}_i^T\gamma)$ is the geometric mean of C_i, and $E(C_i) = \exp(\mathbf{X}_i^T\gamma)E(\exp(e_i)) > \exp(\mathbf{X}_i^T\gamma)$. Geometric means are commonly used for modeling exposure data, but may not always be appropriate for PKPD modeling.

Transformations are also used for nonlinear models. The error structure of the model is a key factor to consider in selecting an appropriate transformation. We take the Emax model (2.3) as an example to show how to select the transformation. Suppose that Y_i is positive (e.g., the tumor size or a positive valued biomarker) and its relationship with C_i has a sigmoid-like shape, then the following model may be appropriate:

$$\begin{aligned}\log(Y_i) &= \log(E_{max}/(1 + EC_{50}/C_i)\varepsilon_i) \\ &= \log(E_{max}) - \log(1 + EC_{50}/C_i) + \log(\varepsilon_i) \qquad (2.22)\end{aligned}$$

where $\log(\varepsilon_i) \sim N(0, \sigma_\varepsilon^2)$ is an additive error term. This is a direct application of TBS to the Emax model with a multiplicative error term. The assumption of multiplicative error is reasonable when all $Y_i > 0$. Consider an additive Emax model

$$Y_i = E_{max}/(1 + EC_{50}/C_i) + \varepsilon_i^*. \qquad (2.23)$$

Under constraint $Y_i > 0$, the error term has to satisfy the condition $E_{max}/(1+ EC_{50}/C_i) > \varepsilon_i^*$ that makes the distribution of ε_i^* depend on $E(Y_i)$ in an awkward way, although this may not be a serious practical problem if σ_ϵ^2 is low. The model (2.22) can be considered as a partial linear model, since the parameter $\log(E_{max})$ is linear with respect to Y_i.

From model (2.22) we can derive

$$E(Y_i) = E_{max}/(1 + EC_{50}/C_i)\exp(\sigma_\varepsilon^2/2) \qquad (2.24)$$

Not that the relationship between $E(Y_i)$ and C_i is still described by the Emax model if σ_ε^2 is constant. E_{max} and EC_{50} are still the maximum effect and the concentration for achieving 50% of the maximum effect. However, the absolute change in $E(Y_i)$ due to C_i depends on σ_ε^2. A constant σ_ε^2 is an important condition for maintaining the Emax relationship between $E(Y_i)$ and C_i, as the geometric mean, denoted by $E^g(Y_i) = E_{max}/(1 + EC_{50}/C_i)$ is proportional to $E(Y_i)$ only when σ_ε^2 is constant. The two may be different functions if σ_ε^2 depends on C_i directly or indirectly.

We note that, with this model, $E(Y_i) = 0$ when $C_i = 0$ and $E(Y_i) = E_{max}$ when $C_i \to \infty$. $E(Y_i) = 0$ may be an unreasonable constraint, as often the baseline of response Y_{i0} (that is, the outcome when $C_i = 0$) may not be zero. Therefore, we may want to model the percent change from baseline or the ratio of the response to the baseline. Multiplicative models are commonly used for this purpose. For example, let Y_i be the tumor size or a biomarker measure, and Y_{i0} the baseline value. We are interested in the treatment effect on Y_i/Y_{i0} or more specifically the reduction of tumor size or biomarker measure from baseline. In this case, we want the geometric mean $E^g(Y_i) = Y_{i0}$ when $C_i = 0$. In this situation, a variant of model (2.22) is

$$Y_i/Y_{i0} = (1 - E_{max}/(1 + EC_{50}/C_i))\varepsilon_i \tag{2.25}$$

where Y_{i0} is the baseline and $\log(\varepsilon_i) \sim N(0, \sigma_\epsilon^2)$. This model leads to $E^g(Y_i|Y_{i0}, C_i = 0) = Y_{i0}$, as we want. Note that often a constraint $E_{max} \leq 1$ should be applied as the tumor or biomarker values should be non-negative. A further extension may allow fitting Y_{i0} in the model as a covariate:

$$Y_i = Y_{i0}^{\alpha}(1 - E_{max}/(1 + EC_{50}/C_i))\varepsilon_i \tag{2.26}$$

where α is a new parameter representing the impact of Y_{i0} on Y_i. With a log transformation on both sides, the model

$$\log(Y_i) = \alpha \log(Y_{i0}) + \log(1 - E_{max}/(1 + EC_{50}/C_i)) + \log(\varepsilon_i) \tag{2.27}$$

can be fitted as a partial linear model. A numerical problem may occur when $1 - E_{max}/(1 + EC_{50}/C_i)$ is too close to zero. Often making E_{max} bounded away from 1 can avoid this problem. However, E_{max} can be negative if the exposure effect increases Y_i from Y_{i0}.

Finally, it is important to note that dealing with zero exposures (e.g., exposure of the control group) is difficult for log-transformation in a model with $\log(C_i)$, e.g., $\log(Y_i) = \beta \log(C_i) + \log(\varepsilon_i)$. An ad hoc approach of replacing the zero value with a small value may work fine. However, the sensitivity of the model to the imputed value should be examined. If the purpose is to extrapolate the exposure-response relationship to a lower exposure range than the observed exposure range, one should ensure the model fits well in the extrapolation range, as the imputed value may not affect the overall model fitting but have a strong impact on prediction for the lower exposure range.

2.4 Semi-parametric and non-parametric models

Models for a ER relationship are often empirical in nature (in contrast to compartmental popPK models derived from a pharmacological mechanism). Therefore, the modeler may be less certain on the correctness of the model and may not be able to take advantage of using a model with clear pharmacological meaning. Sometimes parametric models may not fit the data well, hence more flexible models are useful alternatives. There are many non- and semi-parametric approaches described in the literature. We will concentrate on the approach using spline functions [De Boor, 1978]. This approach has a number of advantages over the other approaches, the most important being its ease of use with implementations in R and SAS.

Spline functions have been widely used to approximate a function with known or unknown analytical form in computational mathematics, with well-developed algorithms for calculating them [De Boor, 1978]. Without going into details, we simply state that spline functions are piecewise polynomial functions connected at a number of points (knots) where their value and derivatives up to a certain order are continuous, so that the curve they generated is sufficiently smooth. The most commonly used are cubic spline functions consisting of cubic polynomials with continuous values and up to the second order derivatives.

Using regression with spline functions is straightforward. We use B-splines as an example to introduce this approach. Suppose that we would like to construct a smoothed ER curve in the exposure range (0, 1). The simplest B-splines are those with knots at 0 and 1 only (known as boundary knots). In this case, the B-splines are expressed in terms of $C_n^k x^n (1-x)^k, k = 0, ..., n$, with C_n^k the number of combinations to take k balls from a total of n. With only boundary knots, the cubic B-spline has n=3+1=4 such terms. Using the function bs() in the R [R Core Team, 2013] library splines, we can construct

```
> x=(0:10)/10
> cbind(x,bs(x,degree = 3,intercept=T))
        x     1     2     3     4
 [1,] 0.0 1.000 0.000 0.000 0.000
 [2,] 0.1 0.729 0.243 0.027 0.001
 [3,] 0.2 0.512 0.384 0.096 0.008
 [4,] 0.3 0.343 0.441 0.189 0.027
 [5,] 0.4 0.216 0.432 0.288 0.064
 [6,] 0.5 0.125 0.375 0.375 0.125
 [7,] 0.6 0.064 0.288 0.432 0.216
 [8,] 0.7 0.027 0.189 0.441 0.343
 [9,] 0.8 0.008 0.096 0.384 0.512
[10,] 0.9 0.001 0.027 0.243 0.729
[11,] 1.0 0.000 0.000 0.000 1.000
```

gives the value of the function at different x. For each interior knot, there is one more term

```
> bs(x,degree = 3,knots=0.5,intercept=T)
          1     2     3     4     5
 [1,] 1.000 0.000 0.000 0.000 0.000
 [2,] 0.512 0.434 0.052 0.002 0.000
 [3,] 0.216 0.592 0.176 0.016 0.000
 [4,] 0.064 0.558 0.324 0.054 0.000
 [5,] 0.008 0.416 0.448 0.128 0.000
 [6,] 0.000 0.250 0.500 0.250 0.000
 [7,] 0.000 0.128 0.448 0.416 0.008
 [8,] 0.000 0.054 0.324 0.558 0.064
 [9,] 0.000 0.016 0.176 0.592 0.216
[10,] 0.000 0.002 0.052 0.434 0.512
[11,] 0.000 0.000 0.000 0.000 1.000
```

```
attr(,"degree")
[1] 3
attr(,"knots")
[1] 0.5
attr(,"Boundary.knots")
[1] 0 1
```

However, one of the terms is redundant since $C_n^k x^n(1-x)^k$s are the probability of having k events in n trials when x is the probability. Therefore, $\sum_{k=1}^n C_n^k x^n(1-x)^k = 1$. Therefore, to fit the B-spline to, e.g., $\sqrt{x}$, one should use the bs() function without the option intercept = T, which defaults not to produce the first term:

```
lm(sqrt(x)~bs(x,degree=3))
```

Otherwise, the intercept cannot be fitted. The algorithm for constructing B-splines [De Boor, 1978] is very efficient, but the details will not be discussed here. The coefficient C_n^k is not needed from a practical point of view as for each term a parameter will be fitted. Therefore, we may simply note each term as $B_k(x)$. There are other types of spline function; among them, natural spline functions are also commonly used.

When using spline functions in a ER regression model one can simply include them as covariates:

$$Y_i = \sum_{k=1}^{K} B_k(C_i)\eta_k + \varepsilon_i. \tag{2.28}$$

where $B_k(C_i)$ is evaluated at exposure level C_i. Construction of B-spline functions is very efficient with software such as R-library splines(.). For example, using the argatroban data at the 6-hour time point and predicted exposures, which will be discussed in Chapter 4, we can use function bs() together with function *lm*() to fit the spline functions to log(APTT):

```
fittedModel1=lm(log(resp)~bs(pred,3),data=data240),
```

in which data240 is the 6-hour dataset, pred and resp are the predicted exposure and log(APTT) respectively, and $bs(pred, 3)$ produces a matrix of B-spline functions. It produces the model fit

```
lm(formula = log(resp) ~ bs(pred, 3), data = data240)

Coefficients:
 (Intercept)  bs(pred, 3)1  bs(pred, 3)2  bs(pred, 3)3
      3.7845        0.4710        0.2907        0.8023
```

One can also generate the B-spline functions outside of the model fitting function lm(), and then use the matrix as covariates. The following function call gives exactly the same fit.

```
Bspline=bs(data240$pred,3)
fittedModel1=lm(log(data240$resp)~Bspline)
```

Spline functions can be used to construct semi-parametric models such as

$$Y_i = \mathbf{X}_i^T \boldsymbol{\beta} + \sum_{k=1}^{K} B_k(C_i)\eta_k + \varepsilon_i. \tag{2.29}$$

where $\mathbf{X}_i^T \boldsymbol{\beta}$ is the parametric part. For example, in the argatroban analysis we may adjust for log-baseline values ("base") in the model

```
fittedModel2=lm(log(resp)~log(base)+bs(pred,3),data=data240)
```

which gives

```
lm(formula = log(resp) ~ log(base) + bs(pred, 3), data = data240)

Coefficients:
 (Intercept)      log(base)  bs(pred, 3)1  bs(pred, 3)2  bs(pred, 3)3
      1.2619         0.7671        0.3914        0.3924        0.7522
```

The coefficients for the spline functions are difficult to interpret directly. However, since the B-spline functions are basis functions between the knots, an increasing trend of the coefficient indicates the same trend in the ER relationship. This can also be seen from the previous B-spline examples in (0,1).

The sample approach can be used to model the DR relationship. However, when there are only a few dose levels, the complexity of spline functions is limited by the number of dose levels. This issue in regression splines is not alone; any non-parametric approach has the same issue and a complex DR relationship cannot be identified with DR data alone.

In a semi-parametric model, it could be that the non-parametric part is of the primary interest. For example, to explore the dose-response relationship in argatroban data, one may fit a model with spline functions for the time profile, while using dose as a covariate. Since this analysis involves repeated measurements and needs a linear mixed model, it will be postponed until the next chapter.

Semi-parametric methods can also be used to extend GLMs with a smoothing method on the linear predictor. For example, one can add spline functions for exposure to a GLM model and obtain

$$g(E(Y_i)) = \mathbf{X}_i^T \boldsymbol{\beta}_x + \sum_{k=1}^{K} B_k(C_i)\eta_k \tag{2.30}$$

This type of model is known as a generalized additive model, as the spline function part is additive in the linear predictor. We have seen a large difference between the fitted logistic models with and without placebo data, indicating a more complex ER relationship than a linear model can describe. Fitting a logistic model with natural cubic spline functions using

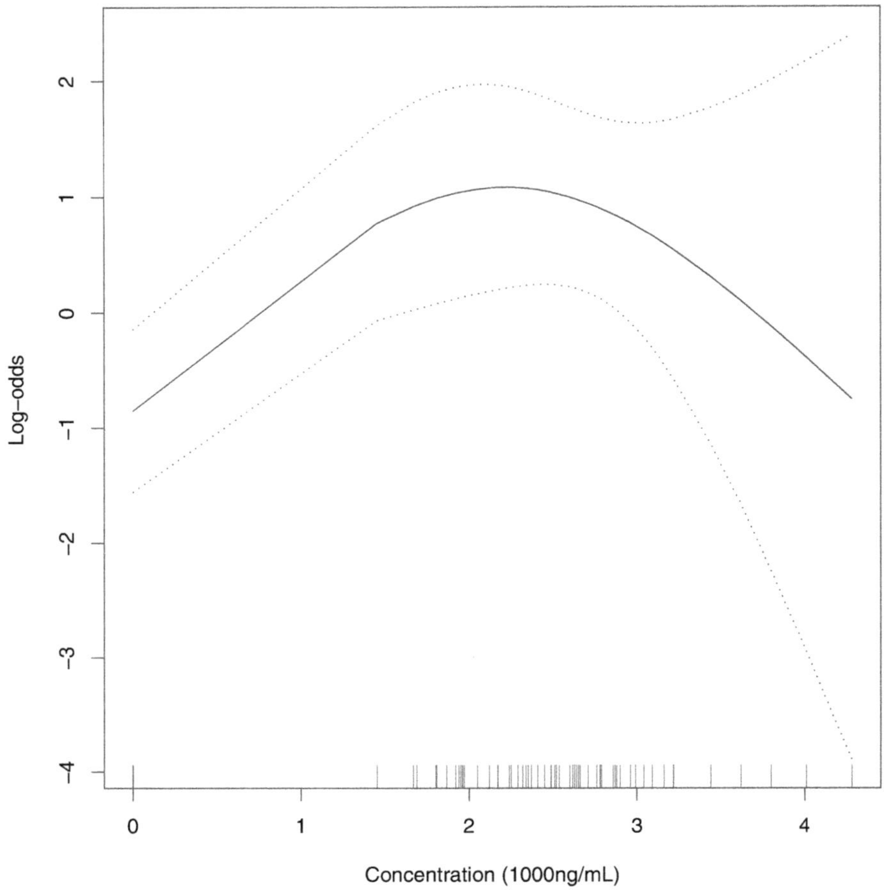

Figure 2.1
Non-parametric estimate of the relationship between moxifloxacin concentration and logOR of 20 ms prolongation in QTcF at 2 hours post dosing using natural cubic spline functions. The dotted lines are 95% CI.

```
fit=gam(qtp~ns(conc,3),family=binomial,data=moxi[moxi$time==2,])
```

where conc and qtq are the moxifloxacin concentration and response, respectively, at 2 hours, giving a bell-shaped curve for the relationship between the concentration and logOR (Figure 2.1).

The results indicate a nonlinear relationship between moxifloxacin exposure and QT prolongation globally. The estimated ER curve has a bell shape, while the lower and higher ends of the curve are very uncertain as there was no event between concentration ranges of zero and 1870ng/mL and higher than 3000ng/mL. Although there is an initial increase in risk along with an increase in exposure, the left part of the curve cannot be quantified. There is no evidence of an ER relationship in the higher concentration range. In summary, there is not sufficient information to quantify the overall ER relationship based on the parametric and semi-parametric models. We will show other approaches that use more information in the data in later parts of the book.

Using spline functions in SAS [SAS Institute Inc., 2011] is also easy for some procedures such as proc GLIMMIX. The following EFFECT statement

```
EFFECT bs = spline(exposure / knotmethod=percentiles(3));
```

creates B-spline function effects with two knots at the lower and upper bounds and internal knots at the median of the exposure data. Then, in the model statement, the effects bs are included as covariates. This statement can be used in a number of other SAS procedures.

As a general approach, creating B-spline functions as covariates outside of a procedure or function for model fitting can be used in almost all software including R/Splus functions *lm* (as shown in the previous example), library *lme4*, SAS and NONMEM. For NONMEM this is slightly more complex since it involves appending the original dataset with extra columns and has to be done outside of the NONMEM run itself. For simple spline functions (e.g., the basic cubic spline functions as generated by R function bs(.)) it is also possible to program them in NONMEM.

The main purpose of using spline functions in an ER model is to predict the response at different exposure levels. Some SAS procedures have prediction facilities, and hence the prediction and graphic presentation of the fitted model are ready after the model is fitted. Some software does not have this function, e.g., R library *lme4*. As a general method, prediction based on the fitted model is always possible. For this, one needs to evaluate the spline function at a given exposure level, which may not be one of the observed exposure levels. The *splines* library has a function *splineDesign* to evaluate the design matrix for the B-splines defined by knots at a given exposure level. There is also a short cut using the generic *predict* function. The following command generates a matrix of B-spline functions evaluated at exposure levels 200, 500 and 1000

```
splinePred=predict(bs(data240$pred,3),newx=c(200,500,1000)).
```

The predicted APTT at these concentration levels and a given baseline value can be calculated using splinePred and the coefficients in the fitted model, e.g., with code fittedModel2 above. Note that if the exposure range for prediction, as specified with "newx=", is outside of the data distribution range, a warning "some 'x' values beyond boundary knots may cause ill-conditioned bases" will occur. It warns the user of the fact that spline functions are developed as a tool for interpolation rather than extrapolation.

There are a number of parameters to choose in the spline functions. In general, the higher the order, or the more knots, the more flexible the functions. A recommendation for the number of knots that works well in common situations is to add one knot for every 4 data points, with an upper bound set at 35 [Ruppert et al., 2003]. The knots can be distributed at equally spaced percentiles of the exposure data. We will come back to this topic in later chapters, where further applications of spline functions can be found.

2.5 Comments and bibliographic notes

There are a number of books about PKPD modeling. As a textbook, Bonate [2006] covers most of important topics, is easy to read with a large number of worked examples, hence is highly recommended to statisticians and modelers. Senn [2008] gives an excellent summary for statistical issues in drug development. McCullagh [2019] and Bates and Watts [1988] are the classical texts for GLMs and nonlinear regression models, respectively. Many examples of using GLMs and their extensions can be found in Lindsey [2000]. Details about count data including over-dispersion and zero-inflated models can be found in Cameron and Trivedi [2013]. Details about transformation can be found in Carroll and Ruppert [2017], although quite some are far beyond our scope. For model fitting using spline functions, Ruppert et al. [2003] provided a good introduction to statisticians and modelers. For readers who want to know mathematical details, De Boor [1978] is a classical text for spline functions.

3

Dose-exposure and exposure-response models for longitudinal data

This chapter introduces the most commonly used models in dose-exposure (DE) and exposure-response (ER) modeling for repeated measures from multiple individuals [Davidian and Giltinan, 2017; Fitzmaurice et al., 2008]. For ER models we assume that the response and exposures are measured at the same time. The role of the exposure model in the ER modeling may not be obvious at this stage, but in the following chapters its importance will be seen clearly. This chapter will cover several common types of response measures, including longitudinal continuous measures and categorical outcomes such as tumor sizes, biomarker measures, and the occurrence of adverse events (AEs).

3.1 Linear mixed models for exposure-response relationships

A linear mixed model (LMM) is a linear model with some factors considered as fixed and some others considered random, often referred to as fixed and random effects, respectively. It can also be considered as an extension of the simple liner model (2.9) to allow the parameters to be random variables. We use theophylline and PEFR data described in Chapter 1 as an example to show the structure of linear mixed models. In the data, both theophylline concentrations and PEFR were measured repeatedly from each patient. Let Y_{ij} and C_{ij} be the PEFR and concentration at time $t_j, j = 1, ..., r$ of patient i. Assuming a linear relationship between them, one may write

$$Y_{ij} = \beta_0 + \beta_c C_{ij} + \varepsilon_{ij}, \tag{3.1}$$

where ε_{ij} represents the within-patient variation in PEFR, β_0 is the mean PEFR and β_c measures the change in mean PEFR for 1mg/L theophylline increase. However, some patient baseline characteristics, such as lung function, that affect PEFR may not be observed. Taking them into the model, we can write

$$Y_{ij} = \beta_0 + \beta_c C_{ij} + U_i + \varepsilon_{ij} \tag{3.2}$$

DOI: 10.1201/9781003457008-3

where U_i is a latent variable representing individual's variability in PEFR. If r is sufficiently large, further assumptions on U_i may not be necessary since U_is can be considered unknown parameters and estimated when fitting the model. However, in many cases r is not large enough to estimate U_is individually. In these cases, an LMM has the advantage of borrowing information between patients and can provide better inference for both β and U_is. For this purpose, we need to assume that U_i is a random variable, e.g., following a normal distribution, so $U_i \sim N(0, \sigma_u^2)$. The issue of specifying the distribution for the random effects will be discussed later. The distribution of ε_{ij} is generally less important but we also assume that $\varepsilon_{ij} \sim N(0, \sigma_e^2)$. When ε_{ij}s are independent of C_{ij}, model (3.2) is among the simplest linear mixed models, but it does contain key features of LMMs. Based on this model one can calculate the correlation between Y_{ij}s in the same patient as $\sqrt{\text{cov}(Y_{ij}, Y_{ij'})/\text{var}(Y_{ij})} = \sqrt{\sigma_u^2/(\sigma_u^2 + \sigma_e^2)}$. The correlation does not depend on the assumed normality. Note that the same correlation occurs between any pair of Y_{ij} and $Y_{ij'}$. The PEFRs from different patients remain independent. This structure is known as compound symmetry and is among the simplest and widely used correlation structures in LMMs.

The basic model (3.2) can be extended in a number of ways. Intuitively, two PEFR measures 5 minutes apart probably have a higher correlation than those measured 5 hours apart. Therefore, it is often reasonable to assume that the correlation between ε_{ij} and $\varepsilon_{ij'}$ at t_j and $t_{j'}$ respectively, denoted by $\rho(\varepsilon_{ij}, \varepsilon_{ij'})$ is a function of $t_j - t_{j'}$, for example, $\rho(\varepsilon_{ij}, \varepsilon_{ij'}) = a|t_j - t_{j'}|^b$ where a and b are parameters to be estimated when fitting the model. This type of correlation is known as serial correlation, with the simplest case being the auto-regressive error of order 1 (AR(1)) given by $\varepsilon_{ij+1} = a\varepsilon_{ij} + \varepsilon_{ij}^*$, where ε_{ij}^*s are independent. Serial correlation and correlation due to patient-level random effects may co-exist and can be modeled if data are sufficient (e.g., when the number of repeated measures is not small). Models with both correlations can be easily fitted by SAS proc MIXED [SAS Institute Inc., 2011] and the R library lme4 [Bates et al., 2015]

In model (3.2) we have assumed that a common slope β_c represents the effect of the concentration on PEFR for **all** patients. This may not be the case, as often the treatment effects (e.g., increase in PEFR per increase in 1 mg / L concentration) may be different between patients. Another extension of the model (3.2) is to allow β to be a random variable. This extension leads to a random coefficient model [Longford, 1995]

$$Y_{ij} = \beta_0 + \beta_i C_{ij} + U_i + \varepsilon_{ij} \tag{3.3}$$

where $\beta_i \sim N(\beta, \sigma_\beta^2)$ is a random coefficient with mean β and variance σ_β^2. A general model form can be written as

$$Y_{ij} = \mathbf{X}_{ij}^T \boldsymbol{\beta}_i + \mathbf{Z}_{ij}^T \mathbf{U}_i + \varepsilon_{ij} \tag{3.4}$$

where $\mathbf{X}_{ij}$ and $\mathbf{Z}_{ij}$ are vectors that may include C_{ij}, additional covariates and a constant, and $\mathbf{U}_i \sim N(0, \mathbf{\Sigma}_u)$ are random subject effects. In the rest of the book we will follow this general model form, and only write the C_{ij} term separately when needed. When $\mathbf{Z}_{ij} = \mathbf{X}_{ij}$ the model is a random coefficient model. $\mathbf{Z}_{ij}$ may only contain a constant, e.g., to form model (3.3). In most mixed model texts, the model is written in vector form

$$\mathbf{Y}_i = \mathbf{X}_i \boldsymbol{\beta}_x + \mathbf{Z}_i \mathbf{U}_i + \boldsymbol{\varepsilon}_i \tag{3.5}$$

where $\mathbf{Y}_i = Y_{i1}, ..., Y_{ir}, \boldsymbol{\varepsilon}_i = \varepsilon_{i1}, ..., \varepsilon_{ir}$ and $\mathbf{X}_i$ and $\mathbf{Z}_i$ are matrices formed by stacking $\mathbf{X}_{ij}^T$s and $\mathbf{Z}_{ij}^T$s. Elements in $\mathbf{\Sigma}_u$ are called variance components, which are important parameters in a mixed model. Based on normality and model structure, the marginal model has a simple form

$$\mathbf{Y}_i = \mathbf{X}_i \boldsymbol{\beta} + \boldsymbol{\varepsilon}_i^* \tag{3.6}$$

with $\boldsymbol{\varepsilon}_i^* \sim N(0, \mathbf{\Sigma}_i)$ where $\mathbf{\Sigma}_i = \text{var}(\boldsymbol{\varepsilon}_i^*) = \mathbf{Z}_i \mathbf{\Sigma}_u \mathbf{Z}_i^T + \sigma_e^2 \mathbf{I} = \mathbf{Z}_i \mathbf{\Sigma}_u \mathbf{Z}_i^T + \sigma_e^2 \mathbf{I}$ and $\mathbf{I}$ is the r-dimensional identity matrix.

With the marginal model (3.6), we can estimate the parameters $\boldsymbol{\beta}$ using MLE. An alternative estimate for $\boldsymbol{\beta}$ (which is also based on the marginal model and is equivalent to the MLE approach) is the generalized LS estimate as the solution to

$$S(\boldsymbol{\beta}) = \sum_{i=1}^{n} \mathbf{X}_i^T \mathbf{\Sigma}_i^{-1} (\mathbf{Y}_i - \mathbf{X}_i \boldsymbol{\beta}) = 0. \tag{3.7}$$

The variance components can be estimated in multiple ways. The MLE may underestimate them, since it does not take into account the impact of estimating $\boldsymbol{\beta}$. A correction for this impact is to use the residual (or restricted) maximum likelihood (REML), particularly when the sample size is small. The REML approach uses a penalty term for the estimation of $\boldsymbol{\beta}$ to correct the bias. All software packages we use in this book can fit LMMs with a complex structure, using MLE or REML and more options for the estimation of the variance components. R and SAS example codes for fitting LMMs of different correlation structures can be found in the online Appendix.

Since in LMMs U_i is an unknown random variable rather than a parameter, a key role of using the model for DER modeling is to predict U_i. To understand the role of distributional assumptions on U_i, let us consider a simple model

$$Y_{ij} = U_i + \varepsilon_{ij}. \tag{3.8}$$

If U_i is considered an unknown parameter, its estimate is the individual mean $\bar{Y}_{i.} = \sum_{j=1}^{r} Y_{ij}/r$, in which the model and data from other patients were ignored. However, with the assumption $U_i \sim N(0, \sigma_u)$, a better estimation for U_i is

$$\hat{U}_i = \bar{Y}_i \sigma_u^2 / (\sigma_u^2 + \sigma_e^2). \tag{3.9}$$

Therefore, the assumption of random U_i centered at zero makes the estimate (or prediction) shrink toward zero. Based on the general model with normally distributed $\mathbf{U}_i$ and ε_{ij}, the conditional mean of $\mathbf{U}_i$ is

$$E(\mathbf{U}_i|\mathbf{Y}_i) = \mathbf{\Sigma}_u\mathbf{Z}_i^T\mathbf{\Sigma}_i^{-1}(\mathbf{Y}_i - \mathbf{X}_i\boldsymbol{\beta}). \tag{3.10}$$

Therefore, the right-hand side with unknown parameters replaced by their estimates can be used for the prediction of $\mathbf{U}_i$. With estimated parameters, (3.10) is no longer an unbiased conditional mean, but is often a good estimator, if the overall sample size is large. The mixed model software usually gives a prediction $\mathbf{U}_i$ on this basis.

The LMM can accommodate complex structure in ER models, e.g., when the ER relationship depends on covariates, by properly constructing the matrices $\mathbf{X}_i$ and $\mathbf{Z}_i$. For example, the response to an increase in exposure may be different among males and females, hence the model becomes

$$Y_{ij} = \beta_0 + \beta_{1i}C_{ij} + Male_i\beta_{2i}C_{ij} + U_i + \varepsilon_{ij}, \tag{3.11}$$

where $Male_i = 1$ for male patients and $Male_i = 0$ otherwise, and $Male_i\beta_{2i}C_{ij}$ is often called an interaction term. In this model β_{1i}s are the exposure coefficients for females and β_{2i} are the coefficients for males/female difference, respectively, and $\beta_{ki} \sim N(\beta_k, \sigma_b^2)$. This model can be written in the form of (3.4) by adding interaction terms between covariates and C_{ij} in $\mathbf{X}_i$. In the previous model two variables in $\mathbf{X}_i$ are the concentration in males and the other the concentration in females. Both R and SAS can form interactions between variables automatically with similar syntax, such as Male*conc in the model statement, but in NONMEM interaction terms have to be formed explicitly. Special attention should be paid to the interpretation of these models. For example, to estimate the effect of 1 unit increase in C_{ij} in a population, the male/female proportion of this population is needed and the effect is a weighted average of β_1 and β_2 based on this proportion. In general, including the interaction term reduces the random variation in $\mathbf{U}_i$ since the variation between genders now becomes explained by β_2.

Apart from parameter estimation, we also need statistical inference tools for model comparison, hypothesis test and constructing CIs for parameters in the model. Among them, hypothesis testing is a key one since it can be used for the other purposes, such as constructing a CI. Hypothesis testing for LMMs in principle is not much different from that for other models, with one exception: the testing of variance components. Since ML or REML is the main tool for model fitting, it is natural to base statistical inference on one of them. A hypothesis can be tested using one of the three tests: Wald test, likelihood ratio (LR) test and score test. The Wald test for a parameter is based on the assumption that $(\hat{\beta} - \beta)/SE(\hat{\beta}) \sim N(0, 1)$ which can be used for testing $\beta = \beta_0$ under H_0. The LR test requires models fitted under the null and alternative hypotheses. The -2log-LR of the model under the alternative to that under the null hypotheses follows approximately a chi-square distribution with degrees of freedom equal to the difference in the numbers of parameters included in the two models. The score test needs the calculation of the score function (i.e., the derivatives of the likelihood function with respect to β, Section 10.2.1) based on the model under the null hypothesis only, which is often a big advantage when the model under the alternative is much more complex. Both Wald and LR tests can be implemented easily using any of the three software, but interestingly none of them offers an option for the score test.

There are more alternative models to an LMM than to a simple linear model, hence model selection is also a key task. Some may prefer to use a hypothesis test for model selection following the principle that to use a complex model with extra parameters, it should show a statistically significant difference to a simpler one at, e.g., the 5% level. Some other model selection indices such as the Akaike information criterion (AIC) [Akaike, 2003] or the Bayesian information criterion (BIC) [Schwarz, 1978] are also widely used. Both criteria are a simple index (the smaller the better) that combines the goodness of fit and the penalty of complexity of the model. All three software packages used for this book provide these indices. Note that the LR test cannot be based on REML since the penalty term may change with different models.

Applying the LMM approach to the theophylline dataset we use the R library lme4. The results of the fit of the basic model are, where THEO and ID are the theophylline concentration and the patient's ID, respectively,

```
Linear mixed model fit by REML
Formula: PEFR ~ THEO + (1 | ID)
   Data: theo
  AIC  BIC logLik deviance REMLdev
 6895 6913  -3444     6893    6887
Random effects:
 Groups   Name        Variance Std.Dev.
 ID       (Intercept) 4055.6   63.683
 Residual             7267.6   85.250
Number of obs: 574, groups: ID, 153

Fixed effects:
            Estimate Std. Error t value
(Intercept) 204.0624     9.5036  21.472
THEO          2.9877     0.5255   5.686
```

where we find that the effect of the concentration on PEFR is 2.99L/(1mg/L) with SE=0.526. The residual variance is 7268 and between-patient variance is 4056. Adding random effects to β seems to have only a small impact with an estimate of σ_β^2 equal to 2.82, and the LR test results in the test statistic $\chi^2 = 3.33$ with 1 d.f.

Adding all covariates to the model leads to the conclusion that all but race are significant at the 5% level. The between-patient variance is reduced to 2007.

```
Linear mixed model fit by REML
Formula: PEFR ~ THEO+AGE+WT+factor(SEX)+factor(RACE)+factor(DIAG)+(1|ID)
   Data: theo
  AIC  BIC logLik deviance REMLdev
 6788 6836  -3383     6808    6766
Random effects:
 Groups   Name        Variance Std.Dev.
 ID       (Intercept) 1541.5   39.262
 Residual             7252.2   85.160
Number of obs: 574, groups: ID, 153

Fixed effects:
              Estimate Std. Error t value
(Intercept)   192.7639    27.0525   7.126
THEO            3.1088     0.4957   6.271
AGE            -1.5694     0.3543  -4.429
WT              0.7961     0.3310   2.405
factor(SEX)1   35.7653    11.1587   3.205
factor(RACE)1  29.3233    17.4045   1.685
factor(RACE)2  -8.0572    19.3195  -0.417
factor(DIAG)2 -73.0507    17.7482  -4.116
factor(DIAG)3  19.2605    38.7723   0.497
```

The covariates are coded as Sex : Male=1 Female=0; Race: Caucasian=1, Polynesian=2, Other=3 and Diag(diagnosis): Asthma=1, COPD=2, Asthma +COPD=3.

The scatter plot (Figure 1.3) suggests that a log-normal distribution may better fit the PEFRs, as does the nature of the PEFR being positive. Fitting log-PEFR to a model with concentration and all the covariates gives AIC=586. Note that this model cannot be compared with the model fitting PEFR using the LR test or the AIC or BIC, since they are not nested (i.e., one includes the other). We have to judge which model fits the data better empirically. We can refine this model by applying transformations to the concentration and covariates. We used the TBS technique to fit the following multiplicative model and it shows a significantly better fit to the data with a 29.2 increase in 2log-likelihood, and with no additional parameter.

```
Linear mixed model fit by REML
Formula: log(PEFR) ~ log(THEO) + log(AGE) + log(WT) + factor(SEX)
    + factor(RACE) + factor(DIAG) + (1 | ID)
   Data: theo
   AIC BIC logLik deviance REMLdev
 579.3 627 -278.6    520.8   557.3
Random effects:
 Groups   Name        Variance Std.Dev.
 ID       (Intercept) 0.032747 0.18096
 Residual             0.124930 0.35345
Number of obs: 569, groups: ID, 152
```

```
Fixed effects:
                Estimate Std. Error t value
(Intercept)      4.41107    0.45412   9.714
log(THEO)        0.15016    0.01601   9.380
log(AGE)        -0.24731    0.05427  -4.557
log(WT)          0.35052    0.11029   3.178
factor(SEX)1     0.13419    0.04891   2.744
factor(RACE)1    0.11214    0.07507   1.494
factor(RACE)2   -0.04028    0.08420  -0.478
factor(DIAG)2   -0.36011    0.07507  -4.797
factor(DIAG)3    0.11500    0.16880   0.681
```

To use the fitted model one has to transform it back to the original scale. Doing so we have

$$\begin{aligned}\text{PEFR}_{ij} &= \exp(4.41)\text{THEO}_{ij}^{0.150}\text{AGE}_i^{-0.247}\text{WT}_i^{0.397}\exp(0.121)^{\text{Male}} \\ &\exp(0.112)^{\text{Caucasian}}\exp(0.040)^{\text{Polynesian}}\exp(-0.360)^{\text{COPD}} \\ &\exp(0.115)^{\text{Athma+COPD}}\exp(U_i+\varepsilon_{ij}) \qquad (3.12)\end{aligned}$$

where the reference category is a female with asthma only and the categorical variables take value 1 if the ith patient belongs to that category, e.g., Male=1 and COPD=1 if patient i is a male with COPD but no asthma. Although the random effect U_i makes the mean PEFR $\exp(\sigma_u^2/2)-1$ higher than the geometric mean of PEFRs, in our case, it is only $\exp(0.033/2)-1$ (1.7%) higher, so it has almost no impact.

3.2 Modeling exposures with linear mixed models

In many situations, longitudinal exposure measures can also be modeled by an LMM. The exposure measure may be an index of air pollution in occupational epidemiology or drug prescriptions in pharmacoepidemiology, and typically drug concentrations or a summary measure of them. We will use modeling drug concentrations as an example to develop models and approaches, but they are also applicable to other areas.

Sometimes, PK samples may be taken repeatedly under the same conditions. These data are not sufficient to fit a complex popPK model. These situations typically occur in a Phase II or III study, in which only the trough PK samples taken before the next dose in a repeated dosing scheme, also known as Cmin, are taken just before the next dose in a repeated dosing scheme. Although one may combine them with external data to fit a popPK model, the value of this approach is often limited, since with trough samples only, the estimated full PK profile is mostly driven by external data. In this case, Cmin is widely used as a surrogate exposure measure for PKPD modeling. Since the samples are taken under the same conditions, an LMM is sufficient to model them.

A commonly used model is the power model, that is, an LMM for log-concentration and log-dose and covariates. Let C_{ij} be the PK sample with corresponding D_{ij}, which may be a constant dose $D_{ij} = D_i$, at visit j from subject i, the power model can be written as

$$\log(C_{ij}) = \mathbf{X}_{ij}^T\gamma + \mathbf{Z}_{ij}^T\mathbf{V}_i + e_{ij} \tag{3.13}$$

where $\mathbf{X}_{ij}$ and $\mathbf{Z}_{ij}$ are sets of covariates including a constant as well as log-dose $\log(D_{ij})$, and $\boldsymbol{\gamma}$ are parameters for the covariates and dose and $\mathbf{V}_i \sim N(0, \boldsymbol{\Sigma}_v)$ are random subject effects. This model is exactly the same as the model (3.4) and the interpretation of its components is also the same, although in the PK context. It can also be written in vector form (3.5).

To understand how this general model (3.13) is used, consider the following example:

$$\log(C_{ij}) = \gamma_1 + \gamma_2 Male_i + \gamma_3 \log(Age_i) + \gamma_4 \log(D_{ij}) + v_{1i} + e_{ij}, \tag{3.14}$$

in which we have $\mathbf{X}_{ij} = (1, Male_i, Age_i, \log(D_{ij}))^T$, $\mathbf{Z}_{ij} = \mathbf{X}_{ij}$ and $\mathbf{V}_i = (V_{1i}, 0, 0, 0)$, or equivalently $\boldsymbol{\Sigma}_v$ only has one non-zero parameter at the position of (1,1). Of course, the term $\mathbf{Z}_{ij}\mathbf{V}_i$ can also be written directly as v_{1i}. The model can be used to predict the concentration for subject i at a given dose d,

$$\hat{C}_i(d) = \exp(\hat{\gamma}_1)\exp(\hat{\gamma}_2)^{Male_i} Age_i^{\hat{\gamma}_3} d^{\hat{\gamma}_4} \exp(\hat{v}_{1i}). \tag{3.15}$$

where $\hat{\gamma}_k, k = 1, ..., 4$, are the estimated parameters and $\hat{v}_{1i}$ is the predicted subject effect v_{1i}.

A special case of these models is for drugs with dose-proportional exposure, i.e., $\gamma_4 = 1$. In this case, often one chooses to directly model the dose-normalized exposure C_{ij}/D_{ij}. Even when $\gamma_4 \neq 1$, the relationship between C_i and dose is simple since $C_i(D) \propto D^{\gamma_4}$. However, this simple relationship is based on the assumption of constant $\text{var}(V_{1i})$. Recall that when modeling C_{ij} directly, one almost always needs to consider the variance as a function of the mean. Using a log-transformation helps stabilize the variance, hence it is often assumed that $\text{var}(V_{1i})$ is a constant. However, it is worthwhile to check whether this assumption holds in an individual dataset. The impact of variance heterogeneity on the estimation of model parameters and the prediction of $\log C_i(D)$ is often small and can be ignored. However, it may have a large impact on the prediction of C_i, since $E(C_i(D)) \propto \exp(\text{var}(V_{1i})/2)$. Furthermore, if $\text{var}(V_{1i})$ depends on, e.g., the dose, the simple relationship of $E(C_i(D)) \propto D^{\gamma_4}$ no longer holds and the exposure is not long dose proportional even if $\hat{\gamma}_4 = 1$. Its impact will be clear when we consider the PKPD model using predicted concentrations as exposure.

3.3 Nonlinear mixed ER models

Nonlinear mixed models (NLMM) describe nonlinear relationships in data with repeated measures from multiple subjects [Davidian and Giltinan, 2017]. These repeated measures can be exposure or response.

3.3.1 Nonlinear mixed ER models

Let $Y_{ij}, i = 1, ..., n, j = 1, ..., r$, be the response (e.g., a biomarker measure) and C_{ij} be the exposure measured (e.g., the trough concentration) at time t_{ij} (e.g., on day 1 of treatment cycle j) from subject i. A general additive NLMM for Y_{ij} can be written as

$$Y_{ij} = g(C_{ij}, \boldsymbol{\beta}_i) + \varepsilon_{ij} \tag{3.16}$$

where $g(C_{ij}, \boldsymbol{\beta}_i)$ is a nonlinear function based on a pharmacological mechanism or as an empirical model, $\boldsymbol{\beta}_i$ is a set of parameters for subject i and $\varepsilon_{ij} \sim N(0, \sigma_\varepsilon^2)$ is a within-subject measurement error.

$\boldsymbol{\beta}_i$ may also depend on covariates. A more general model for β_i is

$$\boldsymbol{\beta}_i = \mathbf{X}_i \boldsymbol{\beta} + \mathbf{Z}_i \mathbf{U}_i \tag{3.17}$$

where $\mathbf{X}_i$ and $\mathbf{Z}_i$ are matrices of categorical and/or continuous covariates, and $\boldsymbol{\beta}$ is a vector of population parameters for $\boldsymbol{\beta}_i$. Often we assume a joint normal (or log-normal) distribution for $\mathbf{U}_i$: $\mathbf{U}_i \sim N(0, \boldsymbol{\Sigma}_u)$. In practice, the most commonly used one is

$$\boldsymbol{\beta}_i = \boldsymbol{\beta} + \mathbf{U}_i \tag{3.18}$$

where $\boldsymbol{\beta}$ is the population mean of $\boldsymbol{\beta}_i$ for the whole population.

One typical NLMM for ER modeling is the Emax mixed effect model

$$Y_{ij} = E_{maxi}/(1 + (EC_{50i}/C_{ij})^{\rho_i}) + \varepsilon_{ij} \tag{3.19}$$

where E_{maxi}, EC_{50i} and ρ_i are, respectively, the maximum effect, exposure to reach 50% of maximum effect and the Hill parameter for subject i. To write the Emax model in the form of (3.16), we define $\boldsymbol{\beta}_i = (E_{maxi}, EC_{50i}, \rho_i)^T$, which may follow the simple model (3.18), or the complex one (3.17). If, e.g., EC_{50i} depends on sex, then we need (3.17) and a binary variable (e.g., $Male_i = 1$ for males) in $\mathbf{X}_i$. Some parameters such as EC_{50i} should be positive; hence a log-normal distribution is more appropriate for all or a part of the elements of $\boldsymbol{\beta}_i$. With this example, we may write $\boldsymbol{\beta}_i = (E_{maxi}, \log(EC_{50i}), \rho_i, \log(EC_{50iMale}))^T$, where the last is the difference between male and female in $\log(EC_{50})$, and

$$\mathbf{X}_i = \begin{pmatrix} 1 & 0 & 0 & 0 \\ 0 & 1 & 0 & \text{Male}_i \\ 0 & 0 & 1 & 0 \end{pmatrix}. \tag{3.20}$$

The model can be written in the form of (3.17) with $\mathbf{Z}_i = \mathbf{X}_i$ if all parameters are random, or in the form of $\mathbf{X}_i\boldsymbol{\beta} + \mathbf{U}_i$ if the gender effect is fixed. Note that the model for EC_{50i} is a multiplicative model with females as the baseline,

$$EC_{50i} = \exp(\beta_{2i}) \exp(\text{Male}_i \beta_{4i}). \tag{3.21}$$

The model is similar to that for the trough concentrations.

Fitting a NLMM is more difficult than fitting an LMM, as it generally does not have a simple marginal model such as model (3.6) for LMMs. To find the MLE, we can write the likelihood function as

$$L(\boldsymbol{\beta}, \boldsymbol{\Sigma}_u) = \prod_{i=1}^{n} \int_u f_y(\mathbf{Y}_i|\mathbf{U}_i) f_u(\mathbf{U}_i|\boldsymbol{\Sigma}_u) d\mathbf{U}_i \tag{3.22}$$

where $f_y(\mathbf{Y}_i|\mathbf{U}_i)$ and $f_u(\mathbf{U}_i|\boldsymbol{\Sigma}_u)$ are the densities of $\mathbf{Y}_i$ and $\mathbf{U}_i$, respectively. To calculate it, however, we need a numerical integration method, such as Gaussian quadrature.

As an alternative to (3.22), we can use approximate marginal models based on

$$\mathbf{Y}_i \approx g(\mathbf{C}_i, \mathbf{X}_i\boldsymbol{\beta}) + \frac{\partial g(C_{ij}, \mathbf{X}_i\boldsymbol{\beta} + \mathbf{Z}_i\mathbf{U}_i)}{\partial \mathbf{U}_i}|_{U_i=0}\mathbf{U}_i + \varepsilon_{ij}, \tag{3.23}$$

where $\mathbf{C}_i = (C_{i1}, ..., C_{ir})$, $f(u)|_{u=u_0}$ denotes $f(u)$ evaluated at $u = u_0$. Then the MLE or generalized LS approaches can be based on the approximate marginal model. As it is based on a first-order Taylor expansion of the mean function around $\mathbf{U}_i = 0$, this model is often called the first-order approximation [Beal and Sheiner, 1982]. The approximation is poor when var$(\mathbf{U}_i)$ is large. A better approximation in this situation is proposed by Lindstrom and Bates [1990]

$$\mathbf{Y}_i \approx g(\mathbf{C}_i, \mathbf{X}_i\boldsymbol{\beta} + \mathbf{Z}_i\hat{\mathbf{U}}_i) + \frac{\partial g(\mathbf{C}_i, \mathbf{X}_i\boldsymbol{\beta} + \mathbf{Z}_i\mathbf{U}_i)}{\partial \mathbf{U}_i}|_{U_i=\hat{U}_i}(\mathbf{U}_i - \hat{\mathbf{U}}_i) + \varepsilon_{ij}. \tag{3.24}$$

where $\hat{\mathbf{U}}_i$ is a prediction of $\mathbf{U}_i$. Since the approximation needs $\hat{\mathbf{U}}_i$, the algorithm involves alternately estimating $\mathbf{U}_i$ and the model parameters. However, its performance heavily depends on sufficient numbers of repeated measures. Both approximations have been implemented in NONMEM and SAS proc NLMIXED, but R library lme4 only has the second one. SAS proc NLMIXED and NONMEM also have the option to use quadrature to calculate the likelihood directly.

3.3.2 Nonlinear mixed population PK model

Population PK modeling has been widely used to determine the relationship between drug exposure and dose and other factors in a population with repeated measures from multiple subjects using NLMMs. Technically, they are similar to using NLMMs for ER modeling, but have a number of specific characteristics. Predicted exposures based on exposure models are commonly used in PKPD modeling. One reason is that population PK modeling is often needed to understand the characteristics of PK in the target population. Therefore, a popPK model may already be well developed at the stage when PKPD analyses are needed. Typical popPK models are compartmental models such as (2.6), but we need to introduce random effects into the parameters, since these parameters vary between subjects. For example, the model (2.6) with random variations in the parameters can be written as

$$C_i(t) = \frac{DK_{ai}F}{V_i(K_{ai} - Cl_i/V_i)}(\exp(-Cl_i/V_it) - \exp(-K_{ai}t)) \tag{3.25}$$

In general, we can write a model for $C_i(t)$ as

$$C_i(t) = h(t, \boldsymbol{\gamma}_i) \tag{3.26}$$

where $\boldsymbol{\gamma}_i$ is a set of parameters specifically for this subject. The parameters may depend on factors such as age, body weight, etc., hence one may write

$$\boldsymbol{\gamma}_i = \mathbf{X}_i\boldsymbol{\gamma} + \mathbf{Z}_i\mathbf{V}_i \tag{3.27}$$

where $\mathbf{X}_i$ and $\mathbf{Z}_i$ are factors that include the intercept and $\boldsymbol{\gamma}$ are population parameters. $\mathbf{V}_i$ represents the remaining variability in $\boldsymbol{\gamma}_i$, after taking into account those explained by factors in $\mathbf{X}_i$, and it is often assumed that $\mathbf{V}_i \sim N(0, \boldsymbol{\Sigma}_v)$. This structure is the same as that in model (3.13), except that here it applies to parameters in an NLMM. This model may be extended to include time-varying covariates in $\mathbf{X}_i$ and $\mathbf{Z}_i$, but they are not common in popPK models.

A transformation may be needed to keep $\boldsymbol{\gamma}_i$ in a valid value range. For example, all the three parameters K_{ai}, V_i and Cl_i in model (3.25) should be positive for any subject, hence a log-transformation is often used to enforce the correct value range. Taking Cl_i as an example, one may write

$$\log(Cl_i) = \gamma_1 + \gamma_2 Weight_i + \gamma_3 \log(Age_i) + v_{cli} \tag{3.28}$$

where $Weight_i$ and Age_i are the weight and age of subject i, often centered on reference values, e.g., 75 kg and 40 years for adults. This is equivalent to

$$Cl_i = \exp(\gamma_1)\exp(\gamma_2)^{Weight_i} Age_i^{\gamma_3} \exp(v_{cli})) \tag{3.29}$$

where $\exp(\gamma_1)$ is the clearance of the reference subject of, e.g., 75 kg in weight and 40 years old. Categorical factors can also be included in the model. If clearance depends on sex, with $Male_i = 1$ for males and $Male_i = 0$ otherwise, an additional term $\gamma_4 Male_i$ in model (3.28) represents the impact of sex on clearance. In model (3.29) $\exp(\gamma_4)$ is multiplied to the right hand side if subject i is a male. We can write a model for $\boldsymbol{\gamma}_i^T = \log(K_{ai}, V_i, Cl_i)$ in the general form (3.27), using the same approach as writing the parameters in the Emax model in the form of (3.17).

The concentration can only be measured by bioassay using a PK sample in the blood. Therefore, we can only observe $C_i(t)$ with an error; and we can add an error in the model to accommodate it. Let C_{ij} be the concentration measure under dose D_i at time t_j from subject i, with the model for γ_i that

$$C_{ij} = h(t_j, D_i, \gamma_i) + e_{ij} \tag{3.30}$$

where e_{ij} contains assay errors but may also include within-subject variations in $C_i(t)$ not described in the model. At this stage, we have reached a model of the same type as the model (3.16). In fact, model fitting and statistical inference including prediction based on this model, model selection, and goodness of fit are the same as model (3.16). However, it is worthwhile to emphasize here that the purpose of exposure modeling in here is mainly exposure prediction for ER models, hence a good prediction rather than, e.g., correct estimation of PK parameters, is the primary objective. Therefore, it may not be necessary to use a compartmental model for exposure modeling. A semi-parametric or non-parametric approach as a more robust alternative sometimes is a better option, even when a popPK model has been developed.

3.3.3 The moxifloxacin example

We consider modeling moxifloxacin concentration data using a popPK model. Figure 3.1 shows the individual PK profiles in this dataset. Florian et al. [2011] has used a one-compartment model with first-order absorption to model moxifloxacin concentrations. Here we follow the same approach using model (3.25), but parameterize the model in terms of K_a, K_e and Cl.

$$C_i(t) = \frac{DK_{ai}K_{ei}}{Cl_i(K_{ai} - K_{ei})}(\exp(-K_{ei}t) - \exp(-K_{ai}t)) \tag{3.31}$$

We do not fit covariates in the model parameters, as subjects in this trial were healthy volunteers and were expected to have similar PK characters. Although all three parameters may vary among subjects, it may not be necessary or even possible to fit a model with random effects on all parameters. Because moxifloxacin has a quick absorption phase, the first sampling point was unable to capture the absorption (ascending) phase of the profile for most subjects. Therefore, it is difficult to fit a model with random effect on K_a. Models with random effects on log-K_e and log-Cl have been fitted, but the final model only needs a random effect on log-Cl. The other two parameters were also modeled on the log-scale. One advantage of this parameterization is that the parameter estimates on the log-scale in this situation often have a distribution closer to normal and confidence intervals based on a normal approximation are more accurate. The fitted model is

```
Random effects:
 Formula: lcl ~ 1 | Subject
              lcl Residual
StdDev: 0.1850413 472.6988
```

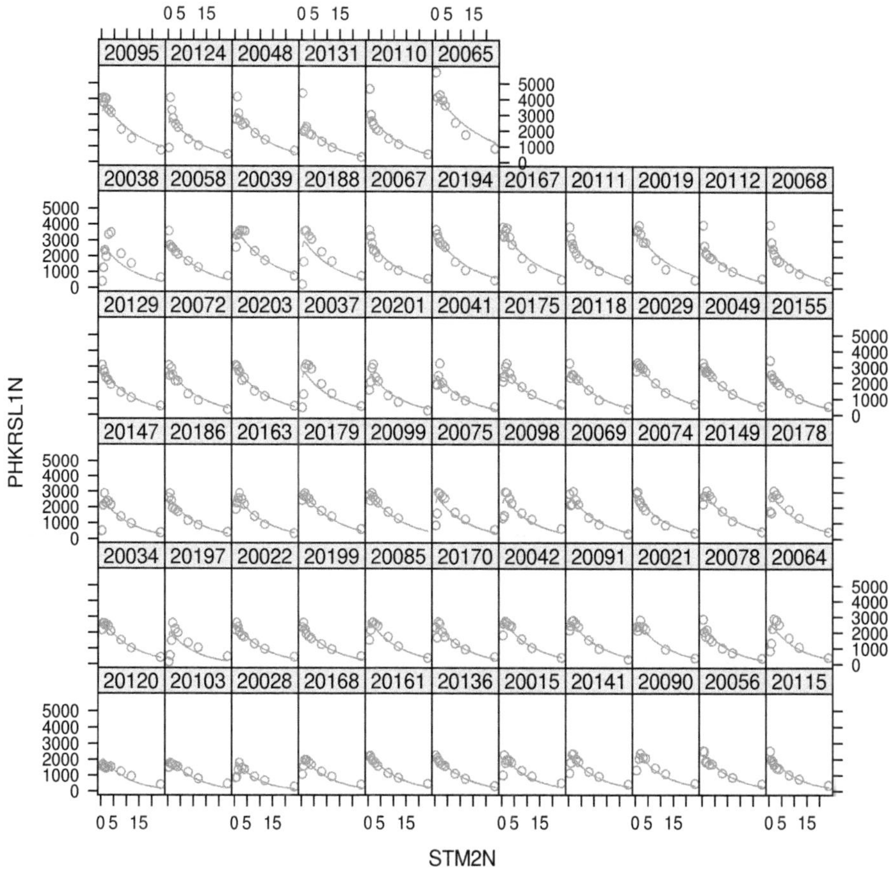

Figure 3.1
Observed and predicted individual moxifloxacin concentration profiles using a one-compartment model with first order absorption.

```
Fixed effects: lka + lke + lcl ~ 1
          Value  Std.Error  DF    t-value
lka    1.332993 0.08766193 474   15.20607
lke   -2.537591 0.04551668 474  -55.75079
lcl -10.489785 0.04369915 474 -240.04550.
```

The variation in clearance is better measured by the coefficient of variation (CV). Using the fact that if $\log(\gamma_i) \sim N(\mu, \sigma^2)$ then $CV = \sqrt{\exp(\sigma^2) - 1}$, we can estimate it for clearance. The CV is $\sqrt{\exp(0.185^2) - 1}$=18.7%, which is quite moderate by pharmacological standards. It also reflects the fact that the subjects in this trial are healthy volunteers of similar ages and had similar PK characteristics.

With the fitted model, we can predict the individual curves as

$$\hat{C}_i(t) = \frac{D\hat{K}_a\hat{K}_eF}{\hat{Cl}_i(\hat{K}_a - \hat{K}_e)}(\exp(-\hat{K}_et) - \exp(-\hat{K}_at)) \tag{3.32}$$

where only $\hat{Cl}_i$ is an individual prediction. The individual time profile prediction based on the fitted model is also presented in Figure 3.1. The plots show well-fit individual PK profile curves to the observed data.

3.4 Mixed-effect models specified by differential equations

Many DER models, particularly mechanistic models, can be specified by ordinary differential equations (ODE). Compartmental PK models such as the open one-compartment model with first-order absorption (2.4) are typical examples for DE models, and model (2.1) is an example for mechanistic PKPD models.

For repeated measurement data with multiple subjects, we need to extend the ODE in a way similar to the extension from nonlinear regression models to NLME. We take the model (2.4), as an example, with random K_a, K_e and Cl and their values for the ith subject as K_{ai}, K_{ei} and Cl_i. Let $A_{2i}(t)$ be the amount of drug in the central compartment of subject i. We can write the sample observed from subject i at time t_j as $C_{ij} = C_i(t_j) + e_{ij}$. In summary, the open-one compartment model specified by the ODEs for repeated measurement data is

$$\begin{aligned} \frac{dA_{1i}(t)}{dt} &= -K_{ai}A_{1i}(t) \\ \frac{dA_{2i}(t)}{dt} &= K_{ai}A_{1i}(t) - K_{ei}A_{2i}(t) \\ C_{ij} &= A_{2i}(t_j)K_{ei}/Cl_i + e_{ij} \end{aligned} \tag{3.33}$$

These equations are an example of a general class of models known as stochastic differential equations (SDEs), or particularly ODEs with random coefficients. The theory of SDEs can be technically very involved even at the introductory level [Oksendal, 2013]. However, in practice, we can use numerical approaches described to find a solution of the ODE system for any set of K_{ai}, K_{ei} and Cl_i values, assuming that conditions for well-behaved solutions are met. Therefore, the model can be considered as NLMM without an analytical form. In this way, we can avoid dealing with the theory of SDEs, which concerns how the solution behaves. We note that more complex SDEs may also find application in DER modeling. See, e.g., Overgaard et al. [2005].

For drugs with linear kinetics, their models are linear ODEs with constant coefficients, and the solutions to these ODEs have analytical form. Therefore, fitting these models is not different from fitting an ordinary NLMM as described in this chapter. However, ODEs without analytical solutions are far more common than those with an analytical solution. In this case, a straightforward solution is to solve the ODEs numerically and to feed the solution into software for fitting NLMMs. NONMEM has a built-in ODE solver and one can specify the ODE as a part of the model. There is also an R-library nlmeODE that provides an interface between an ODE solver and the NLMM fitting software. Note that both NONMEM and nlmeODE use the same Fortran routine "lsoda" in ODEPACK [Hindmarsh, 1982]. The computational efficiency of model fitting using ODE solvers is much lower than that of using an analytical function because of the much heavier computational burden. Another problem is numerical accuracy and stability when ODEs form a stiff system. It is not possible to give details about stiff systems, but as an easy concept for compartmental models, a stiff system consists of very quick and very slow systems which makes solving such a system numerically difficult since the two systems need different step sizes in the ODE solver. Some ODE solvers, such as lsoda, have adaptive selection of the step size to control the accuracy, but there is no guarantee that it works in all situations. In particular, the ODE solver is called for fitting models to individual curves for each subject, and some may have extreme parameter values. It is important to examine individual fits to check if there is any numerical problem in the finally fitted model. However, problems during the search for the MLE are difficult to detect, as it is not feasible to track the accuracy individually because of the huge number of calls on the ODE solver.

The following program uses the R function nlmeODE() [R Core Team, 2013] to fit the moxifloxacin PK data. The function nlmeODE(.) is an interface from the NLMM function nlme(.) to the ODE solver, taking the ODE and initial value specifications from Onecomp.

```
bdata=bdata[order(bdata$Subject,bdata$Time),]
gdata=groupedData(conc~Time|Subject,bdata)

OneComp <- list(DiffEq=list(
      dy1dt = ~ -ka*y1 ,    #Absoption dynamic
      dy2dt = ~ ka*y1-ke*y2), #Central comp. with elimination rate ke
  ObsEq=list(
      c1 = ~ 0,           #No measure for absorption
      c2 = ~ y2/Cl*ke),   #Observe concentration c2=y2/volume
                          #volume=ke/Cl, y2=amount
  Parms=c("ka","ke","Cl"),
  States=c("y1","y2"),
  Init=list(0,0))  #Initial states for the ODE

moximodel=nlmeODE(OneComp,gdata) #generate function for nlme() call
```

```
jk=nlme(conc~moximodel(ka,ke,Cl,Time,Subject)  ,fixed=ka+ke+CL~1,
   random=pdDiag(Cl~1), start=c(ka=2,ke=-1,Cl=-3.5), data=gdata,
   control=list(returnObject=TRUE,msVerbose=TRUE),
   verbose=TRUE)
```

It produces a fitted model:

```
Nonlinear mixed-effects model fit by maximum likelihood
  Model: conc ~ moximodel(ka, ke, Cl, Time, Subject)
 Data: gdata
       AIC      BIC    logLik
  9094.531 9116.483 -4542.266

Random effects:
 Formula: Cl ~ 1 | Subject
              Cl Residual
StdDev: 0.186819 445.4036

Fixed effects: ka + ke + Cl ~ 1
        Value  Std.Error  DF    t-value p-value
ka   1.333360 0.08211898 534   16.23692       0
ke  -2.536335 0.05378410 534  -47.15772       0
Cl -10.487757 0.04901029 534 -213.99091       0
 Correlation:
   ka     ke
ke -0.609
Cl -0.471  0.846
```

Note that in nlmeODE, designed for the purpose of PK modeling, parameters are log-transformed as a default. Hence the three parameters labeled as ka, ke and Cl are on the log-scale. The parameter estimates are very similar to those using the analytical form, as given previously. But when the starting values are far away from the estimated values, the nlmeODE fitted model may be different. These scenarios show that the ODE solver based approach might have numerical issues and may go wrong during the model fitting.

Although using the ODE format in a model is very convenient, it is far less efficient than using the analytical format. For the above example, the CPU time was 29.92 seconds for the nlmeODE run, while it was only 0.17 seconds when using the analytical format.

3.5 Generalized linear mixed model and GEE

A class of models similar to, but not included in the NLMM framework is the generalized linear mixed models (GLMM), which are developed from generalized linear models (GLM) [McCullagh, 2019]. Based on a GLM model, a

GLMM can be constructed to fit longitudinal data by introducing random components in the linear predictor. Taking the Poisson regression model as an example, let $Y_{ij} \sim \text{Poisson}(\lambda_{ij})$ be the count of events on patient i at visit j, the linear predictor for a mixed Poisson model is

$$\log(\lambda_{ij}) = \mathbf{X}_{ij}^T \boldsymbol{\beta} + \mathbf{Z}_{ij}^T \mathbf{U}_i \tag{3.34}$$

where $\mathbf{U}_i$ is a set of random variables representing variations in baseline risk between subjects. In this model $\mathbf{X}_{ij}$ will include C_{ij} with or without a transformation, as well as covariates. A general form of GLMM can be written as

$$g^{-1}(Y_{ij}|\mathbf{U}_i) = \mathbf{X}_{ij}^T \boldsymbol{\beta} + \mathbf{Z}_{ij}^T \mathbf{U}_i \tag{3.35}$$

where Y_{ij} follows a distribution belonging to the exponential family, conditional on $\mathbf{U}_i$. In other words, a GLMM is a GLM for any given value of $\mathbf{U}_i$. Apart from a few exceptions, a GLMM does not have an analytical marginal likelihood function (i.e., the likelihood after averaging over $\mathbf{U}_i$). Therefore, approximations have been widely used since the early development of GLMMs and have been implemented in, e.g., SAS proc GLIMMIX [SAS Institute Inc., 2011]. Alternatively, numerical calculation of the marginal likelihood has become a feasible method, thanks to the rapid increase in computer power in recent years.

The analysis of longitudinal data may not require a full model specification. The generalized estimating equation (GEE) method is a convenient way to analyze longitudinal data based on a model of the mean of the response only. Taking the Poisson regression as an example, and with $\mathbf{Y}_i$ and $\mathbf{X}_i$ as in the LMM (3.5), a GEE estimate $\hat{\boldsymbol{\beta}}_{GEE}$ is the solution to the following estimating equation

$$S(\boldsymbol{\beta}) = \sum_{i=1}^{n} \mathbf{X}_i^T (\mathbf{Y}_i - \exp(\mathbf{X}_i \boldsymbol{\beta})) = 0. \tag{3.36}$$

A general form of GEE is

$$S(\boldsymbol{\beta}) = \sum_{i=1}^{n} \mathbf{X}_i^T \dot{\boldsymbol{\mu}}_i \mathbf{W}_i (\mathbf{Y}_i - \mu(\mathbf{X}_i \boldsymbol{\beta})) = 0, \tag{3.37}$$

where $\mu(\mathbf{X}_i\boldsymbol{\beta}) = E(\mathbf{Y}_i|\mathbf{X}_i\boldsymbol{\beta})$ and $\dot{\boldsymbol{\mu}}_i$ are its derivatives with respect to $\mathbf{X}_i\boldsymbol{\beta}$. $\mathbf{W}_i = \boldsymbol{\Sigma}_i^{1/2}\mathbf{R}\boldsymbol{\Sigma}_i^{1/2}$ is a weight matrix in which $\boldsymbol{\Sigma}_i = \text{diag}(\text{var}(\mathbf{Y}_i))$ and $\mathbf{R}$ is known as the working correlation matrix, which should be chosen as close to the real correlation matrix of $\mathbf{Y}_i$ as possible, but is not necessary for consistent estimation of $\boldsymbol{\beta}$. For a consistent estimation of $\boldsymbol{\beta}$, only $\mu(\mathbf{X}_i\boldsymbol{\beta}) = E(\mathbf{Y}_i)$ has to be correctly specified, in addition to some technical conditions.

Without random effects, the GEE approach is often equivalent to the ML approach. In the above example, (3.36) is also the score function of the Poisson model ($\mathbf{U}_i = 0$ in model (3.34)), so the estimate of GEE is also MLE. However, when the mixed Poisson model is assumed, $E(\mathbf{Y}_i) = \exp(\mathbf{X}_i\boldsymbol{\beta})E(\exp(\mathbf{Z}_i\mathbf{U}_i))$.

Therefore, when fitting a model with $E(\mathbf{Y}_i) = \exp(\mathbf{X}_i\boldsymbol{\beta})$ with GEE, the $E(\exp(\mathbf{Z}_i\mathbf{U}_i))$ part causes an overestimation of the baseline risk if it is included in $\mathbf{X}_i^T\boldsymbol{\beta}$ as a constant. In fact, the baseline estimate for GEE is the population-average baseline. In general, the GEE method uses the marginal mean model $\mu(\mathbf{X}_i\boldsymbol{\beta})$, while GLMMs are subject-specific models. It is important to distinguish the two types of model for longitudinal data. GLMMs are subject-specific models since the linear predictor is explicitly a function of subject-specific effects for a specific $\mathbf{U}_i$, while the GEE uses a marginal or population-average model to describe the population-average ER relationship. For the Poisson model, the difference is in the baseline risk estimate while the effect of treatment can be consistently estimated. This property also holds for multiplicative models that are linear after a log-transformation.

The difference is more problematic for some other models as, e.g., if a logit link function is specified for the GLMM. The marginal model does not have the same link function, as $E_u(1/(1 + \exp(-\mathbf{X}_i\boldsymbol{\beta} - \mathbf{Z}_i\mathbf{U}_i)))$ is not a logistic function with respect to $\mathbf{X}_{ij}^T\boldsymbol{\beta}$. A different example is the mixed probit model

$$E(Y_{ij}|\mathbf{X}_i, \mathbf{U}_i) = \Phi(\mathbf{X}_i\boldsymbol{\beta} + \mathbf{Z}_i\mathbf{U}_i). \tag{3.38}$$

When $\mathbf{U}_i$ follows the normal distribution, averaging over $\mathbf{U}_i$, the marginal model remains a probit model. Although the coefficients for $\mathbf{X}_i$ are no longer $\boldsymbol{\beta}$, the coefficients in the two models can be converted. This property will be used to examine the efficiency of the DR model and DER model approaches in Chapter 8.

The difference between the population-average and subject-specific models should not stop us from using any of them. However, it is important to interpret the results correctly. For example, in the mixed logistic model with $\mathbf{X}_i^T\boldsymbol{\beta}$ containing an exposure measure term $\beta_c C_{ij}$, β_c is the subject-specific log-odds ratio. The population odds ratio will be lower than the subject-specific one $\exp(\beta_c)$, as the variation in $\mathbf{U}_i$ dilutes the individual effects. As a consequence, with the same dataset, the estimate of the population odds ratio is lower than the subject specific one. Both models have their own merits and could provide more relevant results than the other for specific situations. For example, the subject-specific odds ratio is more relevant when considering the dose for individual patients, as it represents the consequence of changing individual dose or exposure. The population odds ratio is more relative when evaluating the effect in a population, hence more suitable for global policy making.

These GLMM approaches can also be used to analyze longitudinal zero-inflated models. Let Y_{ij}, λ_{ij} and ρ_{ij} be those in (2.16) and (2.17) at time t_j. Since model (2.17) has two parts, each of which may depend on a random effect, we may construct models

$$\begin{aligned} \text{logit}(\rho_{ij}) &= \mathbf{X}_{ij}^T\boldsymbol{\beta}_a + C_{ij}\gamma_a + a_i \\ \log(\lambda_i) &= \mathbf{X}_{ij}^T\boldsymbol{\beta}_b + C_{ij}\gamma_b + b_i \end{aligned} \tag{3.39}$$

where $(a_i, b_i) \sim F(\mathbf{\Sigma})$ are random subject effects. The most common choice is a multivariate normal distribution $F(\mathbf{\Sigma}) = N(0, \mathbf{\Sigma})$. The likelihood function for subject i, conditional on a_i and b_i, can be written according to the distribution (2.16) and the overall likelihood function in principle can be obtained by averaging it over a_i and b_i. SAS proc NLMIXED can be used to fit these models.

3.6 Generalized nonlinear mixed models

We have presented models for a continuous response with a linear or nonlinear relationship and for other types of responses that follow distributions belonging to the exponential family, but with the mean connected to the linear predictor as a function of dose or exposure and covariates. One situation we have not covered is when a single linear predictor is not sufficient or inappropriate. For example, let the response Y_{ij} be the number of asthma attacks and λ_{ij} be the risk within the jth period of patient i, $Y_{ij} \sim Poisson(\lambda_{ij})$. Suppose that the effect of exposure on logarithmic risk follows the Emax model:

$$\log(\lambda_{ij}) = \mathbf{X}_{ij}^T \boldsymbol{\beta}_i + \frac{E_{maxi}}{1 + EC_{50i}/C_{ij}} \tag{3.40}$$

which is a simple combination of a GLMM and an Emax model. There are two sources of random effects, one in the linear part $\mathbf{X}_{ij}^T \boldsymbol{\beta}_i$ and another in the Emax part. The parameters in that model. $\boldsymbol{\beta}_i = (\boldsymbol{\beta}_{xi}, E_{maxi}, EC_{50i})^T$ or its transformation can be written in the general form as $\boldsymbol{\beta}_i = \mathbf{X}_i\boldsymbol{\beta} + \mathbf{U}_i$. However, these parameters cannot be linked to λ_{ij} by a single linear predictor.

The major technical consequence is that algorithms for fitting GLMMs cannot be used anymore. Therefore, the fitting of (3.40) needs general algorithms for fitting a NLMM specified by the likelihood function conditional on $\mathbf{U}_i$. For some distributions of Y_{ij}, SAS proc NLMIXED can be used without explicitly specifying the likelihood function. For example, to fit model (3.40), the following dummy codes can be used

```
proc nlmixed;
parms b0=3, b1=1, Emax=0, EC50=0, sigu=1,siguv=0,sigv=1;
Emaxi=exp(Emax+ui);
EC50i=exp(EC50+vi);
linp = b0 + b1*x +conc*Emaxi/(conc+EC50i);
mu = exp(linp);
model y ~ poisson(mu);
random (ui, vi) ~normal([0,0],[sigu,siguv,sigv]) subject=i; run;
```

where, for simplicity, we assume that the random effects are only in the Emax model part.

3.7 Testing variance components in mixed models

Variance components (VC) are key elements in all types of mixed-effects models. Due to the complexity of these models, in particular GLMMs and NLMMs, using a model with fewer random effects is technically beneficial. Therefore, testing variance components is an important tool for model selection. With regard to software for fitting mixed models, the commonly used hypothesis testing tools are the Wald and likelihood ratio tests (LRT). Although score tests are often more efficient to calculate, they have not been implemented in common software for mixed models.

The most common test for VCs is its existence, i.e., we can test H_0 : $\sigma^2_{uk} = 0$ vs. $\sigma^2_{uk} > 0$ to decide if the kth VC in $\mathbf{U}_i$ should be included in the model. The σ^2_{uk} value under H_0 is at the boundary of the parameter space since σ^2_{uk} cannot be negative. This constraint may be enforced during model fitting. The LRT statistic is also affected by the boundary constraint, since forcing $\hat{\sigma}^2_{uk} \geq 0$ changes its distribution. In some simple situations, the distribution of the LRT statistic can be derived under the boundary constraint. In general, the LRT statistic for testing models with K VCs vs. that with $K + 1$ VCs follows a mixture distribution of one χ^2_K and one χ^2_{K+1} with probability 1/2 each [Stram and Lee, 1994]. A special case is the test for no random effect versus one random effect, for which the LRT statistic has a mixture of χ^2_0 and χ^2_1 distributions with 1/2 probability each. Since χ^2_0 has a unit mass at 0, the type I error in the situation of $\hat{\sigma}^2_1 > 0$ is 1/2 of the tail probability of χ^2_1. Therefore, in this situation, the p-value given by the distribution χ^2_1 for LRTs should be halved if the variance estimate is positive. Otherwise, the p-value is 0.5. SAS proc GLIMMIX has adapted these simple rules for VC tests. However, it should be noted that these simple rules may not be accurate for complex models, particularly models with nonlinearity. For other situations, often simulation is needed to find the distribution or to calculate accurate p-values. Recent research has proposed score tests for VCs with boundary constraints, but some also require simulations. Practical applications are limited due to difficulties in implementation in commonly used software.

Now we return to the test in Section 3.1 where the LR test resulted in the test statistic $\chi^2 = 3.33$ with 1 df. Without considering the boundary constraint, it is equivalent to a p-value 0.188. However, with the approximate formula under constraint, the p-value becomes 0.188/2=0.094.

3.8 Non-parametric and semi-parametric models with random effects

The regression spline approach introduced in Chapter 2 can be easily extended to model repeated measure data. To this end, we need to write model (2.28) in a mixed model format and allow the coefficients to be random. A simple extension of model (2.28) is

$$Y_{ij} = \sum_{k=1}^{K} B_k(C_{ij})\eta_{ik} + \varepsilon_i. \tag{3.41}$$

where the $B_k(c)$s are the base spline functions as defined for model (2.29) and $\boldsymbol{\beta}_i = (\eta_{i1}, ..., \eta_{iK})^T \sim N(\boldsymbol{\eta}, \boldsymbol{\Sigma})$ are the random coefficients for subject i. In fact, it is not necessary to use the same bases $B_k(c)$s for fixed and random parts. A general model is

$$Y_{ij} = \sum_{k=1}^{K} B_k(C_{ij})\eta_k + \sum_{k=1}^{K_2} R_k(C_{ij})U_{ik} + \varepsilon_i. \tag{3.42}$$

where $\mathbf{U}_i = (U_{i1}, ..., U_{iK_2})^T \sim N(0, \boldsymbol{\Sigma})$ and $R_k(c)$ is another set of spline functions. This model can be written in the same form as model (3.5) by stacking the $\sum_{k=1}^{K} B_k(C_{ij})$ part to form $\mathbf{X}_i$ and the $\sum_{k=1}^{K_2} R_k(C_{ij})$ part to form $\mathbf{Z}_i$. Most statistical software allows a different design matrix for the fixed and random parts of the model, so the general model can be fitted as easily as the simple model (3.41).

The semi-parametric models using spline functions can also be extended to include mixed effects. For example, model (3.41) can be extended to model longitudinal data

$$Y_{ij} = \mathbf{X}_{ij}^T\boldsymbol{\beta}_i + \mathbf{B}(C_{ij})^T\boldsymbol{\eta}_i + \varepsilon_{ij}, \tag{3.43}$$

where $\boldsymbol{\eta}_i \sim N(\boldsymbol{\eta}, \boldsymbol{\Sigma}_\eta)$ are random coefficients and $\mathbf{B}(C_{ij})$ is a vector of spline functions, as in model (3.41), but evaluated at the exposure level C_{ij}. The spline functions used here can be constructed in the same way as in (3.41). For longitudinal models, the part of the spline function may represent an ER relationship, or a common time profile in a model such as:

$$Y_{ij} = \mathbf{X}_{ij}^T\boldsymbol{\beta}_i + \mathbf{B}(t_{ij})^T\boldsymbol{\eta}_i + \varepsilon_{ij}. \tag{3.44}$$

where $\mathbf{X}_{ij}$ may include the exposure variable.

For the argatroban dataset, one may assume a common time profile for APTT but the magnitude depends on the dose. This assumption leads to the following power model

$$\log(Y_{ij}) = \beta_1 \log(Y_{i0}) + \beta_2 \log(D_i) + \mathbf{B}(t_{ij})^T\boldsymbol{\eta} + u_i \tag{3.45}$$

and the fitted model is

```
Formula: log(resp)~log(base)+bs(time,3,knots=c(240))
              +log(dose)+(1|subject)
   AIC    BIC logLik deviance REMLdev
 -200.1 -169.6  109.1   -245.2  -218.1
Random effects:
 Groups   Name        Variance Std.Dev.
 subject  (Intercept) 0.013317 0.1154
 Residual             0.014424 0.1201
Number of obs: 219, groups: subject, 37

Fixed effects:
                            Estimate Std. Error t value
(Intercept)                  0.15322    0.65377   0.234
log(base)                    0.89956    0.19748   4.555
bs(time, 3, knots = c(240))1  0.91317    0.05241  17.423
bs(time, 3, knots = c(240))2  0.77683    0.07071  10.986
bs(time, 3, knots = c(240))3 -0.25797    0.07300  -3.534
bs(time, 3, knots = c(240))4  0.11119    0.11316   0.983
log(dose)                    0.17640    0.04099   4.304
```

where β_1, β_2 and $\boldsymbol{\eta}$ are labeled as log(base), log(dose) and the coefficients for the spline functions, respectively. Note that this model shows a low between-patient variation (a variance=0.0133 is equivalent to 12% CV), and a similar size of within-patient variation. Figure 3.2 gives the predicted response profiles by dose levels.

To allow more flexibility for the dose level, we can fit a model:

```
lmer(log(resp)~ log(base)+bs(time,3,knots=c(240))+bs(log(dose),3)
                +(1|subject),data=gpd2)
```

in which a smoothed exposure effect is fitted as bs(log(dose),3) and is multiplicative to the other components. One can decide if extra flexibility is needed by comparing the two models, which turns out to be unnecessary here($\chi^2 = 0.18$ for d.f.=2).

As said in Section 2.4, the smoothness of the curves (now there are curves of the fixed and the random parts) is controlled by the number and location of the knots of the spline functions. Compared with those used for the model (2.28), they may be more difficult to choose as the observed points are not well designed. In general, the knots should cover the entire range of observed C_{ij}. However, the equal percentile locations may not work well, particularly when the distribution of C_{ij} varies significantly among subjects. It is advisable to examine the distribution carefully for knot selection rather than using a predetermined approach. This may cause problems in clinical trial reporting for which the analysis should be pre-planned and timelines are tight, making extensive data dependent changes in analysis methods difficult to perform in practice. There are, however, smoothing approaches with much less dependence on the choice of knots, as will be shown in Chapter 4.

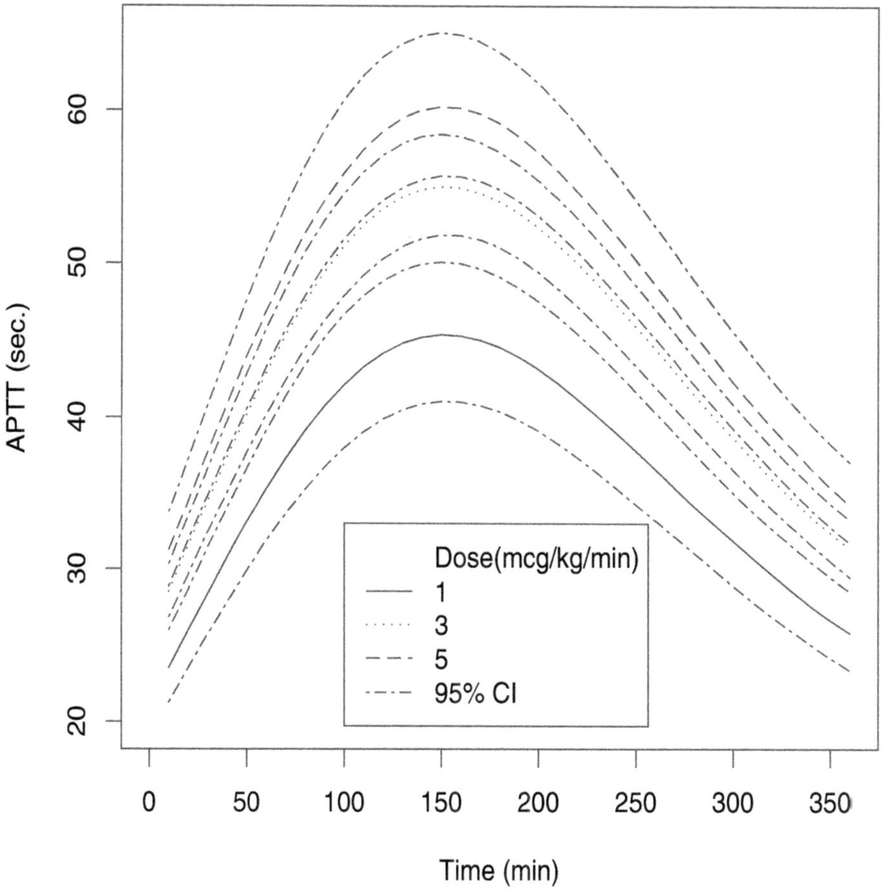

Figure 3.2
Predicted APTT for patients with baseline APTT=25 sec. and argatroban dose at 1, 3, and 5 mg.

We can also construct a semi-parametric GLMM by including a spline function part in the linear predictor

$$g^{-1}(Y_{ij}|\mathbf{b}_i) = \mathbf{X}_{ij}^T\beta + \mathbf{B}(t_{ij})^T\boldsymbol{\eta}_i + \mathbf{Z}_{ij}^T\mathbf{U}_i \tag{3.46}$$

where the $\mathbf{B}(t_{ij})^T\boldsymbol{\eta}_i$ part can be split into the $\mathbf{X}_{ij}^T\boldsymbol{\beta}$ and the $\mathbf{Z}_{ij}^T\mathbf{U}_i$ part. But we write this part explicitly to emphasize the existence of the non-parametric part. One can also fit semi-parametric models using a GEE similar to

$$S(\boldsymbol{\beta},\boldsymbol{\eta}) = \sum_{i=1}^{n}\begin{pmatrix} \mathbf{X}_i^T \\ \mathbf{B}_i^T \end{pmatrix}\dot{\boldsymbol{\mu}}_i\mathbf{W}_i(\mathbf{Y}_i - \mu(\mathbf{X}_i\boldsymbol{\beta} + \mathbf{B}_i\boldsymbol{\eta})) = 0, \tag{3.47}$$

where $\mathbf{B}_i = \mathbf{B}(\mathbf{t}_i)$ is a matrix of the spline functions evaluated at $\mathbf{t}_i = (t_{i1}, ..., t_{ir})$. Note that the GEE approach fits a model with fixed $\boldsymbol{\eta}$, while a GLMM may allow for random $\boldsymbol{\eta}_i$, and hence random individual curves represented by $\mathbf{B}(t)\boldsymbol{\beta}_i$.

The GEE approach can fit a non-parametric model to model the relationship between the moxifloxacin concentration and the probability of a more than 20 ms prolongation in QTcF using the QT data. The event of having such prolongations at all the time points can be considered as a repeated measure of a binary outcome, which can be fitted with a logistic model with spline functions for unspecified individual exposure-response curves and correlations between the repeated measures taken care of with the robust variance estimate. We can use the gee(.) function in R in combination with spline function generators:

```
fit3=gee(qtp~bs(conc,3),family=binomial,id=SID1A,data=moxi).
```

The model was fitted separately to all data and only data from the moxifloxacin period. The fitted model to all data gives the estimated ER curve (Figure 3.3) with 95% CI based on the robust variance estimate for $\boldsymbol{\beta}$. The two fitted models show uncertainty at both high and low exposure ends. But both models suggest that the maximum risk seems occurring when the concentration is around 3000ng/mL but the data could not determine whether a further exposure increase will further increase the risk, nor quantify the risk at a very low exposure level. Therefore, the repeated measure data did not provide much more information than the analysis of events and exposure at 2 hours in Chapter 2. One reason is that extreme QT prolongation occurs mostly around the peak of exposure, and hence the majority of subjects who had no event at 2 hours also had no event at other time points.

3.9 On distributions of random effects

In almost all models that we have introduced, univariate or multivariate normal distributions for random effects are assumed. In fact, these models were initially developed under this assumption. Often in practice, we cannot verify this assumption; hence questions have been asked by methodology researchers and modelers as well about the consequences of misspecified distributions and alternatives to the assumed distributions.

3.9.1 The impact of misspecified random effects

Suppose that the true distribution of the random effects in a LMM, NLMM or GLMM is $\mathbf{U}_i \sim F(\mathbf{U})$, where $F(\mathbf{U})$ is a general distribution function, rather than $\mathbf{U}_i \sim N(0, \boldsymbol{\Sigma})$ as we assumed. Our main interest is in how the difference between the true and assumed distributions affects the fitted model and the estimated parameters. To this end, we need to know how the fitted model behaves if a part of the model (in our case, it is $F(\mathbf{U})$) is misspecified. In

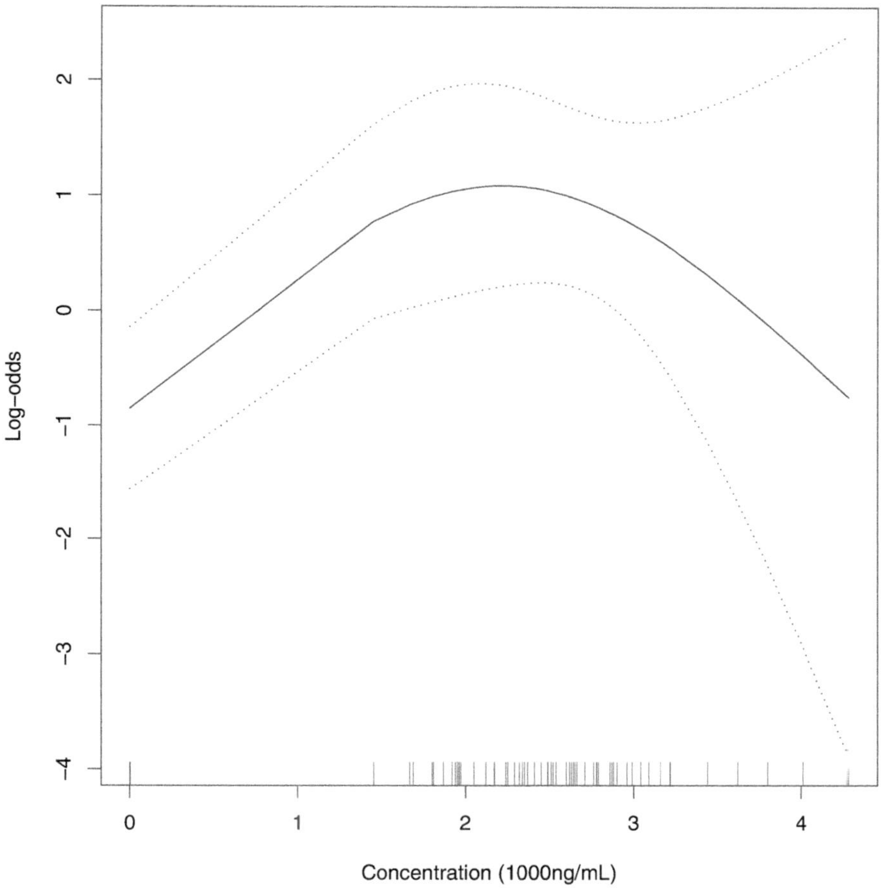

Figure 3.3
Non-parametric estimate of the relationship between moxifloxacin concentration and logOR of the probability of 20 ms prolongation in QTcF using natural cubic spline functions. The dotted lines are 95% CI.

fact, results for general model misspecification are available [White, 1982] and are readily applicable to our situation. Putting his results in an intuitive form and omitting technical conditions, we can say that the estimated parameters in the misspecified model converge to the values that minimize the difference between the misspecified and true models (Appendix). The results seem to be not practically useful since to assess the impact of the misspecification we have to know the true model. However, some general results can be used as a guide in practice, and we summarize them as follows.

For LMMs, $\hat{\boldsymbol{\beta}}$ by MLE or REML is consistent when the number of repeated measures per subject $r \to \infty$, regardless of the true distribution $F(\mathbf{U})$ [Verbeke and Lesaffre, 1997]. In the context of White [1981], for LMMs, $\hat{\boldsymbol{\beta}}$ converges to the true value as long as the model for the $\boldsymbol{\beta}_i^T \mathbf{X}_i$ part is not misspecified. However, statistical inference based on the likelihood function, in particular the CI constructed using the LRT or score test, needs correction.

For NLMMs, with a small r, $\hat{\boldsymbol{\beta}}$ is not consistent due to nonlinearity in the model. Although an approximate evaluation of the impact of misspecified $F(\mathbf{U})$ can be based on the conditional first-order approximation, it is quite complex and therefore has limited practical use. However, when $r \to \infty$, either the exact MLE or the conditional first-order approximation leads to $\hat{\boldsymbol{\beta}} \to \boldsymbol{\beta}$, regardless of $F(\mathbf{U})$, as long as the model for $\boldsymbol{\beta}_i$ is correctly specified.

The same conclusion applies to most GLMMs. For example, to obtain a consistent $\hat{\boldsymbol{\beta}}$, r needs to be very large for a logistic model, if the random effects are misspecified.

3.9.2 Working with misspecified models

In the situation where a misspecified model may still give a valid estimate for $\boldsymbol{\beta}$, we still need correct estimates of its SE and CI for statistical inference. White [1981, 1982] gives asymptotic normal distribution and variance-covariance matrix for the estimated parameters based on a misspecified model. Therefore, if the misspecification does not affect the consistency of the estimates, the asymptotic variance-covariance matrix can be used in inference of the parameters. In fact, for simple models the variance-covariance matrix can be estimated by a sandwich estimate very similar to that of the GEE estimates. The GEE can be considered as a method using a possibly misspecified model to fit the data, yet still yielding consistent estimates for the parameters of interest. These estimates are typically provided by GEE software such as SAS proc GENMOD and the R function gee(). For LMMs proc GENMOD provides a robust alternative to proc MIXED, which bases statistical inference on MLE or REML. For NLMMs, and most GLMMs, a robust estimate for var($\hat{\boldsymbol{\beta}}$) is complex and is not available in common software. There is not much use for this robust estimate since $\hat{\boldsymbol{\beta}}$ is inconsistent. However, in the case of a Poisson mixed model and other models of similar multiplicative structure, the sandwich estimate for var($\hat{\boldsymbol{\beta}}$) from GEE software (e.g., SAS proc GENMOD) normally is valid and can be used together with $\hat{\boldsymbol{\beta}}$.

3.9.3 Using models with non-normal or flexible distributions

There are many alternatives to the normal distribution for random effects. Although common software for mixed models only allows normally distributed random effects, there are approaches to use these software to fit models with alternative distributions. An approach that can be implemented in, e.g., SAS proc NLMIXED, is the integration transformation. First, we consider the situation of only one random effect U_i. Suppose $U_i \sim F(u, \gamma)$, then the marginal likelihood function for subject i can be written as,

$$\begin{aligned} L_i(\mathbf{Y}_i) &= \int_{U_i} L(\mathbf{Y}_i|\mathbf{X}_i, U_i, \boldsymbol{\beta}) dF(U_i, \gamma) \\ &= \int_{S_i} L(\mathbf{Y}_i|\mathbf{X}_i, F^{-1}(\Phi(S_i), \gamma), \boldsymbol{\beta}) \phi(S_i) dS_i \end{aligned} \quad (3.48)$$

where $\Phi(.)$ and $\phi(.)$ are the distribution and density functions of the standard normal distribution. This approach uses the fact that if $S \sim N(0, 1)$ then $\Phi(S) \sim U(0, 1)$ and $U_i \sim F(u)$ can be generated from a $U(0, 1)$ variable by a simple transformation with its inverse distribution function $F^{-1}(.)$, if it has an analytical form. This approach can be easily implemented by the following statements to fit a model with U_i following a gamma distribution: for SAS proc NLMIXED (adapted from Nelson et al. Nelsen [2006]):

```
pi = CDF(NORMAL,si) ;
ui = quantile(GAMMA,pi,1/theta1) ;
...
random si  normal(0,1) subject=id;
```

where theta1 and pi are the two parameters in the gamma distribution.

For multivariate random effects, we can use a similar approach and specify the correlation between the effects within a multivariate normal distribution. Let $\mathbf{U}_i \sim \mathbf{F}(\mathbf{U}, \gamma)$ where $\mathbf{F}(., .)$ is a vector of marginal distribution functions for each element in $\mathbf{U}_i$. $\mathbf{F}(., .)$ may consist of different marginal distributions. Suppose that U_{1i} and U_{2i} are the random variations in $\log(Cl_i)$ and $\log(V_i)$, respectively, and we may assume that U_{1i} follows a gamma distribution and U_{2i} follows a Weibull distribution. In this case, the likelihood function can be written as

$$\begin{aligned} L_i(\mathbf{Y}_i) &= \int_{U_i} L(\mathbf{Y}_i|\mathbf{X}_i, U_i, \boldsymbol{\beta}) d\mathbf{F}(U_i, \gamma) \\ &= \int_{S_i} L(\mathbf{Y}_i|\mathbf{X}_i, \mathbf{F}^{-1}(\Phi(S_i), \gamma) d\boldsymbol{\Phi}(S_i, \boldsymbol{\Sigma}) \end{aligned} \quad (3.49)$$

where $\boldsymbol{\Phi}(S, \boldsymbol{\Sigma})$ is the distribution function of a zero-mean multivariate normal distribution with variance-covariance matrix $\boldsymbol{\Sigma}$, but here we use a correlation matrix only. It is almost the same as (3.48) but with a multivariate $\mathbf{U}_i$. In fact, $\mathbf{U}_i$ can be considered as constructed by the Gaussian copula [Nelsen, 2006] defined as

$$C(\mathbf{w}) = \boldsymbol{\Phi}^{-1}(\phi(w_1), ..., \phi(w_k), \boldsymbol{\Sigma}) \quad (3.50)$$

where $\mathbf{w}$ is a vector of variables distributed on (0,1). The $\mathbf{U}_i$ is generated by applying $\mathbf{F}^{-1}(.)$ to $\mathbf{w}$. A model with bivariate $\mathbf{U}_i$, all with a gamma marginal distribution, can be fitted with

```
p1 = CDF(NORMAL,s1) ;
```

```
p2 = CDF(NORMAL,s2) ;
u1 = quantile(GAMMA,p1,1/theta1) ;
u2 = quantile(GAMMA,p2,1/theta2) ;
...
random s1, s2 normal([0,0],[1,rho,1]) subject=id;
```

Copula theory provides a practical approach to use of a wide range of non-normal multivariate distributions. A more general class is known as the Archimedean copula [Nelsen, 2006], generated in the same way as the Gaussian ones but using other functions to replace the normal distribution functions. However, its implementation in mixed models is not as easy as the Gaussian one.

3.10 Bibliographic Notes

There is a vast volume of literature on modeling longitudinal data; hence a complete list of books on this topic cannot be fit into this book. The most relevant ones for exposure-response modeling and the software we use are Davidian and Giltinan [2017] for NLMMs, Pinheiro and Bates [2000] for LMMs and NLMMs using the R library nlme and McCulloch and Searle [2004] for an excellent introduction to GLMMs. Bonate [2006] has chapters on mixed models that focus on PKPD modeling using NONMEM. Fitzmaurice et al. [2008] cover almost all the important areas in longitudinal data modeling in one book and is worth reading throughout.

4

Sequential and simultaneous dose-exposure-response modeling

In the previous chapter, we have considered fitting individual DE, ER and DR models. Here, we focus on fitting the DE and ER models as a whole approach to model the DR relationship and response prediction for a given dose. This topic has been a focus in pharmacometrics, in which two main approaches are known as sequential modeling and simultaneous modeling [Zhang et al., 2003]. Similar approaches in statistics are two-stage and joint modeling, although in most cases there is no exact correspondence between these methods in the two fields.

4.1 Joint models for exposure and response

In the previous chapter, we have introduced the following two models separately for C_{ij} and Y_{ij}. However, the time at which Y_{ij} and C_{ij} are measured may not be the same. For simplicity, we use only one sequence t_{ij} as the time of C_{ij} or Y_{ij} with a constant dose D_i. For example, if C_{i1} is measured at time $t_{i1} = 1$ and Y_{i2} is measured at $t_{i2} = 2$, then a DE model can be fitted to the DE data D_i and C_{i1}, then the fitted DE model can predict the exposure at t_{i2}, which can be used to fit the ER model to response data Y_{i2}. Alternatively, both models can be fitted jointly. The choice between them is the main topic of this chapter.

With simplified notation, we can write the models

$$\begin{aligned} Y_{ij} &= g(C_{ij}, \boldsymbol{\beta}_i) + \varepsilon_{ij} \\ C_{ij} &= h(D_i, \boldsymbol{\gamma}_i) + e_{ij}. \end{aligned} \tag{4.1}$$

where we omit t_{ij}. As in the previous chapters, we assume that e_{ij} and ε_{ij} follow normal distributions with variances σ_e^2 and σ_ε^2. The assumption of normality is mainly for simplicity, although it may be utilized in MLE and Bayesian approaches. In the following, we will refer to the first model in (4.1) as the y-part and the second one as the c-part, although the two parts correspond to the DE and ER models in previous sections. When C_{ij} are observed, one may think that the c-part is not needed to fit the y-part. However, this approach results in a biased parameter estimate when $\boldsymbol{\gamma}_i$ and $\boldsymbol{\beta}_i$, or ε_{ij} and e_{ij} are

DOI: 10.1201/9781003457008-4

correlated. We will discuss this issue in detail in Chapter 8. Using the c-part model for prediction is also necessary or beneficial if at some time points C_{ij} is not measured.

The y-part model in (4.1) is based on the key assumption that it is the observed exposure C_{ij} that directly causes the response. This assumption is often questionable. An alternative to the model (4.1) is

$$\begin{aligned} Y_{ij} &= g(C^*_{ij}, \boldsymbol{\beta}_i) + \varepsilon_{ij} \\ C^*_{ij} &= h(D_i, \boldsymbol{\gamma}_i) \\ C_{ij} &= C^*_{ij} + e_{ij} \end{aligned} \tag{4.2}$$

where C_{ij} is the observed exposure. The first model can be written in a more compact form $Y_{ij} = g(h(D_i, \boldsymbol{\gamma}_i), \boldsymbol{\beta}_i) + \varepsilon_{ij}$. This model is often considered more reasonable, especially in pharmacometrics, since we may consider that the unobserved exposure C^*_{ij} at the effect site, described by the c-part, rather than the observed C_{ij} that directly drives the response. Therefore, fitting both c-part and y-part may be necessary or may bring a significant advantage over fitting the y-part only.

In practice, a careful consideration on the selection of the two models is often worthwhile. Consider the argatroban example. The following are PK (concentration) and PD (APTT) data of patient 1 in the dataset (PK=1 for PK measures and PK=0 for PD measures). Although the times of the PK and PD measures are generally different, apart from 240 when PK and PD are measured, the PK measures at time 275 and 295 were only 5 apart from the PD measurement time 270 and 300, respectively. Therefore, one may question whether the use of a model for the prediction of the exposure is a better option than the use of observed ones. Later on we will show that sometimes one may be able to find a compromise that fits the ER model better.

```
Argatroban data from patient 1

Patient Time       PD   PK
      1   30   95.700    1
      1   60  122.000    1
      1   90  133.000    1
      1  160  162.000    1
      1  200  200.000    1
      1  240  172.000    1
      1  245  122.000    1
      1  250  120.000    1
      1  260   60.600    1
      1  275   70.000    1
      1  295   47.300    1
      1    0   26.100    0
      1  120   42.700    0
      1  240   43.000    0
      1  270   35.400    0
      1  300   33.900    0
      1  360   26.300    0
```

There is a technical advantage in using the models in (4.1), because $h(D_i, \gamma_i)$ in model (4.2) has unknown parameters γ_i to be estimated by the c-part. Models (4.2) cannot be fitted separately and normally require simultaneous modeling, with a few exceptions. A large part of this chapter is devoted to discussing these exceptions, as they lead to much easier and more robust model fitting.

The y-part model may also be a GLMM as discussed in Section (3.5), so the joint model can be written as

$$\begin{aligned} g(E(Y_{ij})) &= \mathbf{X}_{ij}^T \boldsymbol{\beta}_{xi} + \beta_{ci} h(D_i, \gamma_i) \\ C_{ij} &= h(D_i, \gamma_i) + e_{ij} \end{aligned} \tag{4.3}$$

where $\boldsymbol{\beta}_i = (\boldsymbol{\beta}_{xi}, \beta_{ci})$ are random parameters and $g(.)$ is a link function. This model is similar to model (4.2). It is straightforward to construct a GLMM similar to model (4.1) by replacing $h(D_i, \gamma_i)$ with C_{ij}. The two types of model need quite different model fitting methods, as we shall see later. Furthermore, we can also extend the model into a generalized nonlinear mixed model by replacing the $\beta_{ci} h(D_i, \gamma_i)$ part with a nonlinear function such as the Emax model: $E_{maxi}/(1 + EC_{50i}/h(D_i, \gamma_i))$.

4.2 Simultaneous modeling of dose-exposure and exposure-response models

4.2.1 Maximizing the joint likelihood function

The most common approach to fitting both models (4.1) or (4.2) simultaneously is to maximize the joint likelihood function for both exposure and response. Using models (4.1) or (4.2) leads to different likelihood functions. For the former, the conditional density for $\mathbf{Y}_i$ given $\mathbf{C}_i$ and $\boldsymbol{\beta}_i$ can be written as $f_y(\mathbf{Y}_i|\mathbf{C}_i, \boldsymbol{\beta}_i, \sigma_\varepsilon^2)$, while for the latter, since we do not observe $\mathbf{C}_i^*$, we have to use the conditional density given γ_i through $\mathbf{C}_i^* = h(D_i, \gamma_i)$, therefore we need to write the conditional density as $f_y(\mathbf{Y}_i|\gamma_i, \boldsymbol{\beta}_i, \sigma_\varepsilon^2)$. We will consider the latter case in the general framework, as model fitting for the former is simpler. We can write formally the joint likelihood as

$$L(\gamma, \boldsymbol{\beta}) = \prod_{i=1}^{n} \int_{\gamma_i} \int_{\boldsymbol{\beta}_i} f_y(\mathbf{Y}_i|\boldsymbol{\beta}_i, \gamma_i, \sigma_\varepsilon^2) f_c(\mathbf{C}_i|\boldsymbol{\beta}_i, \sigma_e^2) dF(\gamma_i, \boldsymbol{\beta}_i|\gamma, \boldsymbol{\beta}, \boldsymbol{\Omega}) \tag{4.4}$$

where $f_c(\mathbf{C}_i|\boldsymbol{\beta}_i, \sigma_e^2)$ is specified by the c-part and $F(\gamma_i, \boldsymbol{\beta}_i|\gamma, \boldsymbol{\beta}, \boldsymbol{\Omega})$ is a joint distribution function of γ_i and $\boldsymbol{\beta}_i$, e.g., a multivariate normal distribution with parameters γ and $\boldsymbol{\beta}$ for the means and $\boldsymbol{\Omega}$ for the variances. Note that this model does not cover the scenario of correlated ε_{ij} and e_{ij}, as in this case, the density function for $\mathbf{Y}_i$ and $\mathbf{C}_i$ cannot be separated even conditionally on γ_i and β_i. In pharmacometrics the main interest is often in models with independent PK and PKPD parts, that is, β_i and γ_i, and ε_{ij} and e_{ij} are all independent. For example, a frequently cited work in pharmacometrics [Zhang et al., 2003], which compares the performance of simultaneous and sequential modeling, only considered this situation.

Fitting the joint model is computationally demanding, but there is software, e.g., NONMEM and SAS proc NLMIXED designed for this purpose. Details about programming and discussion on other technical issues can be found in the next subsection. In the case of independent normal distributions of γ_i and β_i, i.e., when $F(\gamma_i, \beta_i|\gamma, \beta, \Omega) = F(\gamma_i|\gamma, \Omega_\gamma)F(\beta_i|\beta, \Omega_\beta)$, the likelihood function (4.4) can be factorized into two parts corresponding to the c- and y-parts, and the c-part can be maximized separately. However, the y-part model still depends on γ_is. The sequential modeling (SM) method follows this idea to fit the c-part first, then plug in the predicted γ_i s in the PKPD part to estimate the parameters in this part.

An important advantage of joint modeling is that the information matrix gives variance estimates for the MLE $\hat{\gamma}$ and $\hat{\beta}$, taking into account the uncertainties in fitting the other model. In contrast, in the SM approach, the variances of the fitted y-part model parameters given by common software do not take into account the uncertainty in the estimation and prediction of the c-part.

The joint modeling approach estimates both γ and β in one go. Theoretically, the joint model fitting is more efficient in terms of the precision of the estimated parameters than the sequential model fittings, even for the parameters in the PK model, if both models are correctly specified. However, the estimates of parameters in the PK model also depend on the response, a feature that is not often desirable. As the PKPD model is often empirical while the PK model is often mechanism-based, it is prudent not to base the estimation of the PK parameters on assumptions for the PKPD model that are difficult to verify. Consider the following hypothetical situation. Suppose that with a popPK model, patient i's clearance is predicted to be 10L/h, whereas when fitting a joint popPK and PKPD model the estimated clearance is 15L/h. Do we believe that the response data help us better predict clearance? This depends on how certain we are with the PKPD model. This example suggests that when the estimates in the PK part of the joint model are quite different from those when the PK model is fitted separately, the models and assumptions should be examined carefully.

An advantage of the likelihood approach is that the theory and model fitting algorithms apply to a wide range of models for which the likelihood function can be specified. These models include LMM, NLMM, GLMM and GNLMM and software such as SAS proc NLMIXED and GLIMMIX can be used for normally or log-normally distributed random effects. However, numerical problems often occur because of the relatively large number of parameters to be estimated in the joint model.

4.2.2 Implementation of simultaneous modeling

General purpose software is not designed to fit multiple models to multiple responses. However, SAS, R and NONMEM have facilities to maximize joint likelihood functions. The user needs to specify the conditional density function

$$f_y(\mathbf{Y}_i|\boldsymbol{\beta}_i, \gamma_i)f_c(\mathbf{C}_i|\boldsymbol{\beta}_i) \tag{4.5}$$

in (4.4), then the software calculates the marginal likelihood function based on $F(\gamma_i, \boldsymbol{\beta}_i|\gamma, \boldsymbol{\beta}, \boldsymbol{\Omega})$. The likelihood function may be specified implicitly via the mean function or explicitly specified by the conditional density functions. For example, in the code for jointly modeling argatroban concentration and APTT, the following part specifies the models for PK (ind=1) and PKPD (ind=0) parts in SAS proc NLMIXED. Both PK and PD data are in the variable "resp" and flagged by the variable "ind".

```
...
pk=(dose/cl)*(1-exp(-cl*t2/v))*exp(-cl*(1-t1)*(time-tinf)/v);
var=(sig**2)*(pred**(2*0.22));
if ind=1 then pred=pk;
else if ind=0 then do;
   emaxi=exp(emax+u1);
   ec50i=exp(ec50);
   pred=E0+(emaxi-E0)*pk/(pk+ec50i);
   var=sig2;
end;
model resp ~ normal(pred,var);
...
```

Note that both the mean "pred" and variance "var" are needed for each of the models.

The following SAS program is an example of explicit specification of the likelihood function for the same model. Denoting sige and sigv as variances of the PK and PD responses and ci and yi as exposure and response measures, we can specify

```
...sige=(sig**2)*(pred**(2*0.22));
   resc=ci-(dose/cl)*(1-exp(-cl*t2/v))*exp(-cl*(1-t1)*(time-tinf)/v);
   resy=yi-E0+(emaxi-E0)*pk/(pk+ec50i);
    if ind=0 then do;
       if (abs(resy) > 1E50) or (sige < 1e-12) then lly = -1e20;
       else   lly = -0.5*(resy**2 / sige  + log(sige)); llw = -1e20;
    end;
    if ind=1 thendo;
       if (abs(resc) > 1E50) or (sigv < 1e-12) then llw = -1e20;
       else  llw = -0.5*(resw**2 / sigv  + log(sigv)); lly = -1e20;
    end;
  model yi ~general(lly+llw);   *yi here is symbolic;
.....
```

where, in order to prevent numerical problems when the residuals are too large or the residual variances are too small, the contribution of these data to the likelihood is set to a very small value (10^{-20}).

4.2.3 The argatroban example

We use the argatroban dataset to illustrate the applications of joint modeling of longitudinal data. SAS proc NLMIXED is used for the analysis, but the approach of implementation can be applied to similar packages such as NONMEM and R. Detailed example codes can be found in the appendices. In this example, both exposure and response are continuous variables and can be assumed to have a normal distribution. Therefore, we can use the mean and variance in the model switching between the exposure and the response. The following codes run the joint model:

$$\begin{aligned}
C_{ij} &= \begin{cases} D_i(1-\exp(-t_{ij}Cl_i/V_i)) & t_{ij} < t_f \\ D_i(1-\exp(-t_f Cl_i/V_i))\exp(-(t_{ij}-t_f)Cl_i/V_i) & t_{ij} \geq t_f \end{cases} \\
C^*_{ij} &= C_{ij} + e_{ij} \\
Y_{ik} &= E_0 + (E_{maxi} - E_0)C_{ij}/(C_{ij} + EC_{50})
\end{aligned} \tag{4.6}$$

After a number of trial-and-error attempts, the following program and parameter setting leads to a successful fit.

```
proc nlmixed data=arg qpoints=2 ebsubsteps=70 ebsteps=100 ebssfrac=0.8
    ebopt ebtol=1e-4 ebsstol=1e-3 ABSXTOL=1e-5 abstol=1e-5 ftol=1e-5
    gtol=1e-3;
parms beta1=-5.4 beta2=-2.0 E0=30 emax=4.5 ec50=5  logb1=-1 logb2=-3
      sig=17 sig2=23 logu=-2;
bounds  sig sig2>0;
cl=exp(beta1+b1);
v=exp(beta2+b2);
sigu1=exp(logu);
s2b1=exp(logb1);
s2b2=exp(logb2);
pk=(dose/cl)*(1-exp(-cl*t2/v))*exp(-cl*(1-t1)*(time-tinf)/v);
var=(sig**2)*(pred**(2*0.22));
if ind=1 then pred=pk;
else if ind=0 then do;
   emaxi=exp(emax+u1);
   ec50i=exp(ec50);
   pred=E0+(emaxi-E0)*pk/(pk+ec50i);
   var=sig2;
end;
model resp ~ normal(pred,var);
random b1 b2 u1 ~ normal([0,0,0],[s2b1,0,s2b2,0,0,sigu1]) subject=subject;
run;
```

which generates the following outputs:

Parameter	Estimate	Standard Error	DF	t Value
beta1	-5.4329	0.08878	34	-61.19
beta2	-1.9516	0.02707	34	-72.09
E0	29.6918	0.5647	34	52.58
emax	4.4003	0.06318	34	69.65
ec50	6.3800	0.1902	34	33.55
logb1	-1.9051	0.2490	34	-7.65
logb2	-5.0309	1.2982	34	-3.88
sig	23.3031	1.0813	34	21.55
sig2	22.3237	3.6708	34	6.08
logu	-3.7331	0.3140	34	-11.89

with 2×log-likelihood=7044. This fit uses a two-point quadrature (qpoints=2) to evaluate the likelihood function numerically. Note that two key parameters for the ER relationship are emax and ec50, which are on the log-scale in the model.

To use the first-order approximation we replace "qpoints=2" with "method=firo" and obtain similar parameter estimates:

Parameter	Estimate	Standard Error	DF	t Value
beta1	-5.6498	0.03501	34	-161.40
beta2	-1.7763	0.03066	34	-57.94
E0	30.1260	0.5531	34	54.47
emax	4.5060	0.07850	34	57.40
ec50	6.7661	0.1959	34	34.53
logb1	-1.9536	0.2383	34	-8.20
logb2	-4.2040	0.4737	34	-8.88
sig	24.3275	0.9007	34	27.01
sig2	20.7338	2.2675	34	9.14
logu	-3.5179	0.3002	34	-11.72

The estimates are rather similar to those from the previous fit, but some SEs are considerably different.

4.2.4 Alternatives to the likelihood approach

Although fitting the joint model using the MLE approach seems natural, other approaches may be more convenient to fit some types of model jointly. Recall that the GEE approach as an alternative to the MLE approach for mixed models has been used widely for longitudinal data analysis. It is also possible to use a similar approach for joint modeling of the exposure and response data. First, we write the model (4.1) or (4.2) in a compact form. Let $\mathbf{S}_i = (\mathbf{Y}_i, \mathbf{C}_i)$ be the vector containing all the response and exposure measures, $\boldsymbol{\theta}_i = (\boldsymbol{\beta}_i, \boldsymbol{\gamma}_i)$,

$\boldsymbol{\theta} = (\boldsymbol{\beta}, \boldsymbol{\gamma})$, and $E(\mathbf{S}_i|\boldsymbol{\theta}_i) = \mathbf{H}^*(\mathbf{C}_i, D_i, \boldsymbol{\theta}_i)$ be the conditional means of $\mathbf{S}_i$. We assume that the marginal mean $\mathbf{H}(\mathbf{C}_i, D_i, \boldsymbol{\theta}) = E(\mathbf{H}^*(\mathbf{C}_i, D_i, \boldsymbol{\theta}_i))$, where the expectation is taken over the random components in $\boldsymbol{\theta}_i$, can be calculated analytically or numerically, we can write the residuals as

$$\mathbf{R}_i = \mathbf{S}_i - \mathbf{H}(\mathbf{C}_i, D_i, \boldsymbol{\theta}). \tag{4.7}$$

A GEE approach to estimate $\boldsymbol{\theta}$ is to solve the following estimating equation (EE)

$$\sum_{i=1}^{n} \frac{\partial \mathbf{H}(\mathbf{C}_i, D_i, \boldsymbol{\theta})}{\partial \boldsymbol{\theta}} \mathbf{W}_i \mathbf{R}_i = 0, \tag{4.8}$$

where $\mathbf{W}_i$ is a working weight matrix.

The generalized methods of moments (GMM) approach is similar to GEE but more general, and a SAS proc MODEL implements this approach with a number of useful options for, e.g., model fitting approaches and numerical calculation of $\mathbf{H}(\mathbf{C}_i, D_i, \boldsymbol{\theta})$ from $\mathbf{H}^*(\mathbf{C}_i, D_i, \boldsymbol{\theta}_i)$ if it does not have a closed form. The GMM approach estimates $\boldsymbol{\theta}$ by finding $\hat{\boldsymbol{\theta}}_{GMM}$ that minimizes

$$Q(\boldsymbol{\theta}) = \mathbf{R}^T(\boldsymbol{\theta}) \mathbf{A} \mathbf{R}(\boldsymbol{\theta}), \tag{4.9}$$

where $\mathbf{R}(\boldsymbol{\theta})$ in our case can be $\mathbf{R}(\boldsymbol{\theta}) = \sum_{i=1}^{n} \mathbf{W}_i \mathbf{R}_i / n$, or, in general, any set of statistics that have zero means when and only when $\boldsymbol{\theta}$ are the true parameter values. $\mathbf{A}$ is a positive matrix of the user's choice, but the optimal one is $\text{var}(\mathbf{R}(\boldsymbol{\theta}))^{-1}$. It can be shown that the GMM estimate that minimizes $Q(\boldsymbol{\theta})$ is a consistent estimate for $\boldsymbol{\theta}$ if there is only a unique $\boldsymbol{\theta}$ such that $E(\mathbf{R}(\boldsymbol{\theta})) = 0$. Although a formal proof of the consistency is outside our scope, we note that it follows that for large samples $\mathbf{R}(\boldsymbol{\theta}) \to E(\mathbf{R}(\boldsymbol{\theta})) = 0$, hence $Q(\boldsymbol{\theta}) \to 0$. Therefore, $\hat{\boldsymbol{\theta}}_{GMM} \to \boldsymbol{\theta}$ under some technical conditions. The GMM approach has similar advantages to the GEE approach, in particular, robust variance-covariance matrices for $\hat{\boldsymbol{\theta}}_{GMM}$.

As GMM is a big topic, the readers interested in this area are referred to Cameron and Trivedi [2005]. Here, we concentrate on the implementation of this approach. The following is a SAS program that estimates the relative risk for a Poisson model with over-dispersion due to a normally distributed subject effect. We assume that three repeated measures for exposure and event count are taken, together with the dose levels at each time. The mean functions $\mathbf{H}(\boldsymbol{\theta})$ consist of

$$\begin{aligned} E(Y_{ij}) &= \exp(\beta_0 + \beta C_{ij}) \\ E(\log(C_{ij})) &= \gamma_0 + \gamma_d \log(D_i). \end{aligned} \tag{4.10}$$

The following program uses the residuals to form $Q(\boldsymbol{\theta})$, where $\mathbf{A}$ is an inverse empirical variance-covariance of $\mathbf{R}$ estimated based on a preliminary least squares fit. The individual residuals of Y_{ij} are weighted by $1/\exp(\beta_0 + \beta C_{ij})$ to take variance heterogeneity into account.

```
proc model data=simu;
  EXOGENOUS dose1 dose2 dose3;
  parms base=-3 beta=0.2 a=0 b=1;
  eq.c1=a+b*dose1-lc1;
  eq.c2=a+b*dose2-lc2;
  eq.c3=a+b*dose3-lc3;
  means=exp(base+beta*exp(a+b*dose1));
  eq.y1=(means-resp1)/means;
  means=exp(base+beta*exp(a+b*dose2));
  eq.y2=(means-resp2)/means;
  means=exp(base+beta*exp(a+b*dose3));
  eq.y3=(means-resp3)/means;
  fit c1 c2 c3 y1  y2 y3/ gmm;
run;
```

Applying this program to a dataset generated by this code, with correlation between the c- and y-parts,

```
%let nsimu=1; %let nsub=100; %let cdose=log(1.3); %let bound=log(10);
%let base=-2; %let dose1=log(5); %let sigv=0.5; %let sigu=0.3;
%let sige=0.2; %let nsub=100; %let nrep=3; %let beta=0.25;

data simu;
  array conc{&nrep} lc1-lc&nrep;
  array ddose{&nrep} dose1-dose&nrep;
  array  resp{&nrep} resp1-resp&nrep;
 do simu=1 to &nsimu;
  do group=0 to 1;
  do sub=1 to &nsub;
    ui=rannor(1)*&sigu;
    vi=rannor(1)*&sigv;
    nn=0;
    dose=&dose1;
    do i=1 to &nrep;
    lci=dose+ui;
    lce=lci+rannor(12)*&sige;
*    trend=0.1*i-0.4;
    trend=0;
    if group=1 then lmd=exp(&base+&beta*exp(lci)+vi+trend);
    else lmd=exp(&base+vi+trend);
    yi=ranpoi(1,lmd);
    ddose{i}=dose; conc{i}=lce;  resp{i}=yi;
    if lce<&bound then dose=dose+&cdose;
     end;
     output;
  end;
 end;
end; run;
```

we obtain the following estimates which are reasonably close to the parameters used for the data generation. Here, the approximate SEs are from the robust variance-covariance matrix of $\hat{\boldsymbol{\theta}}_{GMM}$.

```
                 Nonlinear GMM Parameter Estimates
                                 Approx                       Approx
Parameter          Estimate     Std Err    t Value      Pr > |t|

base               -2.07026      0.2992      -6.92        <.0001
beta               0.229641      0.0463       4.96        <.0001
a                  0.052874      0.0789       0.67        0.5035
b                   0.96653      0.0412      23.46        <.0001
```

The analysis does not need to specify the form of correlations between the repeated measures. Although the generated data may be considered as an ideal situation, the robustness of GMM approaches has been well documented and verified in practical applications. Minimization of $Q(\boldsymbol{\theta})$ can also be performed using SAS or R using a general purpose optimization software, or SAS proc NLMIXED treating $Q(\boldsymbol{\theta})$ as a quasi-likelihood function. However, robust variance-covariance matrices have to be calculated separately.

4.2.5 Simultaneously fitting simplified joint models

Since $\boldsymbol{\beta}_i$ and $\boldsymbol{\gamma}_i$ are multidimensional, a full joint distribution is difficult to specify and hard to fit. However, general models (4.1) or (4.2) may have simple forms that allow for easier model fitting approaches. For example, the correlation between exposure and response may be in the baseline only. Accordingly, models (4.1) may be simplified to become

$$\begin{aligned} Y_{ij} &= g(C_{ij}, \boldsymbol{\beta}_i) + U_i + \varepsilon_{ij} \\ C_{ij} &= h(D_i, \boldsymbol{\gamma}_i) + V_i + e_{ij} \end{aligned} \tag{4.11}$$

where $\boldsymbol{\beta}_i$ and $\boldsymbol{\gamma}_i$ are independent, U_i and V_i are random subject baselines and may be correlated. To estimate $\boldsymbol{\beta}$, it seems that the second model does not need to be fitted at all. But this is true only when U_i and V_i are independent. When U_i and V_i are correlated, as the exposure C_{ij} depends on V_i, U_i in the first model becomes a confounding factor. The implications of confounding will be discussed in Chapter 8.

When the two models in (4.11) can be easily fitted separately, for example, if they are linear or generalized linear mixed models, the joint model may also be fitted with some standard software, such as SAS proc MIXED or proc GLIMMIX without extra programming. For example, to fit a joint linear mixed model:

$$\begin{aligned} Y_{ij} &= \beta_0 + \beta_c C_{ij} + U_i + \varepsilon_{ij} \\ C_{ij} &= \gamma_0 + \gamma_d D_i + V_i + e_{ij}, \end{aligned} \tag{4.12}$$

The following code shows how to organize the data and use the proc MIXED options

```
data pkpd;
  set pkdata(in=pk) pddata(in=pd);
  if pk then do;
      yv=conc;
   ind="pk";
    conc=0; end;
  else if pd then do;
    yv=QTcF;
 ind="pd";
    dose=0;  end; run;

proc mixed data=pkpd;
  class sid1a  ind;
  model yv=ind dose conc/solution;
  random ind /type=un subject=sid1a;
  repeated /group=ind; run;
```

where pkdata has variables conc and dose and pddata has QTcF and conc. In the data step, a flag "ind" is created and used in proc MIXED to specify if the intercept is γ_0 or β_0 and the corresponding variances to PK and PD (with "group=ind"). For a PD record, the dose is set to 0 so it has no impact on the PKPD model. The same is true for conc in the PK record. This approach also applies to GLMM models.

This linear mixed model approach cannot be applied to the y-part in (4.2) even when both PK and PD models are linear, e.g., when

$$\begin{aligned} Y_{ij} &= (\gamma_i D_i)\boldsymbol{\beta}_i + U_i + e_{ij} \\ C_{ij} &= \gamma_i D_i + V_i + \varepsilon_{ij}, \end{aligned} \tag{4.13}$$

and $\gamma_i = \gamma_d + V_{\gamma i}$ and $\boldsymbol{\beta}_i = \beta_c + U_{\beta i}$ are independent. Note that the first equation can be written as

$$Y_{ij} = \beta_c \gamma_d D_i + U_i^* + e_{ij} \tag{4.14}$$

where $U_i^* = D_i(\beta_c U_{\gamma i} + \gamma_d V_{\beta i} + U_{\gamma_i} V_{\beta_i}) + U_i$ has $E(U_i^*) = 0$. However, both γ_d and β_c appear in the term D_i, so they cannot be estimated in a linear mixed model. One needs to use, e.g., proc NLMIXED to fit it. Alternatively, we can estimate $\gamma_d \beta_c$ as one parameter in this model, then divide it by $\hat{\gamma}_d$ from the c-part separately. But this approach often has bad properties, particularly when $\hat{\gamma}_d$ has a large variation.

4.3 Sequential exposure-response modeling

Sequential modeling (SM) is a routine approach in pharmacometrics to analyze PKPD relationships when a PK model is available. The logic of the SM approach is to replace exposure in the ER model with a prediction based on the PK model. Therefore, this approach is based on the assumption that the y-part model is (4.2), that is, we assume

$$\begin{aligned} Y_{ij} &= g(h(D_i, \boldsymbol{\gamma}_i), \boldsymbol{\beta}_i) + \varepsilon_{ij} \\ C_{ij} &= h(D_i, \boldsymbol{\gamma}_i) + e_{ij}. \end{aligned} \quad (4.15)$$

The SM approach first fits the c-part model, then uses predicted exposures to replace those of the y-part to fit the response data. Specifically in the first stage, the c-part in (4.15) is fitted and $\boldsymbol{\gamma}_i$ is predicted as $\hat{\gamma}_i = \mathbf{X}_i\hat{\gamma} + \mathbf{Z}_i\hat{\mathbf{V}}_i$. Then, in the second stage, we fit a model

$$Y_{ij} = g(h(D_i, \hat{\gamma}_i), \boldsymbol{\beta}_i) + \varepsilon_{ij} \quad (4.16)$$

The model can be fitted in the same way as described in Chapter 3.

The major advantage of this approach is its simplicity as it can be easily implemented with standard software. Another advantage is that the estimates of the parameters of the PK model are consistent as long as the PK model is correct and fitted correctly. Often an intensive popPK modeling may have been carried out and information is available to assess the PK model and model fitting. Therefore, a good prediction of the PK data is likely to be available.

Now we apply the SM approach to the QT dataset based on the PK model fitted in Section 3.3.3. Following the SM approach, we fit a linear mixed model for $Y_{ij} = \Delta\Delta QTcF_i(t_j)$:

$$Y_{ij} = \beta_0 + \beta_c\hat{C}_{ij} + U_i + \varepsilon_{ij} \quad (4.17)$$

where $\hat{C}_{ij}$ is the predicted $C_i(t_j)$ based on the model (2.6) in Chapter 2 with random effects only on clearance. The fitted model is summarized by the following output:

```
Random effects:
 Formula: ~1 | Subject
        (Intercept) Residual
StdDev:     5.11129 7.442359

Fixed effects: dd_tavg ~ pred
               Value Std.Error  DF  t-value p-value
(Intercept) 7.252284 0.9351954 535 7.754832       0
pred        1.726746 0.3298987 535 5.234171       0
```

However, concentrations were also measured at all time points. They might fit the QT data better than the predicted ones. In fact, using the observed moxifloxacin concentration to fit the model (3.16) we get the log-likelihood = 2087, while using the predicted ones we get 2097, showing a better fit and a stronger exposure-response relationship. The following is the fitted model:

```
Random effects:
 Formula: ~1 | Subject
        (Intercept) Residual
StdDev:    5.113733 7.339934

Fixed effects: dd_tavg ~ concmu
                Value Std.Error  DF  t-value p-value
(Intercept) 6.868198 0.8962787 535 7.663016       0
concmu      1.948925 0.2958786 535 6.586909       0
```

Since the true exposure in the PKPD model (denoted by C^*_{ij}) is unknown and both C_{ij} and $h(D_i, \hat{\gamma}_i)$ can be considered as surrogates for C^*_{ij}, subject to a random error, which we will refer to as measurement error. The impact of measurement errors is the main problem in SM. For complete understanding, we will need knowledge of the ME models to be introduced in Section 4.4.

Pharmacometricians have developed several approaches to improve the performance of SM procedures. An approach, referred to as PPP&D [Lacroix et al., 2012] is to fix the population parameters in the model but allow γ_i to be re-estimated when fitting the ER model. This approach is to reduce the complexity of parameter estimation in the joint model, yet still allow for individual random effects in the parameters to be estimated jointly. A few variants of this approach have also been developed. One will be introduced in Section 4.4.

4.4 Measurement error models and regression calibration

Measurement error (ME) models [Carroll et al., 2006] describe the relationship between observed measures with error and the unobserved true value. In ER analysis, although both exposures and responses may be measured with error, we will focus on the first. To see why ME in exposures is an important issue before going into the technical details, consider the following hypothetical example. Suppose a drug, which can increase the response from 0 to 1 units, is compared with placebo in a trial with 20 hypothetical patients. However, two patients, one from each group, have their treatment group recorded incorrectly, which can be considered a measurement error in exposure. Then the mean treatment difference between the two groups as recorded will be 9/10 - 1/10=0.8 units. Therefore, measurement error in exposure can reduce the estimated effect. This example also indicates that, if we know the error rate, we may be able to adjust the bias caused by ME.

4.4.1 Measurement error models

We introduce ME models starting from a simple linear model in which the exposure is measured with errors. Details about ME models can be found in standard texts such as Carroll et al. [2006]. Let $C_i^*, i = 1, ..., n$ be the true exposure in a model for the response Y_i with coefficients β_0 and β_c, and error term ε_i

$$Y_i = \beta_0 + \beta_c C_i^* + \varepsilon_i. \tag{4.18}$$

Suppose that C_i^* cannot be measured directly. Instead,

$$C_i = C_i^* + e_i \tag{4.19}$$

is measured as a surrogate, where e_i is an error term. This model is known as the classical ME model. Another type of ME model is the Berkson model:

$$C_i^* = C_i + e_i, \tag{4.20}$$

in which we also only observe C_i, but in contrast to (4.19), here C_i^* is a random variable conditional on C_i.

If C_i, instead of C_i^*, is used to fit model (4.18) using the least squares (LS) method, in the situation of the classical model, the LS estimate $\hat{\beta}_{cLS}$ is attenuated to $\beta_c\lambda$ where $\lambda = \sigma^2_{C^*}/(\sigma^2_{C^*}+\sigma^2_e)$, and $\sigma^2_{C^*}$ and σ^2_e are the variances of C_i^* and e_i, respectively. There is no attenuation in the same LS estimate if the exposure follows the Berkson model. However, in both situations, the measurement error leads to an increase in the residual variance and therefore in the variance of $\hat{\beta}_{cLS}$. Consequently, the accuracy of the estimation and the power for testing, e.g., $\beta_c = 0$ will be reduced.

A third type of ME model is a combination of the first two types, i.e., a mixture of the classical and Berkson models. For this type of ME model we assume that

$$C_i = S_i + U_{bi}, \qquad C_i^* = S_i + U_{ci} \tag{4.21}$$

are all random variables, conditional on an unknown variable S_i, and U_{bi} and U_{ci} are independent. It is C_i^* that acts directly in model (4.18); but we can only observe C_i. This model includes both the classical model ($U_{ci} = 0$) and the Berkson model ($U_{bi} = 0$) as special cases. If C_i is used for a LS estimate for β_c, the estimate is biased due to U_{bi}, but U_{ci} does not contribute to the bias.

A numerical example is useful to illustrate the difference between the different ME models. In the following, we simulated 1000 samples from a linear regression of unit slope assuming the classical, Berkson, and the mixed ME models separately. The classical ME model leads to a shrinkage to 0.53 from 1.0 in the estimated slope, the Berkson model results in no shrinkage, and the mixed ME model gives almost the same estimated slope as the classical model, since only the classical part of ME causes bias.

```
> nsimu=1000
%Classical ME
> ci=rnorm(nsimu)
> xi=ci+rnorm(nsimu)
> yi=ci+rnorm(nsimu)
> lm(yi~xi)
(Intercept)          xi
   -0.03009     0.53276
%Berkson
> ci=xi+rnorm(nsimu)
> yi=ci+rnorm(nsimu)
> lm(yi~xi)
(Intercept)          xi
    0.03645     0.96008
%Mixed
> ui=rnorm(nsimu)
> ci=ui+rnorm(nsimu)
> xi=ui+rnorm(nsimu)
> yi=ci+rnorm(nsimu)
> lm(yi~xi)
(Intercept)          xi
    0.07416     0.53546
```

We have not specified a DE model for how C_i^* changes with, e.g., dose in the ME model. The model can be used to adjust the bias in sequential modeling using predicted concentrations based on a fitted DE model. For example, when the ER model is linear and $\hat{\lambda}$ is the estimate of λ using the variance estimates from the fitted model, $\hat{\beta}_c = \hat{\beta}_{cLS}/\hat{\lambda}$ is a consistent estimator of β_c. For other types of ER model, the correction may be more complex. Compared with direct adjustment, regression calibration (RC) is a more general and powerful approach than direct correction, as described below.

4.4.2 Regression calibration

RC is a systematic approach to fit the y-part model using expected exposure, conditional on observed data [Carroll et al., 2006] to correct biases due to ME. Taking the linear model

$$Y_i = \beta_c C_i^* + \varepsilon_i, \tag{4.22}$$

as an example, we examine the idea behind the RC approach. Since only C_i is observed, we would like to fit Y_i with its conditional mean $E(Y_i|C_i) = \beta_c E(C_i^*|C_i)$, that is, we fit

$$Y_i = \beta_c E(C_i^*|C_i) + \varepsilon_i^*, \tag{4.23}$$

where $\varepsilon_i^* = \varepsilon_i + \beta_c(C_i^* - E(C_i^*|C_i))$. It is easy to verify that as long as $E(C_i^*|C_i)$ is specified correctly, fitting this model gives a correct estimate for β_c, although ε_i^* depends on β_c. For a Berkson model $C_i^* = C_i + e_i$, $E(C_i^*|C_i) = C_i$, so the RC approach is just to fit the model with C_i as the covariate. With the classical model, when C_i and C_i^* are jointly normally distributed, it is also easy to find $E(C_i^*|C_i) = C_i/\lambda$, following the conditional distribution of C_i^*. Therefore, RC also leads to the correction $\hat{\beta}_c = \hat{\beta}_{cLS}/\hat{\lambda}$.

For the mixture ME model, if the latent exposure measure S_i in (4.21) can be modeled, e.g., as

$$S_i = h(D_i, \gamma), \tag{4.24}$$

the RC approach can be based on $E(C_i^*|D_i, C_i) = E(S_i|D_i, C_i)$. Since given γ, $E(S_i|D_i, C_i) = h(D_i, \gamma)$, we can estimate $E(S_i|D_i, C_i)$ by $h(D_i, \hat{\gamma})$, where $\hat{\gamma}$ is estimated by the exposure data. Again, the RC approach leads to replacing C_i^* with $h(D_i, \hat{\gamma})$, which is the SM approach.

The following example shows that when there are repeated measures for C_i^*, even without a dose-exposure model for C_i^*, the RC still leads to the same approach as SM when the first stage uses a linear mixed model prediction. Suppose that $C_i^* \sim N(0, \sigma_v^2)$ and that it is measured repeatedly with error as $C_{ij} = C_i^* + e_{ij}, j = 1, ..., r$, where $e_{ij} \sim N(0, \sigma_e^2)$. Let $\bar{C}_{i.}$ be the mean of the C_{ij}s, then $\bar{C}_{i.}|C_i^* \sim N(C_i^*, \sigma_e^2/r)$ and unconditionally $\bar{C}_{i.} \sim N(0, \sigma_v^2 + \sigma_e^2/r)$. Therefore, a linear mixed model with only subject effect V_i would predict C_i^* as an estimate of $E(C_i^*|\bar{C}_{i.})$:

$$\hat{C}_i = \lambda \bar{C}_{i.} \tag{4.25}$$

where $\lambda = \sigma_v^2/(\sigma_v^2 + \sigma_e^2/r)$, the correction factor for β_c. The RC approach uses $\hat{\lambda}\bar{C}_{i.}$, which is exactly the SM approach as $\hat{C}_i$ is the prediction of the linear mixed model from the first stage. From here we can also find that when r is large, $\bar{C}_{i.}$ is a very good estimate for C_i^*, and $\lambda \approx 1$, hence we may simply replace C_i^* with $\bar{C}_{i.}$.

The RC approach is based on the prediction $E(C_i^*|C_i)$ or $E(C_i^*|D_i, C_i)$ for C_i^*, so we may write

$$\hat{C}_i^* = E(C_i^*|D_i, C_i) + e_i, \tag{4.26}$$

where e_i is the prediction error. This model can be considered as a Berkson model; therefore, using $E(C_i^*|D_i, C_i)$ to replace C_i^* in a linear model, we obtain a consistent estimate for β_c. However, this is generally not true for nonlinear models.

For a nonlinear model $Y_i = g(C_i^*, \beta)$, RC is more complex since one needs to calculate

$$E(Y_i|C_i) = E(g(C_i^*, \beta)|C_i) \tag{4.27}$$

during the model fitting for different β values. One may use a simulation approach to calculate it, but since C_i^* is univariate, it is often more efficient to use Gaussian quadrature

$$E(g(C_i^*, \beta)|C_i) \approx \sum_{k=1}^{K} w_k g(C_i + x_k, \beta) \tag{4.28}$$

where w_k and x_k are the weights and points that can be found by, e.g., the R package "gaussquad".

For some special nonlinear models, $E(g(C_i^*, \beta)|C_i)$ can be calculated analytically and the RC method is very simple to use. One example is a multiplicative model with conditional mean

$$E(Y_i|C_i^*) = \exp(\beta_0 + \beta_c C_i^*). \tag{4.29}$$

Replacing C^* with the RC estimate $E(C_i^*|C_i) = \lambda C_i$, we have

$$E(Y_i|C_i) = E(\exp(\beta_0 + \beta_c \lambda C_i) + e_i|C_i) = \exp(\beta_c \lambda C_i)K \tag{4.30}$$

where K may have a simple form, e.g., when $e_i \sim N(0, \sigma_e^2)$, e.g., $K = \exp(\beta^2\sigma_e^2/2)$. But if we are only concerned with β_c (not β_0) there is no need to find K. The estimate for β_c remains consistent.

4.4.3 Models for longitudinal data

We consider different mixed models for the analysis of longitudinal data [Carroll et al., 2006], and will not include covariates for simplicity. Let $\mathbf{Y}_i$ and $\mathbf{C}_i^*$ be the repeated response and the true exposure measures, respectively. We first consider the linear mixed model

$$\mathbf{Y}_i = \beta_0 + \beta_c \mathbf{C}_i^* + U_i + \boldsymbol{\varepsilon}_i \tag{4.31}$$

where $\boldsymbol{\varepsilon}_i$ is a vector of IID, zero-mean random errors. We further assume that we observe $\mathbf{C}_i = \mathbf{C}_i^* + \mathbf{e}_i$ with $\mathbf{e}_i \sim N(0, \sigma_e^2\mathbf{I})$ as measurement errors. As before, the approach is to construct a model based on $E(\mathbf{Y}_i|\mathbf{C}_i)$ and takes into account the nature of longitudinal data. For the linear model, this is simple since, as long as $E(\mathbf{C}_i^*|\mathbf{C}_i)$ can be estimated by an unbiased estimate $\hat{E}(\mathbf{C}_i^*|\mathbf{C}_i)$, we can use the following mixed linear model:

$$\mathbf{Y}_i = \beta_0 + \beta_c \hat{E}(\mathbf{C}_i^*|\mathbf{C}_i) + \mathbf{U}_i^* + \mathbf{e}_i^*, \tag{4.32}$$

where $\mathbf{U}_i^*$ and $\mathbf{e}_i^*$ may contain error terms from $C_i^* - \hat{E}(\mathbf{C}_i^*|\mathbf{C}_i)$. This model can be fitted using standard mixed model software such as SAS proc MIXED, or R function lme(), if $\hat{E}(\mathbf{C}_i^*|\mathbf{C}_i)$ is available.

Therefore, the key step in the RC approach is to estimate $E(\mathbf{C}_i^*|\mathbf{C}_i)$. When there are repeated exposure measurements and the exposure is stationary, a mixed model can be used to predict an individual average exposure and replace $\mathbf{C}_i^*$ with it, or with the sample average $\bar{\mathbf{C}}_{i.}$, if appropriate. When $\mathbf{C}_i^*$ depends on the dose through a model with $E(\mathbf{C}_i^*|\mathbf{C}_i, \gamma_i) = h(\gamma_i, \mathbf{D}_i)$, a model-based RC is often a better choice. $E(\mathbf{C}_i^*|\mathbf{C}_i)$ can be estimated by $h(\hat{\gamma}_i, \mathbf{D}_i)$ if repeated exposure measures are available, or by $h(\hat{\gamma}, D_i)$ if there are no repeated exposure measures. This approach works for both dose changes over time within subjects and a constant dose with multiple dose groups, or a mixture of the two situations.

This approach can be extended to some GLMMs and GEEs. For example, for repeated count data with Y_{ij} being the count of events in the time interval j, and risk

$$\boldsymbol{\lambda}_i = \exp(\beta_0 + \beta_c \mathbf{C}_i^*), \tag{4.33}$$

one can simply replace $\mathbf{C}_i^*$ with $\hat{E}(\mathbf{C}_i^*|\mathbf{C}_i)$ in a GEE to obtain a consistent estimate for β. The reason is that the conditional mean of $\mathbf{Y}_i$ after the replacement is,

$$\begin{aligned} E(\mathbf{Y}_i|\mathbf{C}_i) &= E(\exp(\beta_0 + \beta_c \hat{E}(\mathbf{C}_i^*|\mathbf{C}_i) + \mathbf{e}_i)) \\ &= E(\exp(\beta_0 + K + \beta_c \hat{E}(\mathbf{C}_i^*|\mathbf{C}_i))) \end{aligned} \tag{4.34}$$

where $K = \log(E(\exp(\mathbf{e}_i)))$. Therefore, replacing C_i^* with $E(C_i^*|C_i)$ leads to a consistent estimate for β, and a robust SE estimate can be obtained by the sandwich robust variance estimate option in, e.g., SAS proc GENMOD or the R library "geepack". In addition to dose-exposure models, a commonly used model for RC in longitudinal data modeling includes terms for a time profile, e.g., as in Tosteson et al. [1998], where they used a linear time trend for the underlining exposure. Extending the RC approach to fit other models, such as the generalized logistic model, is more complex, as generally $E(\mathbf{Y}_i|\mathbf{C}_i)$ is no longer a logistic function of $E(\mathbf{C}_i^*|\mathbf{C}_i)$, and one has to calculate $E(\mathbf{Y}_i|\mathbf{C}_i)$ numerically.

Measurement errors in NLMMs are more difficult to handle, due to the nonlinearity of the NLMM. Consider the model

$$\mathbf{Y}_i = g(\mathbf{C}_i^*, \boldsymbol{\beta}_i) + \boldsymbol{\varepsilon}_i. \tag{4.35}$$

It is much more difficult to construct a model based on $E(\mathbf{C}_i^*|\mathbf{C}_i)$ for the same reason as for the GLMM above, since in general $E(g(\mathbf{C}_i^*, \boldsymbol{\beta}_i)|\mathbf{C}_i) \neq g(E(\mathbf{C}_i^*|\mathbf{C}_i), \boldsymbol{\beta}_i)$. Higgins et al. (1997) used a time profile model for RC, assuming $E(g(\mathbf{C}_i^*, \boldsymbol{\beta}_i)|\mathbf{C}_i) \approx g(E(\mathbf{C}_i^*|\mathbf{C}_i), \boldsymbol{\beta}_i)$. More complex approaches were investigated by Wang and Davidian [1996] and Ko and Davidian [2000]. Both used linear expansions on the NLMM and derived asymptotic results and corrections for ME. However, this approach has not been widely used, perhaps because of the complexity of the formulae and the lack of software implementation.

In fact, with software for calculating a marginal likelihood exactly or approximately such as SAS proc NLMIXED or NONMEM, one practical approach is to consider $\mathbf{e}_i$ as a random effect in the NLMM. This approach is based on the following approximation:

$$\boldsymbol{\delta}_i \equiv \hat{\boldsymbol{\gamma}}_i - \boldsymbol{\gamma}_i \sim N(0, \mathbf{S}_i) \tag{4.36}$$

so that

$$\mathbf{Y}_i = g(h(t_{ij}, \hat{\boldsymbol{\gamma}}_i - \boldsymbol{\delta}_i), \boldsymbol{\beta}_i) + \boldsymbol{\varepsilon}_i. \tag{4.37}$$

To fit this model, we add $\boldsymbol{\delta}_i$ as jointly normally distributed variables with fixed variance $\mathbf{S}_i$. This approach requires intensive calculation, but the number of parameters to be estimated is not increased. The approach was named IPPSE by Lacroix et al. [2012] and was implemented in NONMEM. They assumed that $\mathbf{S}_i$ is a diagonal matrix of squared SEs of each parameter for subject i. One practical reason is that NONMEM only provides SEs for $\hat{\boldsymbol{\gamma}}_i$. Nevertheless, the approach seems a useful way to address one of the issues and has been shown to perform better than ignoring the estimation error. The approach can be implemented in SAS proc NLMIXED, as shown in the next subsection.

4.4.4 Sequential modeling for argatroban data

We illustrate the use of SM approaches by applying them to the argatroban data. First, we add the time points when PD is measured as additional variables ptime=time, p1=t1 and p2=t2 so that the predicted concentrations can be generated from the fitted model.

```
data pkpred;
  merge arg(where=(ind=1) in=a) arg(where=(ind=0) keep=subject t1 t2
   time resp ind rename=(resp=pd time=ptime t1=p1 t2=p2));
  by subject;  if a;
run;
```

The following program fits the c-part in (4.6):

```
proc nlmixed data=pkpred method=gauss tech=trureg qmax=101 qtol=1e-5;
parms beta1=-5.5 beta2=-2.0 s2b1=0.14 cb12=0.006 s2b2=0.006 sig=23.0;
cl=exp(beta1+b1);
v=exp(beta2+b2);
pred=(dose/cl)*(1-exp(-cl*t2/v))*exp(-cl*(1-t1)*(time-tinf)/v);
var=(sig**2)*(pred**(2*0.22));
id pd;
*The following line generate predicted concentration at PD time points;
predict (dose/cl)*(1-exp(-cl*p2/v))*exp(-cl*(1-p1)*(ptime-tinf)/v) out=pred;
model resp ~ normal(pred,var);
random b1 b2 ~ normal([0,0],[s2b1,cb12,s2b2]) subject=subject;
run;
```

and gives the following parameter estimates.

Parameter	Estimate	Standard Error	DF	t Value
beta1	-5.4220	0.06423	35	-84.41
beta2	-1.9210	0.03242	35	-59.26
s2b1	0.1473	0.03556	35	4.14
cb12	0.005757	0.01170	35	0.49
s2b2	0.01112	0.007969	35	1.40
sig	23.0211	0.8178	35	28.15

The following data step and program take the predicted $C_i(t_j)$ to fit the ER model in (4.6):

```
data pred;  set pred;
  if ind=0;
  rename pred=conc;
run;
```

```
proc nlmixed data=pred qpoints=16 qtol=1e-3 ebtol=1e-7 EBOPT itdetails;
parms E0=30 emax=5 ec50=3  sig=23.0  sigu1=0.2;
    bounds emax  sig  sigu1>0;
   emaxi=exp(emax+u1);
   ec50i=exp(ec50);
   pred=E0+(emaxi-E0)*conc/(conc+ec50i);
model pd ~ normal(pred,sig);
random u1 ~ normal([0],[sigu1]) subject=subject;
run;
```

The estimated parameters in the ER model are

Parameter	Estimate	Standard Error	DF	t Value
E0	29.5821	0.4843	36	61.09
emax	4.3813	0.05641	36	77.66
ec50	6.3204	0.1573	36	40.19
sig	16.9057	1.7844	36	9.47
sigu1	0.03403	0.009881	36	3.44

The estimated key parameters emax and ec50 are very similar to those in the joint model (Section 4.2.3). However, here the SEs are lower: 0.157 (rather than 0.196) for ec50 and 0.056 (rather than 0.079) for emax, since the variation in the dose-exposure fitted model has not been counted.

Next, we implement the IPPSE approach in SAS, in a similar way as in NONMEM. To this end, one needs to predict the individual parameters (here cl and v) for each patient. The SEs of the predicted values are generated in the output dataset. In the proc NLMIXED call for fitting the ER model, the calculation of concentrations is repeated with the predicted parameter values plus random effects b1 and b2. Note that they have a different meaning than in the model for the dose-PK relationship, where they are the random subject effects; here they are the random error terms.

```
proc nlmixed data=pkpred method=gauss tech=trureg qmax=101 qtol=1e-5;
parms beta1=-5.5 beta2=-2.0 s2b1=0.14 cb12=0.006 s2b2=0.006 sig=23.0;
cl=exp(beta1+b1);
v=exp(beta2+b2);
pred=(dose/cl)*(1-exp(-cl*t2/v))*exp(-cl*(1-t1)*(time-tinf)/v);
var=(sig**2)*(pred**(2*0.22));
id pd;
predict beta1+b1 out=cl;
predict beta2+b2  out=v;
model resp ~ normal(pred,var);
random b1 b2 ~ normal([0,0],[s2b1,cb12,s2b2]) subject=subject;
run;

data para;
  merge cl(rename=(pred=lcl StdErrPred=secl)) v(rename=(pred=lv StdErrPred=sev));
run;

proc nlmixed data=para qpoints=16 qtol=1e-3 ebtol=1e-7 EBOPT itdetails;
parms E0=30 emax=5 ec50=3  sig=23.0  sigu1=0.2;
```

```
bounds sig sigu>0;
cl=exp(lcl+b1);
v=exp(lv+b2);
conc=(dose/cl)*(1-exp(-cl*p2/v))*exp(-cl*(1-p1)*(ptime-tinf)/v);
    bounds emax  sig  sigu1>0;
   emaxi=exp(emax+u1);
   ec50i=exp(ec50);
   pred=E0+(emaxi-E0)*conc/(conc+ec50i);
model pd ~ normal(pred,sig);
random u1 b1 b2 ~ normal([0,0,0],[sigu1,0,secl**2,0,0,sev**2]) subject=subject;
run;
```

The fitted model gives similar parameter estimates. The SEs for the two key parameter estimates are only slightly higher: 0.162 (rather than 0.157) for ec50 and 0.059 (rather than 0.056) for emax, but are still considerably lower than the joint modeling estimate.

Parameter	Estimate	Standard Error	DF	t Value
E0	29.4559	0.4739	34	62.15
emax	4.4016	0.05852	34	75.22
ec50	6.3846	0.1620	34	39.41
sig	15.5709	1.7145	34	9.08
sigu1	0.03208	0.009479	34	3.38

In summary, for the argatroban data, the SM approach gave quite similar parameter estimates to those in the joint model, but the variability of the estimates seemed underestimated, even with a procedure taking the SEs in the c-part parameters into account compared with the joint approach.

4.4.5 Simulation extrapolation

Simulation extrapolation (SIMEX) [Carroll et al., 2006] is an approach to estimate the ER model parameter with an extrapolation from artificially biased estimates. This approach seems not widely used in ER modeling, apart from an application to a PK-QT relationship analysis in Bonate [2013]. Consider a simple ME model $C_i = C_i^* + e_i$ with $e_i \sim N(0, \sigma_e^2)$. The idea of SIMEX is to first increase the variance of e_i by adding additional variation to assess the relationship between the increased variation and the estimate of β_c, then extrapolate back to $\sigma_e = 0$. To implement SIMEX, one needs to know σ_e in order to generate e_i' which is independent of e_i with $\text{var}(e_i') = \rho\sigma_e^2$. Then $C_i' = C_i + e_i'$ with variance $\sigma_e^2(1+\rho)$ can be generated to replace C_i in the ER model. Then $\hat{\beta}_c$ can be obtained by the following algorithm. For a grid of ρ values, B sets of $e_{bi}', b = 1, ..., B$ samples are generated to form the exposure with extra variation $C_{bi}' = C_i + e_{bi}'$. Then B estimates $\hat{\beta}_b(\rho)$ can be obtained. With a flexible model, we can extrapolate the $\hat{\beta}_b(\rho)$s to the corresponding value of $\rho = -1$. The corresponding estimate $\hat{\beta}_c(-1)$ is the SIMEX estimate for β_c.

This approach can be easily extended to models with heterogeneous variances, in particular, when $\sigma_{ei}^2(\mu_i)$ is a function of the mean μ_i. To do this, one needs to generate $e'_{bi} \sim N(0, \rho\sigma_{ei}^2(\mu_i))$. Otherwise, the approach applies in the same way as for the constant-variance case. Another case is that $\sigma_{ei}^2(\mu_i)$ is unknown, but there are repeated measures available to construct the variance-inflated exposure. This approach is slightly complex, and the reader is referred to Carroll et al. [2006]. The SE of $\hat{\beta}_c$ is difficult to find analytically. A technically more straightforward way is to use the bootstrap method. An introduction to the bootstrap can be found in the appendix. In short, the bootstrap approach repeats the above steps on each bootstrapped dataset constructed by resampling from the original data to obtain an SIMEX estimate for β_c. This approach forms an empirical distribution for $\hat{\beta}$, from which the SE can be obtained or statistical inference can be made based on the distribution.

4.4.6 A compromised y-models

We have asked the question of which of the two following models is correct:

$$\begin{aligned} Y_{ij} &= g(C_{ij}, \boldsymbol{\beta}_i) + \varepsilon_{ij}, \text{or} && (4.38)\\ Y_{ij} &= g(C^*_{ij}, \boldsymbol{\beta}_i) + \varepsilon_{ij}, && (4.39) \end{aligned}$$

with $C^*_{ij} = h(D_i, \gamma_i)$, particularly when the available data allow fitting both models. As an empirical approach, we may assume that in the second model C^*_{ij} could be a linear combination of the observed and model-based exposures:

$$C^*_{ij} = \rho h(t_{ij}, \gamma_i) + (1-\rho)C_{ij}, \tag{4.40}$$

where, we explicitly include time t_{ij} in the model, and ρ is a parameter. Setting ρ to 1 or 0 we obtain the first or second model. However, other ρ values might lead to a better fit. For linear and generalized linear mixed models, we can easily estimate ρ and test if the linear combination is better than any of them by fitting both $h(t_{ij}, \gamma_i)$ and C_{ij} in the same model. For example, if the true model is

$$Y_{ij} = \beta_0 + \beta_c C^*_{ij} + U_i + e_{ij}, \tag{4.41}$$

where C^*_{ij} is given by (4.40), we can fit

$$Y_{ij} = \beta_0 + \beta_1 h(t_{ij}, \hat{\gamma}_i) + \beta_2 C_{ij} + U_i + e_{ij}, \tag{4.42}$$

and ρ can be estimated as $\hat{\rho} = 1/(1+\beta_2/\beta_1)$. The two models can also be compared with, e.g., a likelihood ratio test (LRT) or a model selection criterion such as the AIC. The same approach can also be used for models with random coefficients. The following model

$$Y_{ij} = \beta_0 + \beta_{1i} h(t_{ij}, \hat{\gamma}_i) + \beta_{2i} C_{ij} + U_i + e_{ij} \tag{4.43}$$

allows different variances for β_{1i} and β_{2i}. This approach can be an empirical tool to explore the role of model-based and observed exposures in the model.

Applying this approach to moxifloxacin-QT data by fitting both observed concentration C_{ij} and its prediction $h(t_{ij}, \hat{\gamma}_i)$, we obtain the model fitted.

```
       AIC      BIC    logLik
  4180.384 4202.335 -2085.192

Random effects:
 Formula: ~1 | Subject
        (Intercept) Residual
StdDev:    5.116812 7.321278

Fixed effects: dd_tavg ~ concmu + pred
                   Value Std.Error  DF   t-value p-value
(Intercept)  7.270901 0.9290171 534  7.826444  0.0000
cij        3.011423 0.7094194 534  4.244912  0.0000
pred         -1.285460 0.7802837 534 -1.647426  0.1001
```

The LRT test gave a p-value=0.099 for the comparison between this model and that with the model for C_{ij} only, but the AIC of this model is 4180, slightly lower than AIC=4181 for the model with C_{ij} only. From the fitted model we can estimate $\hat{\rho} = 1/(1 + \beta_2/\beta_1) = 1/(1 + 3.01/(-1.29)) = -0.75$. The value suggests that the exposure directly relating to the QTcF is not a compromise between $h(t_{ij}, \hat{\gamma}_i)$ and C_{ij}, but is beyond C_{ij}. Although this is mechanically unlikely, the results suggest that using C_{ij} directly seems to be a better choice, which is consistent with the comparison based on AIC.

4.4.7 When measurement error models are useful?

Since dealing with ME increases the complexity in ER modeling, one may ask how much value this approach adds, given that the true exposure is almost never observed? In fact, if the question is, e.g., "how much is the difference in blood pressure between two patients with observed concentration 10ng / ml and 20mg / ml of drug A?", there is no need to use the ME approach. The simple modeling approach using observed exposures can answer this question. However, the ME approach may answer some very important questions, such as: if the true exposure level is increased from 10ng / ml to 20mg / ml, how much reduction in blood pressure will it cause? To help understand the difference between the two, we recall the hypothetical example of a trial with treatment wrongly labeled. The first question asks, in this context, what is the average difference between two patients *labeled* as treated and placebo, respectively. A real example concerns treatment effects in the presence of noncompliance, e.g., some patients who are prescribed a drug may not actually take it. In this case, prescribing a drug can be considered as a surrogate to taking the drug. Therefore, to estimate the effects of *prescribing* treatment, the mean difference between the prescribed and non-prescribed patients is sufficient. But if we ask what the effect is of eliminating non-compliance, then an ME approach is needed. This question is often asked during the dose-finding process within which an appropriate dose is selected by comparing the response between different doses. Note that an increase of dose from, e.g., 10mg to 20mg will increase the *true* exposure from 10ng/mL to 20ng/mL. This question is also valid for adjustment for exposure for individual patients, since repeated PK measures can be taken and used to estimate the true concentration with reasonable precision.

The RC approach may also provide additional interpretation, e.g., DR analysis results. For example, if on average the responses under dose levels 10mg and 20mg were 1 and 2 units, and the two doses produced exposure levels of 10ng / ml to 20ng / ml, assuming a linear relationship between ER, an increase of 10ng / ml would produce a response of 1 unit. If the dose level is randomized, then this difference could serve as a gold standard to check confounding biases in PKPD modeling. Details can be found in Chapter 8.

4.4.8 Biases in parameter estimation by sequential modeling

Although the SM approach is simple to use, due to errors in the prediction of C^*_{ij} in the y-part model, the parameter estimates are generally biased if the y-part is a nonlinear regression model, such as, $Y_i = g(C^*_i, \boldsymbol{\beta}) + \epsilon_i$. Here, a bias assessment method based on model misspecification theory [White, 1981] is described. Although a thorough investigation must take the approach of predicting C^*_i into account, if the c-part model is linear or log-linear, e.g., the power model, the problem can be much simplified. If the c-part model is additive, an unbiased prediction $\hat{E}(C^*_i|C_i)$ for $E(C^*_i|C_i)$ can be obtained and we can write

$$C^*_i = \hat{E}(C^*_i|C_i) + S_i, \tag{4.44}$$

where $S_i \sim N(0, \sigma_s^2)$ represents the prediction error. If the c-part model is log-linear, the prediction has a multiplicative error term. We can write

$$C^*_i = \exp(\hat{E}(\log(C^*_i)|C_i) + S_i). \tag{4.45}$$

In general, neither

$$E(Y_i|C_i) = E_s(g(\hat{E}(C^*_i|C_i) + S_i, \boldsymbol{\beta})) \tag{4.46}$$

and

$$E(Y_i) = E(g(\exp(\hat{E}(\log(C^*_i)|C_i) + S_i), \boldsymbol{\beta})) \tag{4.47}$$

equals $g(\hat{E}(C^*_i|C_i), \boldsymbol{\beta})$, due to the impact of S_i and the nonlinearity of $g(\hat{E}(C^*_i|C_i) + S_i, \boldsymbol{\beta})$. We are interested in the bias when fitting a model with a mean function of the y-part $g(\hat{E}(\log(C^*_i)|C_i), \boldsymbol{\beta})$ or $g(\exp(\hat{E}(\log(C^*_i)|C_i)), \boldsymbol{\beta})$.

A classical approach for bias evaluation is simulation in which the exposure and response data are generated and the ER model is fitted by RC. However, there is a shortcut to evaluating large-sample bias. Using the theory of model misspecification [White, 1981], we can determine the large sample bias in the parameter estimate for $\boldsymbol{\beta}$ if S_i is ignored in the SM. In general, LS estimates based on the model $g(\hat{E}(C^*_i|C_i), \boldsymbol{\beta})$, $\hat{\boldsymbol{\beta}}_{LS} \to \boldsymbol{\beta}^*$ when $n \to \infty$. $\boldsymbol{\beta}^*$ minimizes the squared difference between this model and the true model $E(g(C_i^*, \boldsymbol{\beta}))$ at given C_i^* values:

$$D(\boldsymbol{\beta}^*) = \sum_{i=1}^{n} (E(g(C_i^*, \boldsymbol{\beta})) - g(\hat{E}(C_i^*|C_i), \boldsymbol{\beta}^*))^2. \tag{4.48}$$

Therefore, the bias $\boldsymbol{\beta}^* - \boldsymbol{\beta}$ depends not only on the model parameters but also on the distribution of C_i. In practice, with given $\hat{E}(C_i^*|C_i), i = 1, ..., n$, (4.48) can be calculated numerically and $\boldsymbol{\beta}^*$ can be found with optimization software. The bias when using a multiplicative exposure model can be determined in the same way, after replacing $g(\hat{E}(C_i^*|C_i), \boldsymbol{\beta})$ with $g(\hat{E}(\log(C_i^*)|C_i), \boldsymbol{\beta})$ in (4.48).

The bias can be evaluated by a large number of simulation runs. The calculation of (4.48) is numerically very stable and easy to perform. The large sample bias, together with the assessment of the small sample property by simulation, provides useful information for the evaluation of the SM approach.

We use the combination of the power model and the Emax model to illustrate this approach. Consider the following Emax model

$$Y_i = E_{max}/(1 + EC_{50}/C_i^*) + \varepsilon_i. \tag{4.49}$$

with C_i^* given by a power model. For our purposes, we estimate C_i^* from the predicted conditional mean of $\log(C_i^*)$

$$C_i^* = \exp(\hat{E}(\log(C_i^*)|C_i) + S_i). \tag{4.50}$$

The main computational task is to calculate $E(g(\hat{E}(C_i^*|C_i), \boldsymbol{\beta}))$, for which we use a 10-point Gaussian-Hermite quadrature, assuming that $\log(\hat{C}_i^*)$ has a uniform distribution over (-1,1). Then $\boldsymbol{\beta}^*$ was found for different $\boldsymbol{\beta}$ and σ_s^2 values using the R-function "optim(.)". Figure 4.1 shows the relative bias as a function of σ_s^2 when $EC_{50} = 1$ and 2. In general, in this setting the bias is small to moderate, unless σ_s is very large. Since $EC_{50} = 1$ is at the center of the distribution of $\hat{C}_i^*$, but $EC_{50} = 2$ is far away from it, the impact of the distribution range for $\log(\hat{C}_i^*)$ relative to the value EC_{50} can be clearly seen in the figure.

4.4.9 Instrumental variable methods

The instrumental variable (IV) approach [Cameron and Trivedi, 2005]is another way to eliminate bias due to ME [Carroll et al., 2006]. The same IV approaches have been used for the estimation of causal effects (Chapter 8). To see how the IV approach can eliminate bias due to ME, it is useful to have another look at the simple ER models

$$\begin{aligned} Y_i &= \beta_c C_i^* + \varepsilon_i \\ C_i &= C_i^* + U_i. \end{aligned} \tag{4.51}$$

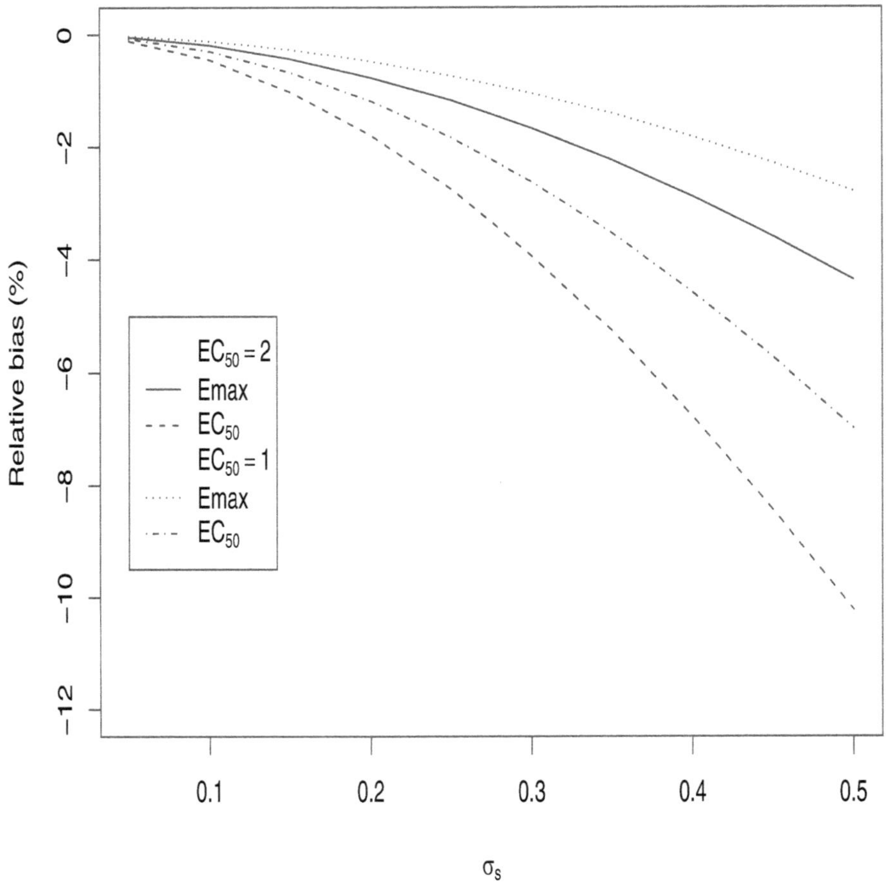

Figure 4.1
Relative asymptotic bias in $\hat{\boldsymbol{\beta}}_{LS}$ in the Emax model as a function of σ_s under different parameter settings.

It seems that the first one can be written as $Y_i = \beta_c C_i - \beta_c U_i + \varepsilon_i$, where $\beta_c U_i + \varepsilon_i$ has zero mean, so we can consider it as a random error. However, the fundamental assumption of independence between C_i and the error terms $\beta_c U_i + \varepsilon_i$ no longer holds, since C_i depends on U_i, and consequently the LS estimate for β_c is inconsistent. In the context of ER modeling, an IV is a variable that correlates with exposure, but not with response, apart from via exposure, that is, it is independent of ε_i. When C_i^* is a function of the randomized dose D_i, e.g.,

$$C_i^* = \gamma_d D_i \tag{4.52}$$

we can use dose D_i as an IV. It is a valid VI since it affects C_i^* via the DE model above, and it is independent of ε_i since it is randomized. An IV estimate is the solution to the following estimating equation

$$\sum_{i=1}^{n} D_i(Y_i - \beta_c C_i) = 0, \tag{4.53}$$

which leads to an estimate:

$$\hat{\beta}_{IV} = \sum_{i=1}^{n} D_i Y_i / \sum_{i=1}^{n} D_i C_i. \tag{4.54}$$

It can be verified that $\hat{\beta}_{IV} \to \beta_c$. Other instrumental variables may include time, if a varying time profile explains a considerable part of the variation in C_i^*. In fact, $\hat{\beta}_{IV}$ is the same as the two-stage IV estimate obtained by the following two steps:

1. Fitting model $C_i = \gamma_d D_i + e_i$ to estimate $\hat{C}_i^* = \hat{\gamma}_d D_i$
2. Fitting model $Y_i = \beta_c \hat{C}_i^* + \varepsilon_i$ to obtain $\hat{\beta}_{IV}$,

which is exactly the RC approaches.

The IV approach can be used for more complex models and its estimate is generally different from the two-stage estimate. In general if $Y_i = g(C_i^*, \boldsymbol{\beta}) + \varepsilon_i$, the optimal IV estimate (with the minimum SE) for $\boldsymbol{\beta}$ is the solution to

$$\sum_{i=1}^{n} \frac{\partial E(g(C_i^*, \boldsymbol{\beta})|D_i)}{\partial \boldsymbol{\beta}}(Y_i - g(C_i, \boldsymbol{\beta})) = 0 \tag{4.55}$$

where D_i are instrumental variables.

This approach can be extended to the situation where Y_i contains multiple repeated measurements. But in this case, the implementation needs substantial programming effort. Here we consider the following linear mixed model

$$\mathbf{Y}_i = \beta_c \mathbf{C}_i^* + U_i + \varepsilon_i \tag{4.56}$$

where $\mathbf{C}_i^* = h(\mathbf{t}_i, \boldsymbol{\gamma}_i)$ and $\mathbf{C}_i = \mathbf{C}_i^* + \mathbf{e}_i$ are measured at time points $\mathbf{t}_i$. In this case, $\mathbf{t}_i$ can be used as IVs if there is sufficient variation in $h(\mathbf{t}_i, \gamma_i)$, and the IV estimate for β_c is the solution to

$$\sum_{i=1}^{n} E(\mathbf{C}_i^*|\mathbf{t}_i)^T \mathbf{W}_i(\mathbf{Y}_i - \beta_c \mathbf{C}_i) \tag{4.57}$$

where $\mathbf{W}_i$ is a matrix that can be chosen based on var$(\mathbf{Y}_i)$ to optimize the IV estimate. $E(\mathbf{C}_i^*|\mathbf{t}_i)$ can be estimated as $h(\mathbf{t}_i, \hat{\boldsymbol{\gamma}}_i)$ after fitting the model for $\mathbf{C}_i$ as a function of $\mathbf{t}_i$. Note that although using $E(\mathbf{C}_i^*|\mathbf{t}_i)$ is optimal, the estimate for β_c is robust to its misspecification. This is in contrast to the SM method, which requires a correct specification of the c-part model. The following simulation example shows the robustness of the IV approach. In the simulation, we generate $\mathbf{C}_i$ based on an exponential model $C_i^*(t) =$

$D_i \exp(-(k+V_i)t)$. Then $\mathbf{C}_i$ are fitted to a model with a linear(rather than exponential) time trend and the fitted model is used to predict $E(\mathbf{C}_i^*|\mathbf{t}_i)$ as IV, hence the IV is generated from a misspecified model $C_i^*(t) = a_i + b_i t$. The following SAS code generates and analyzes the data.

```
%let nsimu=500; %let nsub=50; %let nrep=6; %let sigv=0.2;
%let sigu=0.2; %let ke=-1; %let sig=0.2; %let sigme=0.2;
data simu;
   dose=5;
 do simu=1 to &nsimu;
  do sub=1 to &nsub;
    ui=rannor(12)*&sige;
    vi=rannor(12)*&sigv;
    kei=exp(&ke+ui);
    do rep=1 to &nrep;
      cij=dose*exp(-kei*&nrep);
      csij=cij+rannor(12)*&sigme;
      yij=cij+rannor(12)*&sig;
      output;
    end;
   end;
 end; run;

proc mixed data=simu;
  class sub;
  model csij=rep/outp=pred; *IV in pred;
  random intercept rep/subject=sub;
  by simu;
run;
ods output ParameterEstimates=iv;
proc panel data=pred;
  inst exogenous=(pred);
  id sub rep;
  model yij=csij/ranone gmm;
  by simu;
run;
ods output ParameterEstimates=LSE;
proc panel data=pred;
  id sub rep;
  model yij=csij/ranone;
  by simu;
run;
```

The 500 simulated datasets are analyzed using a linear mixed model with C_i as exposure without adjustment and the IV approach, implemented in SAS proc PANEL in the time series and econometrics (TSE) package. The two estimates for β_c have means (SD) of 0.354(0.058) and 0.982(0.030), respectively. Compared with the true value of 1, and the estimates of the linear mixed model with the true exposure C_i^* as the gold standard, which have a mean (SD) of 1.002(0.022), the IV estimate is almost unbiased with SD lower than the unadjusted, although $E(\mathbf{C}_i^*|\mathbf{t}_i)$ is misspecified. The SD is higher than that of the gold standard but the difference is moderate. Therefore, the IV approach provides a robust alternative to the two-stage approach when the specification of the model for $\mathbf{C}_i$ is uncertain. Furthermore, unlike the two-stage method for which standard software does not directly provide the SE of the estimate, software for IV based estimates gives a valid robust SE. For example, with 50 subjects, the mean of SE estimates from proc PANEL was 0.033, only slightly higher than the SD of the estimates. When the sample size was increased to 100, the mean of the SEs is 0.023, almost the same as the SD of estimates 0.022.

Proc PANEL is not commonly used by biostatisticians, hence it is worthwhile to give some detailed explanations. The "id" statement specifies individual subjects or cohorts and the time variable. The statement "inst exogenous=(pred)" specifies "pred" as the IV, which is exogenous as it is independent of the error terms. The option "gmm" is an important feature in this procedure, as it requests using GMM for parameter estimation. The option "oneran" specifies a one-way random-effects model. The GMM method provides a sandwich robust SE estimate, as the GEE approach does in proc GENMOD. For nonlinear regression models, SAS proc MODEL provides IV estimates. Unfortunately, the procedure does not allow for fitting NLMMs or GLMMs. Special programs are needed to use IV methods for these models. For R-users, there are multiple packages such as ivtools dedicated to IV-based approaches.

4.5 Modeling multiple exposure and response

Sometimes subjects may be exposed to more multiple exposures. A typical example is a clinical trial with two or more drugs used in combination. In clinical practice, it is also common for a patient to be prescribed more than one drug. The impact of exposure of one drug to another is known as a drug-drug interaction (DDI) [Sun et al., 2023], and this DDI is particularly referred to as the exposure interaction. For example, if one drug inhibits the liver enzymes that help the metabolism of the other drug, then the increase of its exposure will also increase the exposure of the other. However, we will focus on simple statistical models rather than mechanistic models such as those in Niu et al. [2019]. Let C_{ik} and D_{ik} be the exposure of the kth drug of subject i. If two drugs are administered together, one may assume that

$$\begin{aligned}\log(C_{i1}) &= \gamma_{01} + \gamma_1 \log(D_{i1}) + \gamma_{12} \log(C_{i2}) + V_{i1} \\ \log(C_{i2}) &= \gamma_{02} + \gamma_2 \log(D_{i2}) + \gamma_{21} \log(C_{i1}) + V_{i2},\end{aligned} \tag{4.58}$$

where γ_{12} and γ_{21} present the DDI effects of the other drug. However, the concentration occurs on both sides of the model. These models are often referred to as simultaneous models. Special modeling procedures have been developed to fit them, e.g., available in SAS proc MODEL. However, since our goal is to predict the concentration and fit ER models, considering the following marginal model derived from (4.58) is sufficient:

$$\begin{aligned}\log(C_{i1}) &= \gamma_{01}+\gamma_1\log(D_{i1})+\gamma_{12}\log(D_{i2})+V_{i1}\\ \log(C_{i2}) &= \gamma_{02}+\gamma_2\log(D_{i2})+\gamma_{21}\log(D_{i1})+V_{i2}.\end{aligned} \tag{4.59}$$

They are almost the same as the model (4.58), except that the interaction term $\gamma_{kk'}C_{ik'}, C_{ik}$ is replaced by $D_{ik'}$. The two models are equivalent in terms of the DE relationship. However, all parameters and V_{ik}s in model (4.59), not only $\gamma_{kk'}$, have different meanings from those of model (4.58). But we do not introduce new names for simplicity. Also, even if V_{i1} and V_{i2} are independent in model (4.58), those in model (4.59) are not. Note that the system described by the model (4.58) may not be stable, unless the $\gamma_{kk'}$s satisfy some conditions. For example, if $\gamma_{12}=1$ and $\gamma_{21}=1$, then the increase in drug 1 exposure stimulates an increase in drug 2 exposure. The increase in exposure of drug 2, in turn, increases that of drug 1. This positive feedback through the other drug leads to the exposure going, in theory, to infinity, although in reality attenuation happens when the exposures are high enough. This note gives a caution for using the two linear models, as often nonlinearity occurs more often when DDI occurs. The model (4.59) is always stable, as it cannot be derived from the model (4.58) if the latter is unstable.

DDIs may also occur in ER relationship in which when two drugs act together, the joint effect may be greater (or lower) than the additive effects of two single drugs. Let Y_i be the response of subject i under the exposure of two drugs 1 and 2, a simple linear model to describe the joint effect of the two exposures is

$$Y_i=\beta_0+\beta_1C_{1i}+\beta_2C_{2i}+\beta_{12}C_{1i}C_{2i}+\varepsilon_i \tag{4.60}$$

where β_1 and β_2 represent the individual drugs additive effect and β_{12} is a measure of the extra joint effect. As in the previous sections, we can introduce ME in counterpart models to model (4.2), in which we assume

$$\begin{aligned}\log(C^*_{ki}) &= \gamma_{0k}+\gamma_k\log(D_{ik})+\gamma_{kk'}\log(D_{k'i}), k\neq k'\\ Y_i &= \beta_0+\beta_1C^*_{1i}+\beta_2C^*_{2i}+\beta_{12}C^*_{1i}C^*_{2i}+\varepsilon_i\end{aligned} \tag{4.61}$$

and we only observe $\log(C_{ik})=\log(C^*_{ki})+e_{ik}$. All models can be extended to include repeated measures by introducing random effects in the β s and γ s. In this case, there are two levels of correlation structure in the exposure model, one between the exposures of different drugs at the same time point, and at the subject level over repeated time points. Other types of ER models can also be introduced to replace (4.60). Possible nonlinearity in the exposure-response relationship may also need flexible models using, e.g., two-dimensional spline functions to replace the linear structure.

4.6 Internal validation data, partially observed and surrogate exposure measures

4.6.1 Exposure measured in a subpopulation

In a study, exposure is sometimes measured only in a subgroup of the study population. For example, in a trial with 500 patients randomized into two dose levels, PK samples may be taken only from 100 patients. In ER modeling, should we use the whole population, and if so, how? We consider two scenarios: when there is only one exposure and one response measure on each subject and when there are repeated measures for both exposure and response. The issue here relates to the approaches to ME models with internal validation data [Carroll et al., 2006].

We start from the simple scenario of one exposure and one response measure with a linear ER relationship. Let Y_i and C_i be the response and exposure of subject $i, i = 1, ..., n$,

$$\begin{aligned} Y_i &= \beta_0 + \beta_c C_i + U_i \\ C_i &= h(D_i, \gamma) + V_i. \end{aligned} \tag{4.62}$$

We are interested in estimating β_c, but C_i is observed only from the first n_1 subsets $i = 1, ..., n_1 < n$. In this case, the complete data analysis using the first n_1 subjects gives an unbiased estimate for β_c. However, data from the other subjects can also be used in the RC approach, with different mean functions for the first n_1 subjects and the rest:

$$\begin{aligned} E(Y_i|C_i) = \beta_0 + \beta_c C_i \quad i \leq n_1 \\ E(Y_i|D_i) = \beta_0 + \beta_c E(C_i|D_i) \quad i > n_1 \end{aligned} \tag{4.63}$$

where $E(C_i|D_i) = h(D_i, \gamma)$. Therefore, we can impute $\hat{\gamma}$ to form $\hat{C}_i(D_i) = h(D_i, \hat{\gamma})$ to predict $E(C_i|D_i)$ for those with missing C_i. To ensure that the β_c estimate can be used for the whole population, we have assumed that the subgroup with PK data is randomly selected. Since

$$\begin{aligned} \text{var}(Y_i|C_i) = \sigma_u^2, \quad i \leq n_1 \\ \text{var}(Y_i|D_i) = \sigma_u^2 + \beta_c^2 \sigma_v^2, \quad i > n_1, \end{aligned} \tag{4.64}$$

a weighted LS estimate for β_c is more efficient than the LS one. It can be obtained by setting weights 1 for those with C_i data, and $1/(1 + \beta_C^2 \sigma_i^2 / \sigma_u^2)$ for those with D_i only. Here, β_c is unknown, but can be replaced with an LS estimate based on the first n_i subjects. We have also ignored the parameter estimation error in the weight, as it is normally much smaller than V_i if n_1 is not very small. Note that σ_v^2 can be estimated from the complete pairs.

Now consider the classical ME model

$$\begin{aligned} Y_i &= \beta_0 + \beta_c C_i^* + U_i \\ C_i^* &= h(D_i, \gamma) \end{aligned} \tag{4.65}$$

in which we observe $C_i = C_i^* + V_i, i = 1, ..., n_1$. With this model, the complete data estimate of β_c obtained by replacing C_i^* with C_i for $i = 1, ..., n_1$ is biased, even when missing C_is are completely at random (MCAR). To eliminate bias, we can use the RC approach to replace C_i^* with $\hat{C}_i^* = h(D_i, \hat{\gamma})$, where $\hat{\gamma}$ is estimated based on $C_i, D_i, i = 1, ..., n_1$, since

$$E(Y_i|D_i) \approx \beta_0 + \beta_c E(h(D_i, \hat{\gamma})). \tag{4.66}$$

However, (4.66) holds for $i = n_1 + 1, ..., n$ too. Therefore, we can replace C_i with $\hat{\gamma}_d D_i$ for all subjects. Note that $\text{var}(Y_i|D_i)$ is the same for all subjects, so we should not weight subjects $i = n_1 + 1, ..., n$ differently from the first n_1 subjects.

If n_1 is sufficiently large, the models (4.62) and (4.65) can be compared to assess which fits the complete data better, using a proper goodness-of-fit criterion, as described in previous sections. It is likely that none of the assumed models (4.62 and 4.65) is correct and that the mixed ME model is more appropriate. In this case, as shown in the previous section, one may select the best combination of predicted and observed exposure measures.

This RC approach does not work for single dose situations, whichever model is assumed, because if $D_i = d$ for all i, everyone would have the same $E(\hat{C}_i|D_i)$. If there are other factors that have a significant impact on $C^*(t)$, in theory, these factors can be used to predict C_i, but the information gain is often much smaller than using dose in multiple dose studies. If these factors are also predictors of the response, using this approach also has the risk of introducing confounding bias.

It is useful to see how much gain can be made by including data from subjects $i = n_1 + 1, ..., n$. For simplicity, we assume that all subjects come from the same population with randomized dose and data Y_i have been centered to eliminate the intercept. Under this assumption, we denote $\sigma_h^2 = \sum_{i=1}^n (h(D_i, \gamma) - \bar{h})^2/n$, where $\bar{h}$ is the average of $h(D_i, \gamma)$s, for the variation of $h(D_i, \gamma)$, and assume that it is the same among the first n_1 subjects as among the rest. For model (4.65), if we use the first subjects n_1 only, we obtain an estimate $\hat{\beta}_{n1}$ with $\text{var}(\hat{\beta}_{n1}) = \sigma_u^2/(n_1\sigma_h^2)$ while when all data are used, the weighted LS estimate $\hat{\beta}_n$ has variance $\text{var}(\hat{\beta}_n) = (\sigma_u^{-2} n_1 + (n - n_1)/(\sigma_u^2 + \beta^2\sigma_v^2))^{-1}/\sigma_h^2$, therefore, the information gain can be measured by the variance ratio

$$\begin{aligned} \frac{\text{var}(\hat{\beta}_{n1})}{\text{var}(\hat{\beta}_n)} &= \frac{\sigma_u^{-2} n_1 + (n - n_1)/(\sigma_u^2 + \beta^2\sigma_v^2)}{n_1\sigma_u^{-2}} \\ &= 1 + \frac{(n - n_1)\sigma_u^2}{n_1(\sigma_u^2 + \beta^2\sigma_v^2)}. \end{aligned} \tag{4.67}$$

Therefore, the increase in information is proportional to the sample size ratio $(n - n_1)/n_1$ and the variance ratio $\sigma_u^2/(\sigma_u^2 + \beta^2\sigma_v^2)$. For the classical ME model, the information gain is simply the sample size ratio, since even for the first n_1 subjects, the predicted $h(D_i, \gamma)$ must be used, just as for the rest. Therefore, there is no difference in the variances. This means that we simply gain the information of additional $n - n_1$ subjects by including them in the modeling, and the increase in information is the sample size ratio.

For a multiplicative model such as a Poisson model with a log-link function, the same approach can be applied. Suppose that $Y_i \sim Poisson(\lambda_i)$ and

$$\begin{aligned} \lambda_i &= \exp(\beta_c C_i) \\ C_i &= h(D_i, \gamma) + V_i \end{aligned} \tag{4.68}$$

and $C_i, i = 1, ..., n_1$, are observed; we can also use $h(D_i, \hat{\gamma})$ to replace the missing C_is to fit the Poisson model. To decide how to weight the data with the predicted C_i, we need to calculate the conditional variances of Y_i. This can be done in the standard way using the well-known formula

$$\text{var}(Y_i) = E(\text{var}(Y_i|V_i)) + \text{var}(E(Y_i|V_i)). \tag{4.69}$$

Note that for those with C_i observed, the Poisson model is fitted conditional on C_i and for those without it, the model is fitted conditional on $h(D_i, \hat{\gamma})$. Ignoring the variability in $\hat{\gamma}$, which is negligible compared to that of V_i, the calculation leads to

$$\text{var}(Y_i|D_i) = \bar{\lambda}_i S(1 + \bar{\lambda}_i(S - 1)), \tag{4.70}$$

where $S = \exp(\beta_C^2 \sigma_v^2)$ and $\bar{\lambda}_i = \exp(\beta_c h(D_i, \gamma))$. As the variance depends on unknown parameter in $\bar{\lambda}_i$, we have to estimate it with, e.g., the first n_1 subject, then pre-calculate the weight in the same way as for linear models. Some software such as SAS proc GENMOD allows specifying the variance as a function of $\bar{\lambda}_i$. Hence, if σ_u^2 is known, it is possible to fit the Poisson model with the variance heterogeneity correctly taken into account. Also note that using the option of calculating the over-dispersion parameter in proc GENMOD gives a robust SE estimate for β_c, even when the variances are wrongly specified. For a general GLM such as the logistic model, the variance cannot be easily calculated, hence a weighted estimate may not be possible. However, the gain in information from weighting is generally small.

Under the assumption of the classical ME model, that is, when $\lambda_i = \exp(\beta_c h(D_i, \gamma))$ and we observe only $C_i = h(D_i, \gamma) + e_i, i = 1, ..., n_1$, the same approach as for the linear model can be used, i.e., $h(D_i, \gamma)$ can be replaced by $h(D_i, \hat{\gamma})$ when fitting the model. Again, there is no need to weight the two sets of subjects differently.

When repeated measures $C_{ij} = C_i + e_{ij}$ for $C_i = C_i^* + V_i, i = 1, ..., n_1$, are available, we can fit the dose-PK model in (4.65) to obtain not only $\hat{\gamma}$ but also $\hat{V}_i$. Therefore, we can replace C_i with

$$\hat{E}(C_i|D_i) = \begin{cases} \hat{\gamma}_d D_i + \hat{V}_i & i \leq n_1 \\ \hat{\gamma}_d D_i & i > n_1 \end{cases}.$$

For the linear model

$$\text{var}(Y_i|D_i) = \begin{cases} \sigma_u^2 + \beta_c^2 \text{var}(\hat{V}_i - V_i) & i \leq n_1 \\ \beta_c \sigma_u^2 + \beta_c^2 \sigma_v^2 & i > n_1 \end{cases},$$

and we can weigh the data accordingly to increase the efficiency. The same or similar approaches may be used for other types of ER models. However, we will postpone the extension to the other model types to the next section, since the approaches are similar.

Two more complex situations, for which we are not going to give the details, are when the ER model is an NLMM. Fitting these models to all the data is less straightforward. However, if it is a classical ME model, fitting all data with the RC approach does not require more effort than fitting the complete data, although the calibration will be based only on the complete data. For a model, e.g., $Y_i = h(C_i, \boldsymbol{\beta}) + \varepsilon_i$, the complete data have exposure measured without error, while for the others, we use the predicted C_i, which can be considered as from the Berkson model. It is possible to apply the approaches in the previous sections to this situation.

4.6.2 Exposure measured in a subpopulation but a surrogate is measured in whole population

Another commonly encountered situation is that the exposure (e.g., C_{max}) can only be measured in a subpopulation, while in the whole population a surrogate (e.g., concentration at a fixed time point close to T_{max}: the time C_{max} occurs) is measured. We consider a simple linear ER model

$$Y_i = \beta_c C_i^* + U_i \tag{4.71}$$

with RC approaches to utilize the surrogate data in order to fit all the data. Let C_i be the surrogate and C_i^* be the true exposure. Obviously, when C_i^* is measured, we use it to fit the model. If only C_i is measured, we replace C_i^* with an estimate of $E(C_i^*|C_i)$. Although we have choices among different ME models. Here we take an empirical model $C_i^* = h(C_i, \gamma) + e_i$. Then, fitting the model in the complete data subgroup, $E(C_i^*|C_i)$ can be estimated by $h(C_i, \hat{\gamma})$ for those with the surrogate measure C_i only. Finally the ER model can be fitted with C_i^* or $h(C_i, \hat{\gamma})$. The weighting to take into account the variation in the prediction of C_i^* may also be used, as shown in the previous subsection.

4.6.3 Using a surrogate for Cmax: an example

As an example, we consider using a surrogate for C_{max} to illustrate the approaches described above and to further develop some relevant approaches. First, we assume that Y_i is a biomarker relating to C_{max} and the exposure follows the open one-compartment model with first-order absorption (2.6). Suppose that we can use the samples C_{i1} and C_{i2} taken at 0.5 and 1 hours, respectively, to obtain C_{max} as the maximum of the two, e.g., $C_{maxi} = \max(C_{i1}, C_{i2})$. Note that this C_{maxi} is only an estimate based on concentrations at the two time points. We assume that only half of the patients have both C_{i1} and C_{i2} (identified by wei=1 in the data), hence C_{maxi} can be calculated, while the other half only have C_{i1} available. We are interested in using, e.g., C_{i1} as a surrogate for C_{maxi} for those with C_{i1} only. Again we assume that Y_is are centered and the relationship between C_{maxi} and Y_i is linear:

$$Y_i = \beta_c C_{maxi} + \varepsilon_i. \tag{4.72}$$

The following program simulates a dataset based on a set of parameter values, in particular $\beta_c = 1$.

```
nsimu=10000
ka=exp(1+0.5*rnorm(nsimu))
ke=exp(-1+0.5*rnorm(nsimu))
v=exp(-1+rnorm(nsimu)*0.03)
pk=function(t) (exp(-ke*t)-exp(-ka*t))/v*ka/(ka-ke)
c1=pk(0.5)
c2=pk(1)
cmax=pmax(c1,c2)
yi=cmax+rnorm(nsimu)*0.1
wei=rep(c(0,1),rep(nsimu/2,2)) #wei=1 if Cmax is measured
```

To examine the performance of using the surrogate to estimate β, we first only use the subgroup with C_{i1} only, and fit the model with C_{i1} rather than C_{maxi}, which results in:

```
> summary(lm(yi~c1,weights=1-wei))

lm(formula = yi ~ c1, weights = 1 - wei)
             Estimate Std. Error t value Pr(>|t|)
c1           0.729696   0.006243  116.87   <2e-16 ***,
```

showing a significant shrinkage in $\hat{\beta}$. To use the RC approach, we first need to estimate $E(C_{maxi}|C_{i1})$ by fitting an empirical model

$$C_{maxi} = a + bC_{i1} + e_i. \tag{4.73}$$

The empirical model can be fitted to those with C_{i1} and C_{maxi}, then used to predict C_{maxi} for those with C_{i1} only. To implement this approach, we use the following R-code:

```
> pcmax=predict(lm(cmax~c1,weights=wei))
> summary(lm(yi~pcmax,weights=1-wei))
```

which uses complete pairs (wei=1) to fit the model between C_{i1} and C_{maxi}, then uses the predicted C_{maxi} in the ER model for those without observed C_{max}. The results show that this approach gives an almost unbiased estimate for β_c.

```
              Estimate Std. Error t value Pr(>|t|)
pcmax         1.023243   0.008755 116.874   <2e-16 ***
```

The performance of this approach depends on how good the linear model is. Other models may be used too.

It might be tempting to predict C_{i2} then reconstruct C_{maxi} from the predicted C_{i2} and C_{i1} based on a model $C_{i2} = a + bC_{i1} + e_i$. This approach yields

```
> pc2=predict(lm(c2~c1,weights=wei))
> pcmax=pmax(c1,pc2)
> summary(lm(yi~pcmax,weights=1-wei))

             Estimate Std. Error t value Pr(>|t|)
pcmax        1.073511   0.009438 113.740  < 2e-16 ***
```

There is a considerable upward bias in $\hat{\beta}_c$ (1.07 rather than 1.00). As we discussed earlier, the performance of this approach depends on the empirical model. But the prediction should be for $E(C_{maxi}|C_{i1})$. Even if the model $C_{i2} = a + bC_{i1} + e_i$ is correct, $\max C_{i1}, \hat{C}_{i2})$ is not an unbiased estimate of $E(C_{maxi}|C_{i1})$, because maximization and expectation are not interchangeable. Therefore, as a general rule of RC, we should predict exactly the term in the y-part model, e.g., if C^2_{maxi} is in the model, then a model between C^2_{maxi} and C_{i1} should be used to predict $E(C^2_{maxi}|C_{i1})$.

Now we include all data in the model fitting and use the weighted LS for those with predicted C_{max} and weight=1 for the true C_{max}.

```
> weic=fitm$sigma^2/(fitm$sigma^2+fitm$coef[2,1]^2*fitc$sigma^2)
> weight=ifelse(wei==1,1,weic)
> ncmax=ifelse(wei==1,cmax,pcmax)
> summary(lm(yi~ncmax,weights=weight))

             Estimate Std. Error t value Pr(>|t|)
ncmax        1.007403   0.004313 233.550   <2e-16 ***
```

Compared with the results of fitting the data with Cmax only below, the SE was about 10% smaller.

```
summary(lm(yi~cmax,weights=wei)) #wei=1 if Cmax is measured

             Estimate Std. Error t value Pr(>|t|)
cmax         1.000413   0.004723 211.795   <2e-16 ***.
```

The key assumption on which this approach is based is the empirical model (4.73). One may ask the question: What if the empirical model is

$$C_{i1} = a + bC_{maxi} + e_i? \tag{4.74}$$

Since this is the classical ME model, an adjustment is needed after replacing C_{maxi} with C_{i1} in the model, as we described in the previous sections. Note that the simulation example is based on a real scenario, and the model (4.73) is used as an empirical model. The example has shown a shrinkage in the estimated β_c. In fact, both models can be correct, e.g., when C_{i1} and C_{maxi} are jointly normally distributed, and model (4.73) is the prediction for RC, if model (4.74) is first assumed.

Now suppose that Y_i is an indicator of an adverse event taking the value 1 if an event occurs and 0 otherwise. We consider fitting a logistic model linking C_{max} with the risk of the event. Let $P(Y_i = 1|C_{maxi}) = 1/(1 + \exp(-\beta_0 - \beta_c C_{maxi}))$. Our goal is to use all the data to estimate β_c. Using all the data is especially important if the event is rare. The major technical problem in using the RC approach is that $1/(1+\exp(-\beta_0 - \beta_c E(C_{maci}|C_{i1}))) \neq E(Y_i|C_{i1})$, due to the nonlinearity in the logistic function. If we are willing to assume a normal distribution for C_{maxi}, then a well-known approximation [Carroll et al., 2006]

$$E(1/(1+\exp(\beta x_i))) \approx 1/(1+\exp(\beta\mu_x/(1+\beta^2\sigma_x^2/1.7^2))), \qquad (4.75)$$

where $x_i \sim N(\mu_x, \sigma_x^2)$, can be used. Therefore, let $\hat{\beta}_c^*$ be the estimate of β_c when C_{maxi} is replaced with an unbiased estimate for $E(C_{maxi}|C_{i1})$. One may find a corrected estimate by solving the equation

$$\hat{\beta}_c^* = \beta_c/(1+\beta_c^2\sigma_c^2/1.7^2)^{1/2} \qquad (4.76)$$

where σ_c^2 is the prediction error for C_{maxi}, which can be estimated when fitting the model for C_{maxi} and C_{i1}. Note that the corrected estimate is no longer an unbiased estimate for β. Its SE can be estimated using either an approximation or a bootstrap approach (Section 10.5). However, $(1+\beta_c^2\sigma_c^2/1.7^2)^{1/2}$ is often close to 1, hence $\hat{\beta}_c^* \approx \beta_c + c$.

4.7 Comments and bibliographic notes

Joint and sequential modeling approaches in pharmacometrics can be found in Bonate [2006]; Ette and Williams [2007]. A systematic comparison was reported in Zhang et al. [2003] and is widely cited. For measurement error theory, Carroll et al. [2006] cover a wide range of models and approaches starting from the very basic concept. Several other books are on the same topic, but mainly on linear ME models. Bennett and Wakefield [2001] applied a Bayesian approach to joint modeling, a topic we have not covered. The use of RC for time-to-event data analysis needs to put the ME theory in the context of survival analysis, hence is postponed to Chapter 5.

The literature in this area comes from both statisticians and pharmacometricians with different focus. Joint modeling, used by the former, and simultaneous modeling, used by the latter, seem to carry the same meaning, but refer to slightly different approaches. Joint modeling refers to modeling multiple outcomes (e.g., longitudinal and survival data) to explore the relationship between them, including using two-stage approaches. Simultaneous modeling means fitting multiple models jointly in one step, in contrast to the sequential modeling procedure, which is the same as the two-stage one. The focus of pharmacometricians is on the direct relationship between the exposure and response, while the statistician's focus is often on the correlation between the outcomes, e.g., time to diagnosed AIDS or death and CD4 counts, tumor size and death.

5

Exposure-risk modeling for time-to-event data

Time-to-event (TTE) is often an important outcome in medical or biological research. The analysis of such data is known as survival analysis [Aalen et al., 2008; Fleming and Harrington, 2013; Kalbfleisch and Prentice, 2002]. For DER analysis with TTE as response, our primary interest is the impact of dose or exposure on the risk of an event, which can be quantified by using a model to fit dose or exposure and time-to-event data. In this chapter, we consider situations where the DER relationship is instant, e.g., the exposure level at a certain time only affects the risk at the same time, and also situations with cumulative dose or exposure effect.

5.1 A hypothetical example

The example comes from a type of study used in drug development. For drugs with highly variable exposures, often therapeutic dose monitoring (TDM) is used to control an individual's exposure in a desired range by adjusting individual doses until the exposure is within this range. For detailed dose escalation approaches, the reader is referred to Chapter 9. The dataset used here is simulated to mimic a real scenario. The dataset contains 100 patients, 50 in the active treatment group and 50 in placebo group. The dose levels in the active group were adjusted by TDM to reach the target concentration of 10ng/mL, at 14-day intervals when the drug concentration is measured to decide if a dose escalation is needed. The endpoint is the time of occurrence of an adverse event (AE). The dose, concentration and event data for each interval, until the end of the study, or until the first event of five patients is given below.

```
  group sub dose  conc start   stop event
1     1   1 1.61  6.30     0  14.00     0
2     1   1 1.87  9.61    14  28.00     0
3     1   1 2.13  8.42    28  30.04     1
4     1   2 1.61  3.97     0   7.78     1
5     1   3 1.61  5.64     0  14.00     0
```

DOI: 10.1201/9781003457008-5

```
6      1   3 1.87  8.33    14  28.00     0
7      1   3 2.13  8.80    28  42.00     0
8      1   3 2.40 12.66    42  56.00     0
9      1   3 2.40 13.75    56  70.00     0
10     1   3 2.40 11.11    70  84.00     0
11     1   3 2.40  9.05    84  98.00     0
12     1   3 2.66 12.60    98 112.00     0
13     1   4 1.61  2.50     0   0.68     1
14     1   5 1.61  2.82     0   4.45     1
```

The probability of no event till a time t and be considered as a function of time, known as survival function. For this data set, it is shown in Figure 5.1, along with the distribution of changes in dose level and concentration over time. From the plots, the dose-exposure relationship is obvious. However, the relationship between the risk of AE and the exposure is not clear, although evidence of the exposure-risk relationship is suggested by the increasing difference in survival curves between the active and controls groups (top panel). We are interested in how drug exposure is related to the risk of AE. Depending on the context, we may be interested in 1) the risk of AE for a given dose level; 2) the risk of AE under cumulative exposure following a complex dynamic; 3) how the risk changes with a dose adjustment? The following gives tools to find answers to these questions from analysis of event time aspects. However, approaches and tools from other chapters may also be needed. A number of variants of this example, including one with recurrent events and another when the recurrent events are known to occur with time intervals but not the exact occurrence time (interval censored) will also be used.

5.2 Basic concepts and models for time-to-event data

5.2.1 Distributions for time-to-event data

We start with the basic survival analysis without linking it to DER modeling. An approach for modeling TTE often starts by specifying its distribution, rather than its mean and variance, as we did in the previous chapters. The distribution of the TTE, T, can be specified by the density and distribution functions $f(t)$ and $F(t)$, respectively. In addition, the hazard function

$$h(t) = \lim_{\Delta \to 0} \frac{P(t < T < t + \Delta | T > t)}{\Delta} \tag{5.1}$$

plays a central role in survival analysis. The hazard is the risk of having an event just after time t, conditional on having no event up to time t. From the definition, we can derive $h(t) = f(t)/S(t)$ where $S(t) = 1 - F(t)$ is called the survival function because it is the probability of not having an event until

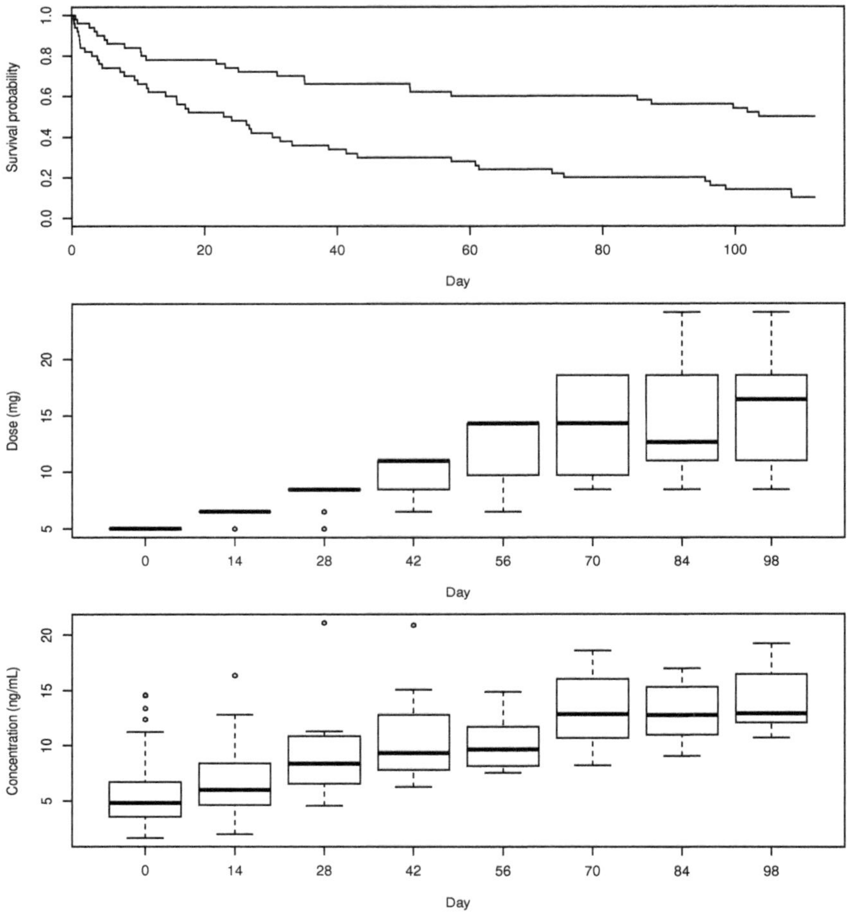

Figure 5.1
Survival curve of time to first AE for active and placebo groups in a hypothetical trial with TDM (top panel), and dose and concentration levels (lower panels).

time t. From $h(t)$ we can define the cumulative hazard function as

$$H(t) = \int_0^t h(\tau)d\tau, \tag{5.2}$$

which links to $S(t)$ with $S(t) = \exp(-H(t))$. The relationships between $h(t)$, $H(t)$, $f(t)$ and $S(t)$ are the key formulas that represent the key concepts in TTE modeling.

One might think of the time-to-event as a positively distributed variable, hence its analysis could use, e.g., a log transformation or a generalized linear model. However, one issue makes the analysis of TTE data a very special topic. Suppose that we are interested in the risk of an adverse event under the exposure of drug X in a clinical trial that runs for 6 months. At the end of the trial, some patients may never have an event, so we only know that the TTE for them is longer than 6 months. In this case, the TTE is (right) *censored* by the end of the study. It may also be censored by another event, such as death. Formally, let T_i^* be the true event time, C_i be the censoring time (e.g., due to the end of the study or death), and observe only $T_i = \min(T_i^*, C_i)$. To identify those who are censored, we also need an event indicator δ_i, with $\delta_i = 0$ if $T_i^* > C_i$ and $\delta_i = 1$, which means that the TTE is observed, otherwise. In previous chapters, we have almost always linked exposure and covariates to the mean of the response. For TTE data, we often link exposure and covariates to $h(t)$, due to reasons that will become clear later.

5.2.2 Parametric models

Some simple models can be constructed by specifying the TTE distribution. See, e.g., Chapter 3 of Kalbfleisch and Prentice [2002]. For example, assume that T follows an exponential distribution: $T \sim Exp(\lambda)$ with $f(t) = \lambda \exp(-\lambda t)$ and $F(t) = 1 - \exp(-\lambda t)$, leading to $S(t) = 1 - F(t) = \exp(-\lambda t)$. Expressing them in $h(t) = f(t)/S(t)$ we get $h(t) = \lambda$, i.e., the hazard function for the exponential distribution is a constant. To link T to covariates $\mathbf{X}_i$, one can assume $T \sim Exp(\lambda_i)$ with $\lambda_i = \exp(\mathbf{X}_i^T\boldsymbol{\beta})$. If a covariate in $\mathbf{X}_i$ is a group indicator, the corresponding $\boldsymbol{\beta}$ element is the log-risk ratio (RR) of this group to that of the reference. Or, if the covariate is a continuous variable, then the $\boldsymbol{\beta}$ element is the log-RR of one unit increase in the covariate. The use of $\exp(\lambda_i)$ is to ensure that the risk at any $\mathbf{X}_i$ value is non-negative. This approach simply replaces λ in $f(t) = \lambda \exp(-\lambda t)$ with $\exp(\mathbf{X}_i^T\boldsymbol{\beta})$. However, in the next section, we will show that this approach is not valid if $\mathbf{X}_i$ has time-varying components.

The exponential distribution is often too restrictive, as it has only one parameter. In principle, any positive distribution can be used for the TTE, and some other distributions can be transformed to a positive distribution. As a simple example, T_i may follow a log-normal distribution, that is, $\log(T_i) \sim N(\mathbf{X}_i^T\boldsymbol{\beta}, \sigma^2)$. With the additional parameter σ^2, this distribution offers more flexibility. The most commonly used distribution for TTE is the Weibull distribution. Its hazard and survival functions are

$$
\begin{aligned}
h(t) &= \gamma a(at)^{\gamma-1} \\
S(t) &= \exp(-(at)^{\gamma}),
\end{aligned}
\tag{5.3}
$$

respectively, where a^{-1} and γ are called the scale and shape parameters, respectively. The density function can be easily found with $f(t) = h(t)S(t)$. To include covariates, one may assume that $\mathbf{X}_i$ has an impact on a, γ or both, but $a_i = \exp(\mathbf{X}_i^T\boldsymbol{\beta})$ is a common choice for a simple model, as a_i is interpreted as an acceleration factor, and $\boldsymbol{\beta}$ is the log-TTE ratio from one category to the other if $\mathbf{X}_i$ is binary. We assume that $\mathbf{X}_i$ includes dose or exposure so that their corresponding elements in $\boldsymbol{\beta}$ represent the DR or ER relationship, conditional on covariates that are also included in $\mathbf{X}_i$.

Based on the observed $T_i, \delta_i, i = 1, ..., n$ we can write the likelihood function as

$$L(\boldsymbol{\beta}) \propto \prod_{i=1}^{n} f^{\delta_i}(T_i, \boldsymbol{\beta}) S^{1-\delta_i}(T_i, \boldsymbol{\beta}) g(\delta_i), \tag{5.4}$$

where $g(\delta_i)$ is the density function of δ_i, and we assume that C_i, and consequently δ_i, are independent of T_i and hence we will ignore the $g(\delta_i)$ part afterwards. This type of censoring is known as non-informative censoring. The MLE maximizes (5.4), which can be done easily in some simple situations. For example, if the exposure is constant and T_i follows the exponential distribution $f(t) = \lambda \exp(-\lambda t)$, and we would like to estimate the risk λ. Taking $f(t)$ and the corresponding survival function $S(t) = \exp(-\lambda t)$ into (5.4) and maximizing it with respect to λ (an easy way is to maximize $\log(L(\lambda))$, we find the MLE for λ is $\hat{\lambda} = n_e / \sum_{i=1}^{n} T_i$, where n_e is the number of events. This estimate is an important measure of the exposure-risk relationship, under the assumption of constant hazard, known as the event rate per person-year exposure. Later on we will find that this measure may not be appropriate for many situations when the exposure or risk is time varying. The MLE for TTE models is almost the same as the MLE elsewhere, except for the extra assumption of independent δ_i. The score equation of MLE can be derived from (5.4) and solved by statistical software. Asymptotic properties, in particular $\sqrt{n}(\hat{\boldsymbol{\beta}} - \boldsymbol{\beta}) \sim N(0, \boldsymbol{\Sigma})$, can also be derived, but the large sample condition must apply to the data after censoring. For example, asymptotic normality of the log-RR estimate based on the exponential model only holds when the number of events after censoring is sufficiently large.

5.2.3 Cox models

The analysis of TTE data is more sensitive to the assumption of the distribution than the analyses described in the previous chapters. Therefore, it is desirable to avoid specifying the distribution by using a semi-parametric model. The most commonly used semi-parametric TTE model is the Cox model [Cox, 1972; Kalbfleisch and Prentice, 2002; Therneau and Grambsch, 2000], which assumes that

$$h(t, \boldsymbol{\beta}, \mathbf{X}_i) = h_0(t) \exp(\mathbf{X}_i^T \boldsymbol{\beta}), \tag{5.5}$$

where $h_0(t)$ is an unspecified baseline hazard function. This model can be fitted by maximizing a partial likelihood function

$$L(\boldsymbol{\beta}) = \prod_{i=1}^{n} \left(\frac{\exp(\mathbf{X}_i^T \boldsymbol{\beta})}{\sum_{j \in R_i} \exp(\mathbf{X}_j^T \boldsymbol{\beta})}\right)^{\delta_i}, \tag{5.6}$$

which consists of the likelihood of event occurrence on subject i at a time point t_i as observed, among R_i: those still at risk at time t_i, for each i who has had an event.

Compared to the ML approach, an advantage is that there is no need to work out $f(t)$ and $S(t)$. Another advantage is that $h_0(t)$ is eliminated, since everyone at risk at time t shares the same $h_0(t)$. The resulting estimating equation by maximizing the partial likelihood is

$$\sum_{i=1}^{n} \delta_i (\mathbf{X}_i - \frac{\sum_{j \in R_i} \mathbf{X}_j \exp(\mathbf{X}_j^T \boldsymbol{\beta})}{\sum_{j \in R_i} \exp(\mathbf{X}_j^T \boldsymbol{\beta})}) = 0. \tag{5.7}$$

Note that the second term in the bracket is a weighted average of $\mathbf{X}_i$. This approach leads to a very efficient algorithm for estimating $\boldsymbol{\beta}$ and has been implemented in common software such as SAS and R. The most important large sample properties of the estimate $\hat{\boldsymbol{\beta}}$ is $\sqrt{n}(\hat{\boldsymbol{\beta}} - \boldsymbol{\beta}) \sim N(0, \boldsymbol{\Sigma})$, where $\boldsymbol{\Sigma}$ is the asymptotic variance of $\boldsymbol{\beta}$ and is routinely provided by software to fit the Cox model. This asymptotic distribution is the basis for statistical inference for $\boldsymbol{\beta}$. The derivation of asymptotic properties and the calculation of $\boldsymbol{\Sigma}$ involve complex formulae, so the reader is referred to textbooks such as Chapter 8 of Fleming and Harrington [2013].

In the example of exposure-safety data in the simulated TDM study, one may be interested in comparing the risks between the two treatment groups, although we know that the risk changes during dose escalation. Fitting a Cox model to the data with R using the function call below, we obtain

```
coxph(Surv(start,stop,event)~group,data=Out)
      coef exp(coef) se(coef)    z       p
group 1.65      5.19    0.286 5.76 8.5e-09
```

which shows log-RR=1.65 (SE=0.286) between the active arm and placebo.

5.2.4 Time-varying covariates

Drug exposure, either as drug dose or concentration, often varies over time. A simple example are the exposure-safety data from the simulated TDM study, in which the dose is piecewise constant. The Cox regression can be easily extended to allow for time-varying covariates including dose or exposure. The corresponding risk function is

$$h(t, \boldsymbol{\beta}, \mathbf{X}_i(t)) = h_0(t) \exp(\mathbf{X}_i^T(t)\boldsymbol{\beta}) \tag{5.8}$$

where $\mathbf{X}_i(t)$ contains time-varying covariates and $h_0(t)$ is the unspecified baseline hazard function. This model can also be fitted by maximizing the partial likelihood function that consists of the likelihood of event occurrence on subject i at a time point t_i as observed, given all those still at risk at this time point. In partial likelihood, $h_0(t)$ is also eliminated. However, for exposure-risk modeling, the effect of an exposure time profile shared by all subjects cannot be estimated, since it is confounded with $h_0(t)$. Estimating $\boldsymbol{\beta}$ for time-varying $\mathbf{X}_i(t)$ follows the approach mentioned above.

The resulting estimating equation for minimizing the partial likelihood is

$$\sum_{i=1}^{n} \delta_i(\mathbf{X}_i(t_i) - \frac{\sum_{j \in R_i} \mathbf{X}_j(t_i) \exp(\mathbf{X}_j^T(t_i)\boldsymbol{\beta})}{\sum_{j \in R_i} \exp(\mathbf{X}_j^T(t_i)\boldsymbol{\beta})}) = 0. \tag{5.9}$$

With time varying $\mathbf{X}_i(t)$, the same large sample properties of $\hat{\boldsymbol{\beta}}$, in particular $\sqrt{n}(\hat{\boldsymbol{\beta}} - \boldsymbol{\beta}) \sim N(0, \boldsymbol{\Sigma})$ also holds, under similar assumptions.

The counting process [Fleming and Harrington, 2013] approach has been used increasingly in TTE modeling, because of its theoretical and practical advantages. A TTE model can be presented as a counting process. For subject i, its counting process $N_i(t)$ is a step function that is zero at the beginning and jumps to 1 when the event occurs. It can be shown, under some technical conditions, that $E(N_i(t)) = h(t)$, if i is at risk. Intuitively one may consider $N_i(t)$ at discrete times t = 0, 1, 2,.... At time t, the probability of $N_i(t) = 1$ is $h(t)$, for those still alive at $t - 1$. This view links the Cox model to a logistic regression model [Efron, 1988] or in a more general setting in Aalen et al. [2008]. The connection between the two will be further explored later.

The counting process approach also provides a convenient way to implement a model with time-varying covariates. To see how the counting process approach helps to implement a TTE model, we consider the following hypothetical example. To accommodate piecewise exposures, the counting process can be split into multiple pieces according to event time and changes in covariates. For example, if subject i has an event at time 10, and $X_i(t) = 1$ when $t \leq 5$ and $X_i(t) = 2$ when $t > 5$, one can write the data in two records: $s = 0, t = 5, N_i(t) = 0, X_i(t) = 1$ and $s = 5, t = 10, N_i(t) = 1, X_i(t) = 2$, where s and t are the beginning and end of an interval. A data structure like this is referred to as a counting process structure and is often used to fit piecewise-constant covariate data. Cox model fitting software such as SAS proc PHREG and R library survival both allow fitting counting process data.

Looking at the example exposure safety dataset in Section 5.1, we find that it is already in the counting process form. It is very easy to fit models with time-varying dose or concentration in the model. The survival library in R provides a function Surv(start,stop,event) in which we specify the start and stop time points (s and t in the example above) of each record and event is an indicator. The following are the function calls for the Cox models that fit the dose and concentration, respectively, and the results.

```
> coxph(Surv(start,stop,event)~dose,data=Out)

      coef exp(coef) se(coef)    z       p
dose 0.806      2.24    0.138 5.84 5.3e-09

Likelihood ratio test=37.1  on 1 df, p=1.1e-09  n= 458, number of events= 63
> coxph(Surv(start,stop,event)~conc,data=Out)
```

```
      coef exp(coef) se(coef)     z       p
conc 0.156      1.17   0.0209 7.46 8.9e-14
```

in which coef is β and exp(coef) is the risk ratio of one unit dose or concentration change.

Since exposures (dose or concentration) change over time, one may also be tempted to fit the same models to the active group only to estimate β based on exposure variations within the group. This approach leads to

```
> coxph(Surv(start,stop,event)~dose,data=Out[Out$group==1,])

     coef exp(coef) se(coef)    z    p
dose 2.09      8.11      1.7 1.23 0.22

Likelihood ratio test=1.77  on 1 df, p=0.183  n= 143, number of events= 45
> coxph(Surv(start,stop,event)~conc,data=Out[Out$group==1,])

      coef exp(coef) se(coef)     z       p
conc 0.133      1.14   0.0344 3.86 0.00011
```

Note that the estimate of β for dose increased more than 100%, indicating a possible confounding between dose changes and risk function, due to the nature of exposure-dependent TDM.

Including time-varying covariates in a parametric model is often more difficult, unless the covariates are among a few types of simple time functions. For example, for the exponential distribution, it is natural to assume that $\mathbf{X}_i(t)$ has an impact on the hazard $h(t)$. Hence we may assume that the hazard of subject i $\lambda_i(t) = \exp(\boldsymbol{\beta}^T\mathbf{X}_i(t))$. However, to use MLE, one also needs to find the corresponding $f(t)$ and $S(t)$. For this, the basic relationships between $h(t)$, $S(t)$ and $f(t)$ are needed. Since $f(t) = h(t)S(t)$ and $S(t) = \exp(-H(t))$, the key step is to calculate $H_i(t, \mathbf{X}_i) = \int_0^t h_i(\tau)d\tau$ for each i. This is trivial when $\mathbf{X}_i(t)$ is constant, but an analytical form of $H_i(t, \boldsymbol{\beta})$ may not exist for a general $\mathbf{X}_i(t)$, even for the exponential distribution. Therefore, the density function $f(t, \boldsymbol{\beta})$ and the survival function $S(t, \boldsymbol{\beta})$ cannot be easily calculated. For some other distributions, we can assume that $h(t) = h_0(t)\exp(\boldsymbol{\beta}^T\mathbf{X}_i(t))$. For example, the Weibull distribution has $h_0(t) = t^{\gamma-1}$. In general, the calculation of $H_i(t, \boldsymbol{\beta})$ is more difficult with a non-constant $h_0(t)$. Common software for fitting parametric survival models, such as SAS proc LIFEREG and the R function survreg do not have the option of counting process structures to support fitting time-varying covariates, probably due to the difficulty of deriving the corresponding distribution function. Therefore, it is not easy to include time-varying covariates even when one is willing to approximate it with a piecewise constant function. In NONMEM and R, a numerical integration algorithm is available, hence one can evaluate $H_i(t)$ numerically. This approach allows for the use of a wide range of exposure models and TTE distributions, at the costs of much more intensive computation and potential numerical instability.

5.2.5 Additive hazard models

The Cox model assumes that the effect of each factor is multiplicative to the hazard function. In contrast, the additive hazard model is based on the assumption that the impact of each factor including the baseline on the hazard is additive:

$$h(t, \mathbf{X}_i) = h_0(t) + \mathbf{X}_i^T(t)\boldsymbol{\beta}, \tag{5.10}$$

where $h_0(t)$ and $\mathbf{X}_i(t)$ have a similar role to play as in the Cox model, except that their effects are additive to the risk. Additive models are less commonly used than the Cox model, for a number of reasons. Since the risk should be non-negative, an additive structure does not fit into this scale naturally. With estimates given for $h_0(t)$ and $\boldsymbol{\beta}$, the predicted risk $h(t, \mathbf{X}_i)$ may not be nonnegative for all possible $\mathbf{X}_i(t)$, unless appropriate range restrictions are applied on $\boldsymbol{\beta}$. Second, the estimations of $h_0(t)$ and $\boldsymbol{\beta}$ cannot be completely separated, as we did in the Cox model. The choice of a baseline function may have a considerable impact on the estimation of $\boldsymbol{\beta}$. Fitting an additive model requires software such as the R library timereg [Martinussen and Scheike, 2006], which is less popular than those for fitting Cox models. The function call for using timereg is almost identical to the coxph function call, which also uses the Surv() function.

However, for an additive model, the calculation of $H_i(t, \mathbf{X}_i) = \int_0^t h_i(\tau)d\tau$ is much easier for a given $\mathbf{X}_i(t)$ since it has an analytical solution as long as $\int \mathbf{X}_i(t)dt$ has one. If appropriate, we may also consider a mixture of additive and multiplicative models

$$h(t, \mathbf{X}_i) = h_0(t)\exp(\mathbf{X}_i^T(t)\boldsymbol{\beta}) + \beta_c C^*(t) \tag{5.11}$$

with additive exposure and multiplicative covariates effects. It can also be fitted with function timereg. If exposure is to increase risk, it is possible to let $\beta_c \geq 0$ to ensure that $h(t) \geq 0$ for all ts. For some typical $C^*(t)$s as a covariate in $\mathbf{X}_i$, $H(t, \mathbf{X}_i)$ can be easily calculated. These include $C^*(t) = \sum_{k=1}^K \theta_k \exp(-C_k t)$ from a linear compartmental model.

5.2.6 Accelerated failure time model

The previous models are mainly specified in terms of the risk function. The accelerated failure time (AFT) model represents another class of TTE models. The most common form for the AFT model can be written as

$$\log(T_i) = \mathbf{X}_i^T\boldsymbol{\beta} + \varepsilon_i, \tag{5.12}$$

where ε_i is a zero-mean random variable. An alternative form to (5.12) is

$$T_i = \exp(\mathbf{X}_i^T\boldsymbol{\beta})T_{i0}, \tag{5.13}$$

where $T_{i0} = \exp(\varepsilon_i)$ is the "baseline" time when $\mathbf{X}_i = 0$. When it is assumed to follow a certain distribution, this AFT model is a parametric model already introduced. Suppose that the survival function for $\exp(\varepsilon_i)$ is $S_0(t)$, since $T_i = \exp(\mathbf{X}_i^T\boldsymbol{\beta} + \varepsilon_i)$, we can derive

$$\begin{aligned} S(t|\mathbf{X}_i) &= P(\exp(\mathbf{X}_i^T\boldsymbol{\beta} + \varepsilon_i) < t|\mathbf{X}_i) \\ &= P(\exp(\varepsilon_i) < t\exp(-\mathbf{X}_i^T\boldsymbol{\beta})|\mathbf{X}_i) \\ &= S_0(t\exp(-\mathbf{X}_i^T\boldsymbol{\beta})). \end{aligned} \tag{5.14}$$

which is $S_0(t)$ with the time scale changed by the acceleration factor $\exp(-\mathbf{X}_i^T\boldsymbol{\beta})$. The corresponding $f(t)$ and $h(t)$ can be easily derived if $S_0(t)$ is known. Therefore, the MLE can be applied to estimate $\boldsymbol{\beta}$ by constructing a likelihood function based on $f(t)$ and $S(t)$ and maximizing it. In general, an AFT model with an arbitrary distribution for ε_i and acceleration factor $\exp(\mathbf{X}_i^T\boldsymbol{\beta})$ does not lead to a proportional hazard model. An exception is the Weibull distribution, which includes the exponential distribution as a special case. Details can be found in textbooks such as Aalen et al. [2008].

For the same reason as for the use of Cox models, we often want to leave the distribution of ε_i unspecified. Recall for linear and nonlinear models of continuous response, we sometimes assume the measurement error as a normally distributed variable. However, the asymptotic properties of the fitted model and estimated parameters do not depend on normality as long as the mean is zero. For the AFT model, the distribution of ε_i plays a far more important role. It is straightforward to introduce a semi-parametric model based on (5.12) by leaving the distribution of ε_i unspecified, giving a model without a parametric assumption. However, a similar approach to deriving a model fitting algorithm for the Cox model leads to a rank regression for $\boldsymbol{\beta}$. A well-known estimate was proposed by Buckley and James [1979]. Although software such as the jm library in R is available, the estimate is much less stable than that of a Cox model.

5.3 Dynamic exposure model as a time-varying covariate

Until now, we have not explicitly considered the effect of exposure on the risk of TTE. If the exposure is available and its impact on the risk is instantaneous, one may simply include it as a time-varying covariate, as discussed before. But often, even when exposure is observed, its impact on the risk of events may not be instantaneous. It is often the case that the risk is built by accumulation of exposures according to a dynamic system. In this section, we assume that latent cumulative exposure $C_i^*(t)$ has an immediate effect on the risk, e.g.,

$$h_i(t) = h_0(t)\exp(\beta_c C_i^*(t)), \tag{5.15}$$

where we drop covariates for simplicity. We also assume that latent exposure $C_i^*(t)$ is related to observed exposures, which may be drug concentration or dose, by means of a mechanistic or empirical model. However, in this section, we concentrate on the situation where there is no need to fit an exposure model separately. The model may have unknown parameters to estimate when fitting the TTE model. A typical exposure dynamic model is given by the effect compartment model in which

$$C_i^*(t) = \int_0^t g(t-\tau, \boldsymbol{\beta}) e_i(\tau) d\tau \tag{5.16}$$

where we use $e_i(t)$ as a general notation for the observed exposure. An example for $g(t, \boldsymbol{\beta})$ is

$$g(t, \boldsymbol{\theta}) = K_{in} \exp(-Kt), \tag{5.17}$$

in which K_{in} and K are unknown parameters. when the exposure is constant, i.e., $e(t) = E$, $C_i^*(t) = EK_{in}(1 - \exp(-Kt)/K)$. This section explores approaches to fitting TTE models when we can determine $C^*(t)$ by a set of parameters, even if it may not be a parametric model.

5.3.1 Semi-parametric models

In some specific cases, we can estimate the exposure dynamic represented by (5.16) with an empirical model approximation while fitting the TTE model. For example, if time t is discrete, taking values 0,1,2,3,..., (5.16) can be approximated by a discrete linear combination of past exposures

$$C_i^*(t) = \sum_{j=0}^{t} g_{t-j} e_i(j) \tag{5.18}$$

where g_js are unknown coefficients. Including $C_i^*(t)$ in the Cox model leads to

$$h_i(t) = h_0(t) \exp(\beta_c \sum_{j=0}^{t} g_{t-j} e_i(j)) \tag{5.19}$$

Note that β_c cannot be distinguished from g_js, unless $C^*(t)$ can be measured. However, $\beta_c g_j$s are sufficient to represent the dynamic relationship between the observed exposure and its impact on the risk. To fit such a model one simply includes lagged exposures as covariates in the Cox model, hence this is the simplest way to explore the exposure dynamic with minimum assumptions on the model. However, the effect of a common time trend in $e_i(t)$ may not be identified, unless it can be identified by, e.g., control subjects with $e_i(t) = 0$.

A simple Cox model can also be used when $g(t)$ in (5.16) is approximated by a set of spline functions. Suppose that $g_i(t) \approx \sum_{k=1}^{K} b_k(t)\theta_{ik}$, where the $b_k(t)$s are spline functions (Chapter 3), we can write (5.16) as

$$C_i^*(t) = \sum_{k=1}^{K} B_k(t)\theta_{ik} \tag{5.20}$$

where $B_k(t) = \int_0^t b_k(t-\tau)e_i(\tau)d\tau$. Since $b_k(t)$ is a piecewise polynomial, for some types of $e_i(t)$, e.g., a sum of exponential functions from a population PK model, $B_k(t)$ can be calculated analytically. This approach has been used in several exposure-risk modeling, e.g., in Sylvestre and Abrahamowicz [2008, 2009]. Fitting these models with standard Cox model software can be made easy by including pre-calculated $B_k(t)$ in the input dataset.

Sometimes, $C_i^*(t)$ may have parameters that are not linear to it, e.g., $C_i^*(t) = D_i(1-\exp(-Kt))$ is not a linear function of K. Although the function is very simple, the technical difficulty is that K cannot be estimated using common software that fits a Cox model. However, these types of exposure models are of particular importance; hence, we discuss model fitting for some simple but typical models. Two typical examples of such models are the K-dynamic models in the PKPD modeling literature, and the models for the relationship between drug prescription and reported adverse events in pharmacoepidemiology [Abrahamowicz et al., 2006]. In both cases, the exposure we observe is the dose. Since often the dose can only be changed at finite time points, one can assume it to be a piecewise constant function of time. Let D_{ik} be the dose level for subject i in the kth time interval from t_{ik} to t_{ik+1}:

$$D_i(t) = D_{ik}, \qquad t_{ik} \le t < t_{ik+1}. \tag{5.21}$$

We assume that the exposure $C_i^*(t)$ follows the effect compartment model (5.16) with $g(t,\beta)$ given in (5.17). In this case, we can calculate

$$\begin{aligned} C_i^*(t) &= K_{in}\int_0^t \exp(-K\tau)D_i(t-\tau)d\tau \\ &= \frac{K_{in}}{K}\Big(\sum_{k:t_{ik}<t} D_{ik-1}[1-\exp(-K(t_{ik}-t_{ik-1}))]\exp(-K(t-t_{ik})) \\ &\quad +D_{ik}[1-\exp(-K(t-t_{ik}))]\Big). \end{aligned} \tag{5.22}$$

For easy computing, the following recursive formula is more convenient:

$$\begin{aligned} C_i^*(t) &= \frac{K_{in}}{K}[C_i^*(t_{ik})\exp(-K(t-t_{ik})) + D_{ik}(1-\exp(-K(t-t_{ik})))], \\ & \quad t_{ik} \le t < t_{ik+1}, \end{aligned} \tag{5.23}$$

where $C_i^*(t_{ik})$ is the cumulative concentration at time t_{ik}.

A familiar example of this general situation is the cumulative exposure after a constant instant dose at level d_0 that gives

$$C^*(t) = d_0K_{in}(1-\exp(-Kt))/K. \tag{5.24}$$

This formula has been widely used as an approximation to the process of reaching steady-state concentration after repeated dosing. It also helps to interpret formula (5.22), as the first term represents the contribution of the

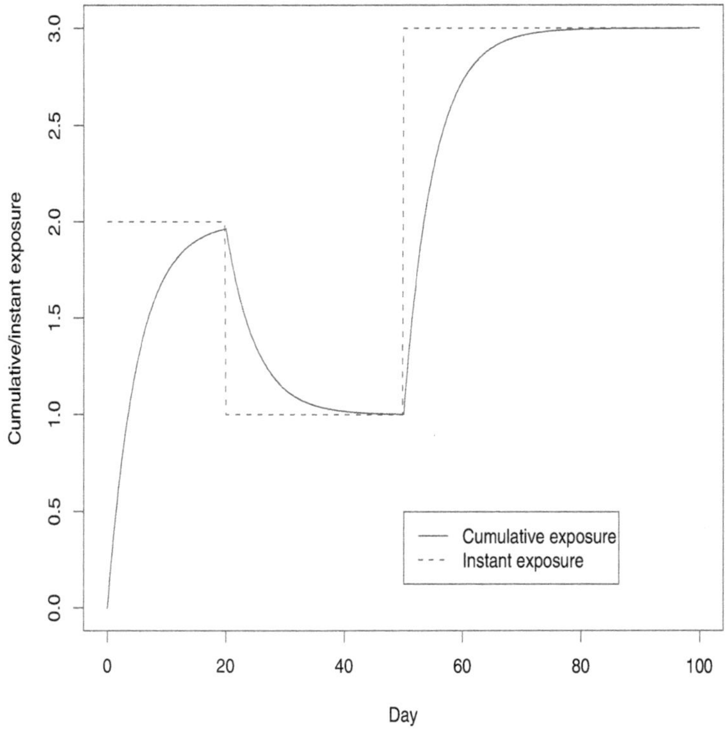

Figure 5.2
The relationship between the cumulative exposure and the piecewise constant instant exposure with an effect compartment model ($K = 0.2$ and $K_{in} = 0.2$).

existing exposure $C_i^*(t_{ik})$ decayed to time t with rate K and the second term is the contribution of additional exposure D_{ik}. Figure 5.2 gives an example of the relationship between $C_i^*(t)$ and piecewise constant $D_i(t)$, in which we set $K = 0.2$ and $K_{in} = 0.2$, so that when steady state is reached, $C_i(t)$ has the same level as $D_i(t)$. Suppose that the TTE follows the Cox model (5.8). Taking $C_i^*(t)$ from model (5.22) or (5.23) into (5.5) we find that K_{in} cannot be distinguished from β_c, hence (5.8) becomes

$$\begin{aligned} h(t) &= h_0(t)\exp[\beta_c(\sum_{k:t_{ik}<t} \frac{D_{ik-1}}{K}[1-\exp(-K(t_{ik}-t_{ik-1}))] \\ &\quad \times \exp(-K(t-t_{ik})) + D_{ik}[1-\exp(-K(t-t_{ik})])))], \qquad (5.25) \end{aligned}$$

where in the exposure accumulation part only K should be estimated.

Fitting model (5.25) directly is not easy with standard Cox regression software, since the log-relative risk is nonlinear with respect to K. However, K can be estimated with a grid search, in which we set K at a number of different values so that we can calculate $C_i^*(t)$ for each of the values. This step involves generating a dataset with precalculated $C_i^*(t)$ for each K value, then fitting the Cox model to the dataset. Then, among the fitted models, we search for the one with the highest partial likelihood value. An alternative is to use a grid of K values in combination with fitting a smooth curve to partial likelihood values at different K values. For example, spline functions are easy to fit and it is also straightforward to find the maximum of the spline functions. This approach can be implemented in standard statistical software such as SAS or R.

As a by-product of the grid search, the partial likelihood values can be used by the profile likelihood [Murphy and Van der Vaart, 2000] approach for statistical inference of K. It is often useful to know if a dynamic system for $C^*(t)$ is necessary. This can be tested by constructing the CI for K using the profile likelihood. It may also be done by comparing the maximum profile likelihood with that without the dynamic system, which is formally equivalent to $K = K_{in} = \infty$, and can be approximated by a very large K value.

Implementation of the grid search in SAS can be made easier, since it allows programming statements within proc PHREG. To this end, we construct a dataset containing one record per subject with time intervals of constant exposure and the corresponding exposure levels recorded in multiple variables. The number of variables needed in the dataset is determined by the one with the maximum number of intervals. The following program calculates $C^*(t)$ given in (5.23) for up to 10 intervals:

```
proc PHREG  data=example;
model Time*event(0)=cstar;
array cc{*} c1-c10;
array tt{*} t1-t10;
  prevc=0; *set start exposure 0;
  do i=1 to nrep;  *nrep is the N of intervals;
  if tt[i] <= Time < tt[i+1] then do;
  cstar= prevc*exp(-&K(Time-tt[i]))+cc[i](1-exp(-&K(Time-tt[i])));
  prevc= exp(-&K(tt[i+1]-tt[i]))+cc[i](1-exp(-&K(tt[i+1]-tt[i])));
end;
run;
```

where the K value is passed on from a macro variable &K. This approach is not computationally efficient for data with a very large number of intervals, particularly when only a few subjects have them.

5.3.2 Parametric models

The approach of including exposure dynamics in the hazard is generally not easy to apply to a model for a parametric baseline density distribution. To derive the density function $f(t)$ with exposure dynamics, one has to follow the route of calculating $H(t)$, then $S(t)$ and $f(t)$ from the baseline density. We may be able to calculate $H(t)$ analytically for certain types of models and distributions. In an additive hazard model (5.10) the baseline hazard and other covariates can be expressed as $h_i(t) = h_0(t) + \beta_c C_i(t) + \boldsymbol{\beta}_z^T \mathbf{Z}_i$, but we will omit the covariates for notational simplicity. In this case,

$$H_i(t) = H_0(t) + \beta_c \int_0^t C_i^*(\tau) d\tau \tag{5.26}$$

In most cases, we can assume that $C^*(t)$ is driven by a linear compartmental model with constant coefficients and can be written as

$$C_i^*(t) = \sum_{l=1}^{L} \theta_{il} \exp(-K_{il} t), \tag{5.27}$$

where θ_{il} and K_{il} are parameters already estimated from the PK data. In this case, we can derive

$$\begin{aligned} H_i(t) &= H_0(t) + \beta_c \int_0^t \sum_{l=1}^{L} \theta_{il} \exp(-K_{il}\tau) d\tau \\ &= H_0(t) + \beta_c \sum_{l=1}^{L} \theta_{il}(1 - \exp(-K_{il}t))/K_{il}. \end{aligned} \tag{5.28}$$

Hence,

$$S_i(t) = \exp(-H(t)) = \exp(-H_0(t) - \beta_c \sum_{l=1}^{L} \theta_{il}(1 - \exp(-K_{il}t))/K_{il} \tag{5.29}$$

and $f(t)$ can also be calculated to form the likelihood function (5.4). Note that for the same $C^*(t)$ but with a multiplicative hazard, $H(t)$ cannot be calculated analytically; hence even for $C^*(t)$ as simple as this, a multiplicative model with a parametric baseline density cannot be easily fitted.

For a complex model, e.g., a model with complex exposure dynamic or TTE distribution, a numerical integration can be used to calculate $H(t)$. Some software such as NONMEM and R has a built-in ODE solver, and can be used to calculate $H(t)$ by specifying a dummy ODE, $dH(t)/dt = h(t)$, although this is not an efficient approach from computational aspects.

5.4 Multiple TTE and competing risks

Often multiple events such as adverse events of different types and death can happen on the same subject. To model the exposure-risk relationship for multiple events, a number of issues should be considered. These include the correlation between the risks of different events, the termination of other events due to one event (e.g., death), and the change of exposure due to the occurrence of an event (e.g., AE leading to dose reduction).

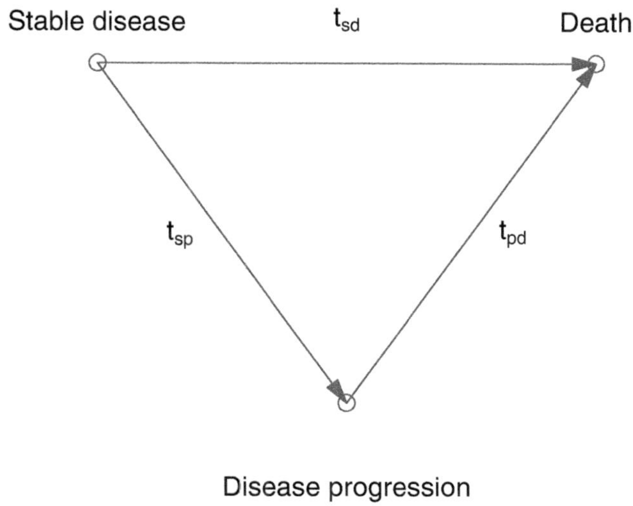

Figure 5.3
A three-state model for stable disease, disease progression and death.

5.4.1 Multi-state models

Multiple TTE can be modeled by multi-state models [Andersen and Keiding, 2002], in which a patient reaches a new state after the occurrence of an event. We are interested in the DER of the TTE from one state to another (known as transit time). Andersen and Keiding [2002] give a short review of multi-state models. For example, a three-state model consists of stable disease (SD) or normal health state, disease progression (DP) and death states, as illustrated in Figure 5.3, in which t_{sp}, t_{sd} and t_{pd} are the times from stable disease to disease progression, to death without disease progression, and from disease progression to death, respectively. For each of them, one can specify a model in a similar way as for a single TTE. For example, the hazard functions of t_{sp}, t_{sd} and t_{pd} can be specified as

$$\begin{aligned} h_{spi}(t, \mathbf{X}_i) &= h_{sp0}(t) \exp(\mathbf{X}_i^T \boldsymbol{\beta}_{sp}) \\ h_{sdi}(t, \mathbf{X}_i) &= h_{sd0}(t) \exp(\mathbf{X}_i^T \boldsymbol{\beta}_{sd}) \\ h_{pdi}(t, \mathbf{X}_i) &= h_{pd0}(t) \exp(\mathbf{X}_i^T \boldsymbol{\beta}_{pd}), \end{aligned} \quad (5.30)$$

respectively, where $\boldsymbol{\beta}_{sp}$,$\boldsymbol{\beta}_{sd}$ and $\boldsymbol{\beta}_{pd}$ are parameters representing the impacts of $\mathbf{X}_i$, including the dose or exposure effect. This model is based on an important assumption that t_{sp}, t_{pd} and t_{sd} are independent, which sometimes may not hold. Under this assumption, fitting such a joint model for three events with shared parameters is straightforward with common software. The first step is to prepare the data so that each subject has records for all possible states along the path he reaches the terminal state or till the end of follow-up.

For example, if patient i had experienced a DP at day 10 then was dead at day 20, with exposure values ci=1.2 before day 10 and ci=2.5 afterwards, then the following records are needed:

Id	start	stop	path	event	ci
i	0	10	SP	1	1.2
i	0	10	SD	0	1.2
i	10	20	PD	1	2.5
i	10	20	PS	0	2.5

The last record is needed only if the model allows transitions from DP to SD. The data contribute an event for models SP and PD, and two censored times for the other two models.

Under the assumption of independent t_{sp}, t_{sd} and t_{pd}, the multi-state models are Markovian with the property of the transition time from one state to another not depending on the history of this subject. The Markovness may not hold due to dependence on the history. However, sometimes we can add states to a model to make it a Markov model. For example, if the number of DPs a patient has experienced may influence the risk of death, the model in Figure 5.3 can be extended to include the states of 1st DP, 2nd DP, ..., to allow for different risks of death from these states. Another easy extension of the Markov model is the semi-Markov model in which the transition time from one state to another depends on the time to reach the current state. Fitting this model one only needs to add this time into $\mathbf{X}_i$.

One may also introduce correlation between the transition times by a joint survival function, e.g., $S(t_{sp}, t_{sd})$ for t_{sp} and t_{sd} and specify a parametric multi-state model. For the three-state model, we can assume that $\mathbf{t}_i = (t_{spi}, t_{sdi}, t_{pdi})^T$ follows a log-multi-normal distribution

$$\log(\mathbf{t}_i) \sim N(\boldsymbol{\mu}_i, \boldsymbol{\Sigma}) \tag{5.31}$$

where $\boldsymbol{\mu}_i = \mathbf{X}_i^T\boldsymbol{\beta}$ and $\boldsymbol{\beta} = (\boldsymbol{\beta}_{sp}, \boldsymbol{\beta}_{sd}, \boldsymbol{\beta}_{pd})^T$. In this model, the correlations between $t_{spi}, t_{sdi}, t_{pdi}$ are determined by $\boldsymbol{\Sigma}$. A simple alternative to this model is the multi-variate exponential model. For distributions without a well-defined correlation structure, the copula function Nelsen [2006] approach is a powerful tool for multivariate TTE analysis, but is outside of our scope due to space limitations. Finally, we note that, depending on the model structure, some correlation structure may not be identifiable due to competing risks in Section 5.4.2.

Statistical inference for individual parameters, e.g., $\boldsymbol{\beta}_{sp}$,$\boldsymbol{\beta}_{sd}$ and $\boldsymbol{\beta}_{pd}$ is straightforward given their estimates $\hat{\boldsymbol{\beta}}_{sp}$,$\hat{\boldsymbol{\beta}}_{sd}$ and $\hat{\boldsymbol{\beta}}_{pd}$, based on their asymptotic properties. But sometimes simultaneous inference for them is also important. For example, one may want to test if there is no exposure effect for overall survival, which can be tested by $H_0 : \boldsymbol{\beta}_{sd} = 0 \cap \boldsymbol{\beta}_{sp} = 0 \cap \boldsymbol{\beta}_{pd} = 0$. In this case, the correlation between the TTEs becomes important, since $\hat{\boldsymbol{\beta}}_{sp}$,$\hat{\boldsymbol{\beta}}_{sd}$ and $\hat{\boldsymbol{\beta}}_{pd}$ are correlated. One may take the correlation into account by explicitly modeling the correlation as above. Alternatively, an estimating equation procedure was developed in Wei et al. [1989] that fits the individual models to obtain the parameter estimates and a robust estimate of their variance-covariance matrix, without specific assumptions on the correlation structure between the transition times. Statistical inference, such as a test of the H_0, can be made based on the estimates and their variance-covariance matrix. This approach has been implemented in SAS [SAS Institute Inc., 2011].

The above has no direct connection to the DER models, apart from that $\mathbf{X}_i(t)$ can include dose or exposure measures and can be fitted to any of the models. Indeed, the exposure dynamic and multiple events may go in parallel and can be modeled as such. For example, if $C_i^*(t)$ is independent of the states and a transition from SD to DP occurs at time t_a, then before t_a, $C_i^*(t)$ may appear in $h_{sp}(t, \mathbf{X}_i(t))$ and $h_{sd}(t, \mathbf{X}_i(t))$, and in $h_{pd}(t, \mathbf{X}_i(t))$ after t_a. It is also possible that a state transition may lead to exposure changes. For example, upon DP, some patients in the placebo arm may be switched to active treatment, known as treatment switching. Therefore, $C_i^*(t)$ changes after t_a. This does not increase the technical difficulty of fitting the model, if $C_i^*(t)$ can be calculated after t_a. However, if the switching depends on a patient's characteristics, confounding bias may be induced. But we leave this topic to Chapter 8.

5.4.2 Competing risks

As shown in the previous section, multiple events can occur in the same patient, and some events may terminate the patient from the study (terminal events) [Pintilie, 2006]. Examples of such events are death from different causes or a severe AE that leads to the subject being withdrawn from a study. These types of events are known as competing events and have been intensively studied in survival analysis. In the 3-state model (Figure 5.3), a patient may die with or without DP. The risks of death of the two types are competing risks as only one can occur in one patient. To avoid the competing risk problem, we can consider a composite outcome, e.g., progression free survival (PFS), and the TTE of PFS is $\min(t_{sp}, t_{sd})$. However, we may also be interested in cause-specific risks, e.g., the risk if direct death and the risk of progression only, that is, the risk of one cause, with all other causes removed. However, this is often not possible, due to the co-existence of the other risks. Let T_k be the time to the event of type k, e.g., the time of death without DP, among all L types and $T = \min(T_1, ..., T_L)$ be the earliest event time, and K be the indicator of the occurred event type, the crude cause-specific risk of type k is defined as

$$h_k(t) = \lim_{\Delta \to 0} \frac{P(t < T < t + \Delta, K = k | T > t)}{\Delta}, \tag{5.32}$$

that is, the risk of having an event of type k, if no terminal event of any type occurred before t. In contrast, the net risk of the event k is defined as the hazard conditioning on no event k happened before

$$h_k^n(t) = \lim_{\Delta \to 0} \frac{P(t < T < t + \Delta, K = k | T_k > t)}{\Delta}. \tag{5.33}$$

We can easily fit the model of the crude risk (5.32), since the risk set at any time t consists of those with $T > t$. A Cox model can be applied to explore the relationship between covariates $\mathbf{X}_i$ and the risk of a specific event, e.g.,

$$h_{ki}(t) = h_{k0}(t) \exp(\mathbf{X}_i^T(t)\boldsymbol{\beta}_k). \tag{5.34}$$

Although one may also write (5.33) in this Cox model form, it is generally not possible to fit such a model, as the risk set of $(T_k > t)$ is not observed. Nevertheless, when the T_ks are independent, assuming no tie in $T_1, .., T_k$, the two risks are the same, since

$$h_k(t) = f_T(t|K = k)/S_T(t) = f_k(t) \prod_{k' \neq k} S_{k'}(t) / \prod_{k=1}^{L} S_k(t) = f_k(t)/S_k(t) = h_k^n(t). \tag{5.35}$$

To link competing risks to the multi-state model, note that the transition times there follow the distributions defined by the net risks, and the competition is between events represented by the model, in the sense that if in (5.3) someone takes the route of SD to death without DP, then he would not be able to take the route SD-DP, hence $h_k^n(t)$ is not generally identifiable. The non-identifiability is also reflected in fitting the multi-state model, since for the example in Figure 5.3, it is not possible to fit the model with random effects in the transition risks. From here we can also see the importance of competing risks in the exposure effect. For example, if exposure reduces the chance of DP, but also increases the risk of safety events such as death and severe AEs leading to treatment discontinuation. Then for those with higher exposure, the competing risk of safety events makes those with prolonged time to DP censored. Hence, adjustment is needed for the estimation of treatment effects on the risk of DP.

An important special case of competing risks is semi-competing risks, referring to the situation that one event time (e.g., death) is always observed but it may censor another event (e.g., disease progression). In this case, it is possible to further explore the relationship between the two events. For example, we can calculate the correlation between the two TTEs.

5.5 Models for recurrent events

Some events, such as asthma attacks and epilepsy seizures, may occur multiple times on one subject. Modeling the relationship between exposure and the risk of occurrence or recurrence provides important information for, e.g., dose selection and adjustment strategies.

5.5.1 Recurrent events as a counting process

We have introduced the counting process $N(t)$ to model TTE [Cook et al., 2007]. It is straightforward to extend it by letting $N(t)$ be the number of recurrent events that occur up to time t. The simplest yet commonly used is the homogeneous Poisson process with two key properties: 1) the number of events occurring within a time interval follows a Poisson distribution and its mean is proportional to the length of the interval, i.e., $N(t) - N(s) \sim Poisson(\lambda(t-s)), t > s$, and 2) the gap time between two events follows an exponential distribution. To model the impact of exposure on $N(t)$, one can follow the Cox regression for time to a single event and assume that the rate function, which is the probability of an event occurring at time t, follows

$$E(dN_i(t)) \equiv h_i(t) = h_0(t)\exp(\mathbf{X}_i^T\boldsymbol{\beta}) \tag{5.36}$$

where $h_0(t)$ is the baseline rate function and the second term represents exposure and covariate effects.

5.5.2 Recurrent events in multi-state models

A simple multi-state model for recurrent events contains states of having had $1, 2, 3,...$ events. The gap time between events can be modeled as the transition time between the state of having k events to that of having $k+1$ events. Let T_{ik} be the time to the kth event after having the $k-1$th, we may assume the hazard of the kth event as

$$h_k(t) = h_{0k}(t)\exp(\mathbf{X}_i^T\boldsymbol{\beta}_k) \tag{5.37}$$

where $h_{0k}(t)$ and $\boldsymbol{\beta}_k$ are state-specific, but some components may be shared. When they are all shared, this model describes a renewal process with completely the same risk of having the next event. This assumption is valid only for very special cases, such as the time to the next failure of a replaced machine part. In biostatics models, the time to the next event often depends on the number of events that have occurred. For example, gastric bleeding, a typical AE of some type of drug, may increase the risk of recurrence of bleeding. The risk of recurrent myocardial infraction follows the same pattern. To avoid using too many parameters, one may assume

$$h_k(t) = h_0(t)\exp(\mathbf{X}_i^T\boldsymbol{\beta}_k + \beta_s\#(k) + \beta_c c(t)) \tag{5.38}$$

where $\#(k)$ is a function of event number k. For example, if the log-baseline risk of recurrent events increases linearly with the number of events that already happened, then using $\#(k) = k$ we can adjust for this effect with only one additional parameter. Alternatively, one can also let the correlation between the transition times remain unspecified and use the approach of Wei et al. [1989] to obtain a robust variance-covariance matrix for the estimates of the $\boldsymbol{\beta}_k$s.

Sometimes an event marks a state change. For example, an infection may last several days, so having an infection should be considered as a state. Therefore, the multi-state model with state 0, 1, 2, 3 events may be extended to 0, 1, 1-, 2, 2-,..., where $k-$ denotes the state of no longer in the kth event state. This model needs another set of transition times from an event to event-free states, in addition to those from event-free to event states. Therefore, one may need to specify several TTE models for these transition times. Under some assumption, it may be simplified to a 2-state model (event on and off), possibly with a counter for the number of events experienced, if the risk of on and off events has the form of (5.38).

5.5.3 Rate and marginal models

The multi-state model approach requires specification of model structure and distribution of transition times. An alternative to modeling the time of events is to model the average number of events $N(t)$ until a given time t directly as a function of time. Here we can consider $N(t)$ as a counting process with mean $m(t) = E(N(t))$, known as the mean function of $N(t)$. This approach has advantages in dealing with recurrent events. One may model $m(t)$ with a non-parametric, semi-parametric, or parametric model. To avoid the complex theory of the stochastic processes of continuous time, we consider discrete time $t = 1, 2, 3, ...$ only, and without loss of generality, we use "day" as a shorthand for the time unit. Let $l_i(t)$ be the indicator that subject i has an event on day t, we have

$$m(t) = E(N(t)), \;\; l(t) = E(l_i(t)) = m(t) - m(t-1). \tag{5.39}$$

Here, $l(t)$ is often called the rate function, since when time is continuous, $l(t)$ is the derivative of $m(t)$. To model recurrent events, we can model $m(t)$ or $l(t)$. We prefer modeling the latter, as it is closer to the modeling of the hazard, although doing so we model the marginal mean of occurrence, that is, we do not condition on the history. For a marginal semi-parametric model for $l(t)$, we may use:

$$l(t|\mathbf{X}_i(t)) = E(l_i(t)|\mathbf{X}_i(t)) = l_0(t)\exp(\mathbf{X}_i^T(t)\boldsymbol{\beta}), \tag{5.40}$$

where $l_0(t)$ is a non-parametric marginal baseline function and $\exp(\mathbf{X}_i^T(t)\boldsymbol{\beta})$ is the parametric part with parameters $\boldsymbol{\beta}$. This model is very similar to the Cox model as they share the same type of model structure.

The model (5.40) can be fitted using an estimation equation (EE) approach. Let C_i be the time of censoring for patient i and denote $\delta_i(t) =$

$I(C_i > t)$, the estimating equations for $l_0(t)$ and $\boldsymbol{\beta}$ can be written as

$$\begin{aligned} U_l(l_0(t), \boldsymbol{\beta},) &= \sum_{i=1}^{n} \delta_i(t)(l_i(t) - l_0(t)\exp(\mathbf{X}_i^T(t)\boldsymbol{\beta})) = 0, \\ U_{\boldsymbol{\beta}}(l_0(t), \boldsymbol{\beta}) &= \sum_{i=1}^{n}\sum_{t=1}^{C_i} \mathbf{X}_i(t)(l_i(t) - l_0(t)\exp(\mathbf{X}_i^T(t)\boldsymbol{\beta})) = 0. \end{aligned} \tag{5.41}$$

With discrete t and the non-parametric setting for $l_0(t)$, one can solve $l_0(t)$ from the first equation and substitute it into the second one and obtain:

$$U_{\boldsymbol{\beta}}(\boldsymbol{\beta}) = \sum_{i=1}^{n}\sum_{t=1}^{C_i} \mathbf{X}_i(t)[l_i(t) - \frac{\sum_{i=1}^{n} \delta_i(t) l_i(t)}{\sum_{i=1}^{n} \delta_i(t)\exp(\mathbf{X}_i^T(t)\boldsymbol{\beta})}\exp(\mathbf{X}_i^T(t)\boldsymbol{\beta})] = 0. \tag{5.42}$$

This EE is also similar to that of the Cox model based on partial likelihood. However, a key difference is that the baseline hazard cannot be completely eliminated, hence the estimation of β also depends on it.

Since $l_i(t)$ and $l_i(t')$ are not independent, for inference on $\boldsymbol{\beta}$, a robust estimate for $\text{var}(\hat{\boldsymbol{\beta}})$ is needed. The covariance matrix of $\hat{\boldsymbol{\beta}}$ depends on the joint distribution of $l_i(t)$s, which we do not specify in the marginal model. However, a robust variance estimate for $\hat{\boldsymbol{\beta}}$ is ready to use [Lawless and Nadeau, 1995]. A more general robust covariance estimate was proposed by Lin and Wei [1989] and has been implemented in SAS PROC PHREG [SAS Institute Inc., 2011].

This approach can also be used to model the cumulative duration of events. The duration is equivalent to state occupancy in an on-off event model and is generally difficult to estimate without a simulation. However, the marginal model provides a straightforward way to model the relationship between the exposure and risk of having an event. To this end, we define $l_i(t)$ as the indicator that subject i is within an event episode. In this case $l(t) = E(l_i(t))$ is the mean prevalence of events and $m(t) = \sum_{j=1}^{t} l(j)$ is the mean cumulative duration of events until time t. For fitting a model for $l(t)$, whether it is the mean incidence or prevalence function, the following pseudo-event approach can generate data based on time to event and duration of event records and then use standard software to fit models such as (5.40) [Wang and Quartey, 2012; Wang, 2012b]. For example, for an event episode starting at day j and end at $j + s$, we generate $s + 1$ "pseudo" event records with $t = j + j', l_i(t) = 1, j' = 0, ..., s$. Here we follow the convention that the days that the event episode starts and ends are all counted as a whole day. The data can then be fed into SAS PROC PHREG using the counting process model formula. Note that this approach also allows exposure or covariate changes during an event, since $\mathbf{X}_i(t)$ values can be different between pseudo-records during an event. Therefore, this approach also allows a dynamic exposure model to be included. One obvious drawback of this approach is the lack of computing efficiency due to the size of pseudo dataset. However, it only leads to practical difficulty for very large and lengthy studies with a long duration of episodes of events. In these cases, t may be discretized in a larger grid to reduce the number of records in the generated data set.

After obtaining $\hat{\boldsymbol{\beta}}$, one can replace it for $\boldsymbol{\beta}$ in (5.40) to obtain the Nelson estimate for $l(t|\mathbf{X}(t))$ for a given $\mathbf{X}(t)$:

$$\hat{l}(t|\mathbf{X}(t)) = \frac{\sum_{i=1}^{n} \delta_i(t) l_i(t)}{\sum_{i=1}^{n} \delta_i(t) \exp(\mathbf{X}_i^T(t)\hat{\boldsymbol{\beta}})} \exp(\mathbf{X}_i^T(t)\hat{\boldsymbol{\beta}}), \tag{5.43}$$

and an estimate for $L(t|\mathbf{X}(t))$ can be calculated based on $\hat{l}(t|\mathbf{X}(t))$. The estimate for $L(t|\mathbf{X}(t))$ and its pointwise confidence band based on a sandwich variance estimate for (5.43) have also been implemented in SAS PROC PHREG.

The following is an example using a dataset generated according to the therapeutic dose monitoring scenario, as discussed in Chapter 1. The dataset is generated by the following SAS program, where the times the AE occurred and resolved are generated alternately according to the drug exposure and the random effects of the subject.

```
%let nsimu=50; %let cdose=log(1.3); %let bound=log(10);
%let base=-8; %let base2=-3;  %let dose1=log(5); %let sigv=0.5;
%let sigu=0.3; %let sige=0.2; %let nsub=50; %let nrep=8;
%let beta=0.25; %let nday=14;
data simu;
  do sub=1 to &nsub;
    ui=rannor(12)*&sigu;
    vi=rannor(1)*&sigv;
    dose=&dose1;
      pevent=0;
    do i=0 to &nrep;
    lci=dose+ui;
    lce=lci+rannor(12)*&sige;
    conc=exp(lci);
    low=i*&nday; up=low+&nday;
      start=low;
      stop=low;
      do k=1 to 30 while (stop < up);
       if pevent in (0 2) then  lmd=exp(&base+&beta*exp(lci)+vi);
       else if pevent =1 then  lmd=exp(&base2-vi);
       ti=ranexp(12)/lmd;
       stop=start+ti;
       if stop le up then do;
          if pevent in (0 2) then event=1;
          else if pevent=1 then event=2;
          output;
          start=stop; pevent=event;
       end;
       else do;
          event=0; stop=up; output;
```

```
      end;
     end;
    if lce<&bound then dose=dose+&cdose;
    end;
  end; run;
```

In the data, off- and on-event periods are indicated by pevent=0 (no previous event) or 2 (off previous event) and pevent=1, respectively, and event=0 means censored. The program assumes that exposure only affects the time to AE, but not the time when the AE is resolved (off-event). For both on- and off-event times, a shared random effect, vi, is added to generate correlation between the recurrent event times, assuming that patients with a higher vi would have a higher risk of AE and would also take longer to resolve the AE. The following programs fit the rate models with the option of robust variance estimates.

```
proc phreg data=simu(where=(pevent in (0 2))) COVS(AGGREGATE);
  model (start, stop)*event(0)=conc;
  id sub; run;

proc phreg data=simu(where=(pevent in (1))) COVS(AGGREGATE);
  model (start, stop)*event(0)=conc;
  id sub; run;
```

The statistics and parameter estimates of the fitted model are:

```
For time to event:
                 Testing Global Null Hypothesis: BETA=0

       Test                       Chi-Square       DF      Pr > ChiSq

       Likelihood Ratio               8.8217        1          0.0030
       Score (Model-Based)            8.8725        1          0.0029
       Score (Sandwich)               5.6290        1          0.0177
       Wald (Model-Based)             8.7452        1          0.0031
       Wald (Sandwich)                7.5404        1          0.0060

               Analysis of Maximum Likelihood Estimates

           Parameter      Standard     StdErr
Parameter   Estimate         Error      Ratio    Chi-Square    Pr > ChiSq

conc         0.24278       0.08841      1.077        7.5404        0.0060

           Test                       Chi-Square       DF      Pr > ChiSq

           Likelihood Ratio               0.1275        1          0.7210
           Score (Model-Based)            0.1270        1          0.7215
```

```
            Score (Sandwich)             0.1209        1         0.7281
            Wald (Model-Based)           0.1269        1         0.7216
            Wald (Sandwich)              0.1202        1         0.7288
```

and for time off event:

```
                Analysis of Maximum Likelihood Estimates

            Parameter      Standard     StdErr
Parameter    Estimate         Error      Ratio    Chi-Square    Pr > ChiSq

conc          0.03560       0.10267      1.028        0.1202        0.7288
```

In the results, the exposure effect estimates for the time-to-event and time-off event are similar to the true values 0.25 and 0 for to event and off event, respectively.

5.6 Frailty: random effects in TTE models

To introduce the concept of frailty, we consider the Cox model

$$h_i(t) = h_0(t)\exp(\mathbf{X}_i^T\boldsymbol{\beta}). \tag{5.44}$$

in which covariates $\mathbf{X}_i$ represent known factors relating to the risk of subject i. Often there are unobserved factors that make subject i different from the others. As we did for mixed models introduced in the previous chapters, we can add a latent subject effect U_i, known as frailty in TTE models, in the hazard function so that conditional on U_i:

$$h_i(t|U_i) = h_0(t)U_i\exp(\mathbf{X}_i^T\boldsymbol{\beta}). \tag{5.45}$$

A common choice for the distribution of U_i is gamma parameterized so that $U_i \sim gamma(\theta)$ with $E(U_i) = 1$ and $\text{var}(U_i) = \theta$, and frailty increases with increasing θ. Since U_i is unobserved, one needs to derive the marginal model in order to use the MLE approach. To this end, we can derive a conditional distribution from the hazard function (5.45), then the marginal distribution can be derived by integrating the conditional distribution over the gamma distribution for U_i [Therneau and Grambsch, 2000]. The resulting marginal likelihood is complex [Klein, 1992] ; hence, is omitted here. Unlike the partial likelihood, the marginal likelihood contains $h_{i0}(t)$ and $H_{0i}(t) = \int h_{0i}(\tau)d\tau$, which must be specified to fit the model. For most other distributions of U_i, the marginal model does not have an analytical form.

Even if the marginal model is simple, frailty models can only be fitted reliably to recurrent event data to identify the frailty, just as a mixed-effects model which can only be fitted to repeated measurement data. To see why, suppose that there is no covariate and $h_0(t) = hU_i$, i.e., the baseline risk is constant but contains frailty U_i. However, those with higher risk (large U_i) will have an event in a short period, and those who did not have an event in a short period are likely to be the low-risk ones. This leads to, on average, a higher risk at the beginning and a trend of reduction later on. Consequently, one cannot distinguish the case of a time-varying baseline risk and a constant risk with frailty. This topic will be discussed further in Sect. 5.9.

Suppose that the risk of the jth event on subject i is

$$h_{ij}(t) = h_{0j}(t)U_i \exp(\mathbf{X}_{ij}^T \boldsymbol{\beta}) \tag{5.46}$$

where $h_{0j}(t)$ is the baseline risk for the jth event and $\mathbf{X}_{ij}$ can include covariates for the jth event specifically, e.g., the history of previous events. This model can be fitted with, e.g., R function survreg with the following codes:

```
rfit2a <- survreg(Surv(time, status) ~ conc + frailty.gaussian(id),
          dist="weibull", data=riskexp )
```

where frailty.gaussian(id) specifies a normally distributed frailty on a Weibull parametric model and id is the subject identity. The same model can also be fitted with SAS proc NLMIXED and NONMEM using the built-in numerical integration function to calculate the marginal likelihood numerically. The following SAS program (adapted from example code in SAS Institute Inc. [2011]) fits a model with a Weibull distribution conditional on U_i and $\log(U_i) \sim N(0, \sigma_u^2)$:

```
proc nlmixed data=mydata qpoints=8;
parms gamma=1 sigu=0.1;
bounds gamma sigu> 0;
linp = a + b ci+ui;
alpha = exp(-linp);
G_t = exp(-(alpha*time)**gamma);
g = gamma*alpha*((alpha*time)**(gamma-1))*G_t;
ll = (status=1)*log(g) + (status=0)*log(G_t);
model time ~ general(ll);
random ui ~ normal(0,sigu) subject=patient; run
```

where we have used the random statement to specify the frailty in the same way as to specify the random effects in a NLMM.

The ML approach can also be used for Cox models by replacing the conditional likelihood given U_i with a conditional partial likelihood function (5.6). One particular model is derived assuming $S_i = \log(U_i) \sim N(0, \sigma_s^2)$, and the joint log-likelihood for T_{ij} and S_i can be written as

$$l(\boldsymbol{\beta}, \mathbf{u}) = l_p(\boldsymbol{\beta}|\mathbf{s}) - \frac{\sum_{i=1}^n S_i^2}{2\sigma_s^2} - n/2 \log(\sigma_s^2) + C. \tag{5.47}$$

where $l_p(\boldsymbol{\beta}|\mathbf{s})$ is the partial likelihood function conditional on frailty $\mathbf{s}$. This is also called penalized partial likelihood since the second term acts to penalize large S_is. To fit the model, we still need to integrate the S_is from (5.47). This can be done by a Laplace approximation [Therneau and Grambsch, 2000] and the algorithm has been implemented in software such as R library survival and SAS proc PHREG. The approximation can be used for other distributions for U_i, with an appropriate penalty term in (5.47). For R the following call fits such a model with log-normal frailty:

```
coxph(Surv(time,status) ~ exposure+ frailty(id, dist='gauss'), data=mydata)
```

where In SAS proc PHREG, the statement RANDOM follows the same syntax as other procedures

```
proc PHREG data=mydata;
model time*status(0)= exposure;
RANDOM id;
```

There are more choices for U_i in the R library but the log-normal distribution is the only one available in SAS. The following SAS codes fit the simulated data to frailty models for times "on" and "off" events.

```
proc phreg data=simu(where=(pevent in (0 2)));
  class sub;
  model (start, stop)*event(0)=conc;
  random sub/solution;
run;
proc phreg data=simu(where=(pevent in (1)));
  class sub;
  model (start, stop)*event(0)=conc;
  random sub/solution;
run;
```

```
Time to event

 Cov          REML     Standard
 Parm     Estimate        Error
 sub        0.1769       0.2728

                Parameter       Standard
 Parameter      Estimate           Error     Chi-Square     Pr > ChiSq
 conc             0.24402        0.08549         8.1470         0.0043

Time off event

Cov          REML     Standard
Parm     Estimate        Error
sub        0.2193       0.3324

                          Analysis of Maximum Likelihood Estimates

                Parameter       Standard
Parameter       Estimate           Error     Chi-Square     Pr > ChiSq
conc            0.00568          0.11350         0.0025         0.9601
```

The β estimates are similar to those in the rate model. In addition, the estimated variances of the frailty are also given together with their SEs, although they are far from statistically significant.

The option "Solution" in the RANDOM statement requires estimation of the random effects. As U_i is a shared frailty, it might be tempting to test the correlation between the predictions of the two models. However, only 30 patients had an estimate for vi, due to the lack of repeated events among other patients. Among the 30 patients, the correlation between the U_is from the two models was 0.11 and the p-value for zero correlation was 0.576, indicating that there is no shared frailty. The reason behind this is the difficulty in estimating random effects. Only when the number of repeated events is large can individual estimates for U_i approximate the true values. In common practical scenarios, this condition is rarely met.

In the general multi-state models discussed in the early section, we have assumed that the risks of transition between the states are independent. This is often not true, since, e.g., the risks of disease-related and non-disease-related deaths are often correlated due to, e.g., age and general health conditions. It might be tempting to include frailty variables to reflect the correlation. However, most of the frailties, e.g., those reflect the correlation between disease-related and non-disease-related deaths on the same subject, cannot be identified, since the two events cannot happen on the same subject. Frailties in sequential states, e.g., those in the risks of disease progression and death after progression, could be identified, but only under some additional conditions, although their correlation can always be estimated.

The frailty model can also be used to model multiple events of different types. Suppose that there are K different types of events, the hazard function of type k event may be specified as

$$h_{ik}(t) = h_{0k}(t)U_i \exp(\mathbf{X}_i^T \boldsymbol{\beta}_k) \tag{5.48}$$

where $h_{0k}(t)$ and $\boldsymbol{\beta}_k$ are the baseline risk and parameters for the type k events and U_i is a shared frailty representing correlation between different events on the same subject i. To fit the model, one needs an indicator of event type and then includes the event type-factor interaction terms in the model to estimate $\boldsymbol{\beta}_k$. However, the model may not be identifiable if the events censor each other, with the case of semi-competing risk as an exception.

5.7 Joint or sequential modeling of exposure and time to event

This section discusses topics similar to those in Chapter 4, but here the response is TTE. In earlier sections, we included the exposure dynamic in the models as a time-varying covariate and estimated the parameters together with the parameters of the TTE model. However, exposure measures are often observed repeatedly at a set of time points $t_1, ..., t_J$, and the use of exposure data can identify a more complex exposure dynamic and obtain better estimates of the model parameters. For the DE model, we assume

$$\begin{aligned} C_i^*(t) &= m(D_i(t), \boldsymbol{\theta}_i) \\ C_{ij} &= C_i^*(t_j) + e_{ij}, \end{aligned} \tag{5.49}$$

where $\boldsymbol{\theta}_i = \mathbf{X}_i\boldsymbol{\theta} + \mathbf{V}_i, \mathbf{V}_i \sim N(0, \boldsymbol{\Sigma}_v)$, and $e_{ij} \sim N(0, \sigma_e^2)$ is the measurement error (ME). This model is the same as the second one in (4.1), except the notation $h(.)$ is changed to $m(.)$ to distinguish it from the hazard function. This model, together with a TTE model

$$h_i(t) = h_0(t)\exp(\beta_c C_i^*(t)) \tag{5.50}$$

forms the classical ME model, that is, $C_i^*(t)$, which directly affects the risk, is measured with error. Therefore, this section follows the structure of Chapter 4 and discusses simultaneous modeling using the ML approach and sequential modeling (SM) using regression calibration approaches. Using exposure data in the modeling also allows the correlation between factors that affect exposure and those that affect the risk of events to be evaluated. However, we postpone this topic to Chapter 8, as it uses approaches dealing with confounding biases. Joint modeling of some special TTE models (e.g., those for recurrent events and interval censored data) is also left to these individual sections. For more details and a wide range of practical background on joint modeling of TTE and longitudinal data, see Rizopoulos [2012].

5.7.1 Simultaneous modeling

Most simultaneous modeling approaches maximize joint likelihood of the TTE and exposure data. The TTE part can use the likelihood or the partial likelihood. But these approaches use a parametric TTE model with the exception of Rizopoulos [2012] where longitudinal models and Cox models are fitted jointly. A major reason is that the partial likelihood is difficult to specify in software such as proc NLMIXED and NONMEM. Formally, we can write the joint likelihood function of TTE and DE models in the same form as (4.4):

$$L(\boldsymbol{\gamma}, \boldsymbol{\beta}) = \prod_{i=1}^{n} \int_{\theta_i} \int_{\beta_i} L_t(\mathbf{t}_i | \boldsymbol{\beta}_i, \mathbf{C}^*(\mathbf{t}_i)) f_c(\mathbf{C}_i | \boldsymbol{\gamma}_i, \sigma_e^2) dF(\boldsymbol{\gamma}_i, \boldsymbol{\beta}_i | \boldsymbol{\gamma}, \boldsymbol{\beta}, \boldsymbol{\Omega}) \tag{5.51}$$

where $f_c(c|.)$ is the density function of the exposure, and we use some general notation so that it can be used for modeling multiple or recurrent events. With this notation $\mathbf{t}_i$ is a set of TTEs, which may be times to multiple or recurrent events, $L_t(\mathbf{t}_i | \boldsymbol{\beta}_i, \mathbf{C}^*(\mathbf{t}_i))$ is the likelihood function of the TTE part, in which $\mathbf{C}^*(\mathbf{t}_i)$ represents $C^*(t)$ at $\mathbf{t}_i$. For example, $L_t(t_i | C^*(t_i)) = f^{\delta_i}(t_i, C^*(t_i)) S^{1-\delta_i}(t_i, C^*(t_i))$, with all parameters omitted. In addition, we use $\boldsymbol{\beta}_i$ to denote both fixed and random coefficients, which we will introduce later, but it can be considered as a fixed coefficient $\boldsymbol{\beta}$ at the moment.

The implementation of the joint modeling approach now relies on maximizing the joint likelihood. To deal with random effects in $\boldsymbol{\gamma}_i$ and $\boldsymbol{\beta}_i$, we can take the same approach as in Chapter 4 by using software such as SAS proc NLMIXED and NONMEM, as both allow specifying the conditional likelihood, conditional on $\boldsymbol{\gamma}_i$ and $\boldsymbol{\beta}_i$, then using an approximation or numerical integration to evaluate (5.51). Here, an additional issue is the calculation of $H_i(t)$. Some situations in which $H_i(t)$ can be calculated analytically have been discussed in earlier sections. They are: 1) constant baseline risk in combination with a wide range of $C^*(t)$ functions, 2) a wide range of baseline risk functions (e.g., for gamma and Weibull distributions) in combination with piecewise constants $C_i^*(t)$, and 3) a wide range of $C^*(t)$ and baseline risk functions with an additive risk model.

For joint modeling with Cox models, Rizopoulos et al. [2009] used the Laplace expansion of the joint likelihood and the EM algorithm. Based on this algorithm, an R library JM was developed, with its details and applications in Rizopoulos [2012]. Although in principle, it can also be implemented in general purposed software e.g., proc NLMIXED, the major problem is the lack of an efficient way to program the partial likelihood, since at one failure time, data from all subjects who are still at risk have to be available. To allow for some flexibility in the baseline risk distribution, the piecewise constant baseline risk has been widely used, which can be programmed in, e.g., proc NLMIXED. Although one can solve the corresponding estimating equation to eliminate parameters for the baseline risk, programming becomes difficult due to the same issue as when using the Cox regression. Therefore, we need to explicitly estimate the baseline parameters.

When exposure is driven by a complex PK model, it is more convenient to calculate $H(t)$ numerically. NONMEM has the facility to model the popPK and TTE model jointly. The following is a sample program for a simple PK model (adapted from a slide set by Nick Holford), but it can be extended to any other PK models specified in terms of ODE (linear or nonlinear). The idea is to calculate $C_i^*(t)$ and $H_i(t)$ by solving the following ODEs with initial conditions $H_i(0) = 0$ and $C_i^*(0) = 0$

$$\begin{aligned} \frac{dC_i^*(t)}{dt} &= -\frac{Cl_i}{V_i} C_i^*(t) \\ \frac{dH_i(t)}{dt} &= \exp(\beta_0 + \beta_c C_i^*(t)) \end{aligned} \tag{5.52}$$

where Cl_i and V_i are random coefficients in the popPK model with variance components estimated in NONMEM as usual.

```
$DES
DCP=A(1)/V
DADT(1)=-CL*DCP
DADT(2)=EXP(BETA0+BETA*DCP)
```

```
$ERROR
CP=A(1)/V
CUMHAZ=A(2) ; cumulative hazard
IF (DV.EQ.0) THEN ; censored
Y=EXP(-CUMHAZ)
ENDIF
IF (DV.EQ.1) THEN ; event
HAZ=EXP(BETA0+BETA*CP)
Y=EXP(-CUMHAZ)*HAZ
ENDIF
```

Here DADT(k) is the kth ODE for A(k) (A(1)=$C_i^*(t)$ and A(2)=$H_i(t)$), HAZ and CUMHAZ are $h_i(t)$ and $H_i(t)$ respectively, and DV is an event indicator. The $ERROR part specifies the likelihood function (5.51). One can also find a very interesting link between the dynamics of $H(t)$ and $C^*(t)$ in Holford et al. [1993b]. The above approach can also be programmed in R, with an ODE solver.

As an example to simultaneously fit the models without the calculation of $H(t)$ by numerical integration, consider the situation of exposure change related to the dose change in which we assume that $C_i^*(t)$ changes instantly with the dose change. We assume the following model

$$C_i^*(t) = \gamma_0 + \gamma_d D_i(t) + V_i \tag{5.53}$$

where $C_{ij} = C_i^*(t_j) + e_{ij}, j = 1, ..., J$ are observed, and $D_i(t)$ is piecewise constant within intervals $t_1, ..., t_j, ...t_J$. For the TTE model we assume

$$h_i(t) = h_0 \exp(\beta_c C_i^*(t) + U_i) \tag{5.54}$$

where we add a random effect U_i, and assume that U_i, V_i have a joint normal distribution. Conditional on U_i, this leads to an exponential distribution with piecewise constant risk, so $H_i(t)$ can be calculated analytically. The constant baseline risk is not an essential restriction and can be replaced with a piecewise function. The following SAS program generates the exposure and TTE paths for 200 patients in a hypothetic TDM trial and fits the exposure and TTE data simultaneously.

```
%let nsimu=3000; %let cdose=log(1.3); %let bound=log(10);
%let base=-6; %let base2=-3; %let dose1=log(5); %let sigv=0.5;
%let sigu=0.3; %let sige=0.2; %let nsub=200; %let nrep=8;
%let beta=0.25;  %let nday=14;
data simu;
  do sub=1 to &nsub;
    fevent=0; retain fevent;
    latent=rannor(12)*0;
    ui=(latent+rannor(12))*&sigu/2;
    vi=(latent+rannor(12))*&sigv/2;
    dose=&dose1;
      pevent=0;
    do i=0 to &nrep;
```

```
    lci=dose+ui;
    lce=lci+rannor(12)*&sige;
    conc=exp(lci);
    low=i*&nday; up=low+&nday;
      start=low;
      stop=low;
      do k=1 to 30 while (stop < up);
       if pevent in (0 2) then  lmd=exp(&base+&beta*exp(lci)+vi);
       else if pevent =1 then  lmd=exp(&base2-vi);
       ti=ranexp(12)/lmd;
       stop=start+ti;
       if stop le up then do;
          if pevent in (0 2) then event=1;
          else if pevent=1 then event=2;
          output; fevent=event;
          start=stop; pevent=event;
       end;
       else do;
          event=0; stop=up; output;
       end;
      end;
     if lce<&bound then dose=dose+&cdose;
     end;
  end; run;

data first;  set simu;  if fevent=0;  run;

proc nlmixed data=first(keep=lci lce dose start stop event sub) qpoints=4 ebopt;
  parm b0=-5 beta=0.25 a=0 b=1 sige=0.02 a11=0.3 a12=0 a22=0.3;
  bounds sige a11 a22 >0;
        lci=a+b*dose+vi;  resc=lce-lci;
    if (abs(resc) > 1E50) or (sige < 1e-20) then llw = 1e-20;
    else  llw = -0.5*(resc**2 / sige  + log(sige)); ll=1e-20;
  hi=exp(b0+beta*exp(lci)+ui);
  Ht=hi*(stop-start);
  ll=event*log(hi+1e-20)-Ht;
*  put sub start stop event lce ll llw;
  model stop ~general(ll+llw);
  random vi ui ~normal([0,0],[a11, a12, a22]) subject=sub; run;
```

Parameter	Estimate	Standard Error	t Value	Pr > |t|
b0	-5.9949	0.3881	-15.45	<.0001
beta	0.2603	0.04650	5.60	<.0001
a	-0.04873	0.05010	-0.97	0.3319
b	1.0189	0.02479	41.10	<.0001
sige	0.04166	0.002475	16.83	<.0001
a11	0.02296	0.003660	6.27	<.0001
a12	0.01541	0.01506	1.02	0.3075
a22	0.08719	0.1816	0.48	0.6317

The results show that β_c is rather well estimated, with the estimated value 0.26 compared to the true value 0.25. Parameters a and b for the PK part are well estimated, as expected. The variance of U_i is estimated to be much worse than that of V_i, due to the difficulty of identifying the frailty. Note that the likelihood for TTE can be written in the form of $L_t(\mathbf{t}_i|\boldsymbol{\beta}_i, \mathbf{C}^*(\mathbf{t}_i))$, as U_i can be considered as a part of $\boldsymbol{\beta}_i$ as it is the random baseline risk. The program takes advantage of built-in multi-normal random effects for "vi" and "ui" in proc NLMIXED.

5.7.2 Sequential modeling and regression calibration

To estimate β, a very intuitive approach is the two-stage method that fits the model (5.49) in the first stage. In the second stage, the fitted model is used to predict $C_i^*(t)$ as $\hat{C}_i^*(t) = m(t, D_i(t), \hat{\gamma}_i)$, which is used as a known covariate varying in time to fit the exposure-risk model. The second stage model can be fitted using the MLE or a semi-parametric approach, depending on the nature of the exposure-risk model. An important advantage of this approach is its simplicity for applied statisticians using common software. For example, for $\hat{C}_i^*(t) = 1 - \exp(-\hat{K}_i t)$ (assuming $D_i = 1$) and constant baseline risk,

$$H_i(t) = \int_0^t \lambda_0 \exp(-\beta_c(1 - \exp(-\hat{K}_i \tau)))d\tau \tag{5.55}$$

needs a numerical calculation. Again, this can be implemented in NONMEM, with individual predicted $\hat{K}_i$s based on the first stage model fitting. This approach can also be used when the popPK model is given by ODEs without an analytical solution. One can provide population parameters in the popPK model, then solve the ODEs of the popPK model together with the ODE for $H(t)$ to provide the prediction for $\boldsymbol{\gamma}_i$ and $C_i^*(t)$. However, the population parameters in the popPK model are not estimated again. Therefore, this is still a two-stage approach and has the pros and cons of such approaches, namely, stability in the estimation but it cannot take the variability of first-stage estimation into account.

The variation in the first stage can be taken into account using an intensive computing approach such as bootstrap to generate bootstrapped samples for $C_i^*(t)$, and in the second stage to fit the Cox model to obtain bootstrapped estimates for β_c. In this way, the variation in $\hat{C}_i^*(t)$ is carried into the bootstrapped estimates and can be evaluated, e.g., to form the confidence interval for β. Here we use the Bayesian bootstrap, which can be considered as a smoothed version of the ordinary bootstrap (Appendix 10.5). The following is a SAS program to fit the power model to the TDM example data and generate bootstrapped predictions $C_{ib}^*(t), b = 1, ..., B$ for a large B.

```
data sub;
  set tdm(where=(group=1));
  keep sub start; run;

data wei;  set sub;
  do simu=1 to 100;
    wei=-log(ranuni(12));
    output;
  end; run;
```

```
proc sort data=wei; by sub start;run;

data all;
  merge tdm0 wei;
  by sub start; run;

proc sort data=all; by simu sub start;run;

proc mixed data=all;
  class  sub dose;
  model lconc=ldose/ outp=pred;
  random sub;
  weight wei;
  by simu; run;

data cox;  set pred;
  pconc=exp(pred); run;

proc phreg data=cox;
  model (start,stop)*event(0)=pconc;
  by simu; run;
```

We use $B = 100$ bootstraps to generate $\hat{\beta}_b, b = 1, ..., 100$. Summary statistics for them are

N	Mean	Std Dev	Minimum	Maximum
100	0.0250844	0.0292990	-0.0544430	0.1069432

As a comparison, the standard two-stage approach gives

Parameter Estimate	Standard Error	Chi-Square	Pr > ChiSq	Hazard Ratio
0.02580	0.00759	11.5513	0.0007	1.026

Although $\hat{\beta} = 0.0258$ is very close to the mean of $\hat{\beta}_b$s, 0.0251, the SE of 0.00759 is much lower than the SD of $\hat{\beta}_b$s. Therefore, using this SE for statistical inference is misleading.

Until now, we have used the plug-in $\hat{C}^*(t)$ without considering the impact of the measurement error discussed in Chapter 4. Although the RC approach of using $E(C_i^*|C_i)$ in place of C_i^* also applies here, as most TTE models are nonlinear, it may lead to inconsistent estimates for β_c without proper adjustment. The problem is similar to that of regression calibration (RC) in Chapter 4, but for TTE models these issues are often more complex.

Given $h_i(t|e_i) = h_0(t)\exp(\beta_c C_i^*(t)) = h_0(t)\exp(\beta_c(C_i^*(t) + e_i))$, the key step for the RC is to find the marginal hazard function,

$$h_i(t|C_i) = h_0(t)E(\exp(\beta_c(C_i^*(t)))|C_i, T_i > t), \tag{5.56}$$

conditional on exposure measures C_i from subject i. Although it can be done, fitting a TTE model based on this marginal hazard function is difficult. However, for rare events $E(\exp(\beta_c(C_i^*(t)))|C_i, T_i > t) \approx \exp(\beta_c E(C_i^*|C_i))$ [Prentice, 1982]. Therefore, if a DE model allows the estimation of $E(C_i^*|C_i)$ by

$\hat{C}_i^*(t)$, $C_i^*(t)$ in the hazard function can be replaced by $\hat{C}_i^*(t)$ and a Cox model can be fitted in the standard way.

When events are not rare, Clayton et al. [1992] proposed a risk set RC that uses RC for each risk set of all failure time T_i, that is, to fit the exposure model to those still at risk to estimate $C_i^*(T_i)$. However, practical experiences show that the difference between the risk set RC and the simple RC using all subjects to fit the exposure model is often small.

5.8 Interval censored data

Although right censoring is the most common type of censoring, interval censoring (IC) is also common [Sun, 2006]. An interval censored TTE refers to the fact that we only know that subject i had an event within a time interval (L_i, R_i), but not the exact time of occurrence. IC includes right-censoring as a special case with $R_i = \infty$, observed event time with $L_i = R_i = T_i$. An example of IC is the time to disease progression (DP) in many types of disease. For solid tumors, DP is defined according to tumor size changes, which can only be measured infrequently. Therefore, the time to DP is always interval censored between the time of the first assessment that classifies the DP and the previous assessment time. To estimate parameters with IC data, one may still use the MLE. Let $S(t|\mathbf{X}_i, \boldsymbol{\beta})$ be the survival function with $\mathbf{X}_i$, and subject i had an IC event (L_i, R_i), we can write $P(L_i < T_i \leq R_i) = S(L_i) - S(R_i)$. The likelihood function can be written as

$$L(\boldsymbol{\beta}) = \prod_{i=1}^{n} (S(R_i|\mathbf{X}_i, \boldsymbol{\beta}) - S(L_i|\mathbf{X}_i, \boldsymbol{\beta})) \tag{5.57}$$

which can be maximized to estimate $\boldsymbol{\beta}$. Note that although $L(\boldsymbol{\beta})$ holds for $R_i = \infty$, the contribution of an observed event time $L_i = R_i = T_i$, if any, to $L(\boldsymbol{\beta})$ must be specified by the density function as in (5.4).

If TTE follows a parametric distribution, the ML approach can be carried out similarly to right-censored data, as long as $S(.|\mathbf{X}_i, \boldsymbol{\beta})$ is given. However, if it follows a semi-parametric model such as the Cox model, the baseline risk function $h_0(t)$ cannot be eliminated by the partial likelihood approach. Let $S_0, ..., S_J$, be all the ordered values of $(L_i, R_i), i = 1, ..., n$. Since the whole $h_0(t)$ is needed to estimate $\boldsymbol{\beta}$, but the $h_0(t)$ values between $S_0, ..., S_J$ cannot be determined, a simple approach is to assume that $h_0(t)$ takes a constant value a_j in the jth interval. Consequently,

$$H_0(t) = \int_{\tau=0}^{t} h_0(\tau) d\tau = \sum_{t < S_{j+1}} a_j \Delta_j \tag{5.58}$$

Then $S(R_i|\mathbf{X}_i, \boldsymbol{\beta})$ can be written as

$$S(R_i|\mathbf{X}_i, \boldsymbol{\beta}) = \exp(-H_0(t)\exp(\boldsymbol{\beta}^T\mathbf{X}_i)) \tag{5.59}$$

and the a_js have to be estimated together with $\boldsymbol{\beta}$. See Chapter 6 in Sun [2006].

For implementation, SAS proc LIFEREG can fit parametric models to interval censored data by maximizing the likelihood (5.57). The following call fits a Weibull model to data with censored interval (lower=L_i, upper=U_i) and exposure conc:

```
proc lifereg data = ic;
  model (lower upper) = conc/ d=weibull;
run;
```

Neither SAS PHREG nor R function coxph (.) can fit a Cox model to interval censored data, although some specialized SAS macros and R libraries are available.

IC may also occur on recurrent events. For example, one may be interested in the effect of an anti-asthma treatment on reducing the risk of asthma attack. In a clinical trial, patients may be asked how many asthma attacks occurred between previous and current visits. The exact time of occurrence may not be recalled and may not be important. Therefore, the times of the events are interval censored between the visit intervals. In this case, IC leads to longitudinal count data (Sun [2006], Chapter 9). In this case, a simple longitudinal model, which still captures important features of the data, can be used to fit the data. Let Y_{ij} and C_{ij} be the number of events and the exposure in the jth interval, we may assume that

$$\begin{aligned} Y_{ij} &\sim Poisson(\lambda_{ij}) \\ \lambda_{ij} &= \exp(C_{ij}\boldsymbol{\beta} + U_i). \end{aligned} \tag{5.60}$$

In addition we can also allow for extra-variation in Y_{ij} for given U_i, either using a negative binomial distribution, or an over-dispersion parameter representing the variance inflation. This model can easily be fitted with, e.g., proc GENMOD or proc GLIMIXED. See Section 3.5 for more details. In fact, one may also consider Y_{ij} as a counting process and λ_{ij} as a rate function. It is also possible to fit the data with proc PHREG, with the option allowing for dependency of events within the same patients. In principle, if we assume that the underlining mechanism of events is a multi-state model with on- and off-states, it is possible to calculate λ_{ij}. But in general, the multi-state model may not lead to a time-constant λ_i even with the simple relationship to $\mathbf{X}_{ij}$ as in (5.60). Therefore, model (5.60) should be considered as an empirical model for IC data.

IC data can also be modeled jointly with exposure data. To this end, we maximize the joint likelihood of the Poisson model (5.60) and an exposure model. Here we use a simulated dataset with generated exposure data from a power model

$$\log(C_{ij}) = \log(D_{ij}) + U_i + e_{ij} \tag{5.61}$$

with the following program:

```
%let nsimu=50; %let nsub=100; %let cdose=log(1.3);
%let bound=log(10); %let base=-3; %let dose1=log(5);
%let sigv=0.5; %let sigu=0.3; %let sige=0.2;
%let nsub=5; %let nrep=8; %let beta=0.25;

data simu0 simu1;
 do simu=1 to &nsimu;
  do group=0 to 1;
  do sub=1 to &nsub;
    ui=rannor(1)*&sigu;
    vi=rannor(1)*&sigv;
    nn=0;
    dose=&dose1;
    do i=1 to &nrep;
    lci=dose+ui;
    lce=lci+rannor(12)*&sige;
    trend=0;
    if group=1 then lmd=exp(&base+&beta*exp(lci)+vi+trend);
    else lmd=exp(&base+vi+trend);
    yi=ranpoi(1,lmd);
    if group=0 then output simu0;
    else if group=1 then output simu1;
    if lce<&bound then dose=dose+&cdose;
     end;
  end;
 end;
end; run;
```

The following SAS program fits the joint models of (5.61) and (5.60) by maximizing the joint likelihood with U_i as the frailty shared with the exposure model:

```
proc nlmixed data=simu(drop=ui vi) qpoints=8 ebsubsteps=100 ebsteps=150
   ebssfrac=0.8 ebopt ftol=1e-12 gtol=1e-12;
  parms base=-3 beta=1 a=0 b=1 sigu=1 sigv=1  siguv=0 sige=1;
  bounds sigu sigv sige >0;
    logci=a+b*dose+ui;
    resc=log(tci+0.0001)-logci;
    if (abs(resc) > 1E50) or (sige < 1e-12) then llw = -1e20;
    else  llw = -0.5*(resc**2 / sige  + log(sige));
    lambda=exp(base+beta*exp(logci)+vi);
   lly = yi*log(max(lambda,0.00001)) - lambda;
  model yi ~general(lly+llw);
  random ui vi ~ normal([0,0],[sigu,siguv,sigv]) subject=sub;
run;
```

which generates the following results:

Parameter	Estimate	Standard Error	DF	t Value	Pr > |t|
base	-3.7550	0.1474	198	-25.47	<.0001
beta	0.3329	0.01203	198	27.67	<.0001
a	0.08036	0.03909	198	2.06	0.0411
b	0.9712	0.01465	198	66.30	<.0001
sigu	0.08622	0.009239	198	9.33	<.0001
sigv	0.2545	0.04903	198	5.19	<.0001
siguv	0.02125	0.01514	198	1.40	0.1620
sige	0.04256	0.001611	198	26.41	<.0001

The result shows reasonably good estimates for almost all parameters including the variance of the frailty.

5.9 Model identification and mis-specification

Model identification is a more important issue for TTE data than it is for other endpoints, particularly for some common types of TTE models. We consider two situations in which model identifiability becomes problematic in ER modeling for TTE data. The following also applies to DR modeling when the dose has features similar to those of the exposure described below. One situation is that the effect of the variation of exposure at the population level cannot be distinguished from the unspecified baseline hazard $h_0(t)$ in the Cox model. Suppose that the exposure at time t for subject i can be written as

$$C_i^*(t) = C_0(t) + C_i'(t) \tag{5.62}$$

where $C_0(t)$ is the common time profile of exposure for all subjects and $c_i'(t)$ represents variations between subjects. In this case, we have

$$h(t) = h_0(t)\exp(\beta_c C_i^*(t)) = h_0(t)\exp(\beta_c C_0(t) + \beta_c C_i'(t)) \tag{5.63}$$

However, the Cox regression will estimate $h_0(t)\exp(\beta_c C_0(t))$ as baseline hazard and $h_0(t)$ and $\exp(\beta_c C_0(t))$ are distinguishable only when $C_0(t)$ is known. Consequently, β_c is only estimated with $C_i'(t)$. Although it is estimable as long as $C_i'(t)$ exists, the estimate could be very poor if this component is small. If $C_0(t)$ forms the major part of the variation in $C_i(t)$, the impact of the measurement error will also be strong and severely dilute the effect of the treatment.

The non-identifiability problem is obvious in the Cox model. But it may also occur even if a parametric model is fitted. The difference is that in a parametric model, the baseline hazard part is not completely separated from the exposure driven hazard part, but for the same reason, a part of the common trend cannot be distinguished from the baseline risk. The shape of the TTE distribution may also reflect the risk changes of natural course, hence, the more flexible the parameter model, the more difficult the identification.

Another situation in which identification becomes problematic is due to the confounding between the baseline function and the change in the risk time profile as a result of frailty. Consider an example where the conditional risk function $h(t|U_i) = U_i a(t)$ with U_i follows a unit mean gamma distribution (hence, we set the scale and shape parameters all equal to γ). This leads to a risk function.

$$h(t) = a(t)/(1 + A(t)/\gamma) \tag{5.64}$$

where $A(t) = \int_0^t a(\tau)d\tau$. It shows that a time-constant frailty causes risk time profile changes. Deriving the corresponding density function involves a lengthy calculation (Chapter 6, Aalen et al. [2008]), so it is omitted here.

Frailty also causes changes in the risk ratio in a proportional risk model. Suppose that two conditional risk functions are risk proportional with $h_1(t|U_i) = U_i a(t)$ and $h_2(t|U_i) = rU_i a(t)$, with U_i following the same distribution as above, then the ratio of the corresponding risk functions is

$$h_2(t)/h_1(t) = r\frac{1 + A(t)/\gamma}{1 + rA(t)/\gamma}, \tag{5.65}$$

hence, the risk ratio also becomes time varying and the model with frailty is no longer risk proportional.

Often in a clinical trial or an observational study, there is a control group that represents the "baseline" disease process, in the context of TTE modeling, $h_0(t)$. It seems reasonable to hope that with the control group, one may be able to eliminate the baseline and frailty in order to identify the exposure effects. However, this is generally not possible. Consider an example such that $h(t, C(t)) = U_i \exp(C(t))$ with U_i following a unit mean gamma distribution. Can we estimate the effect of $C(t)$ on $h(t, C(t))$ by the difference in log-hazard between active and placebo? Figure 5.4 shows the non-parametric estimate and the true $h(t)$ with different values of the shape parameter. It shows that even with this simple model, the true treatment effect cannot be identified in the presence of frailty. This is because the risk sets of the two groups become more and more different over time, if the treatment effects change the risk. Therefore, the two groups are not comparable at all times.

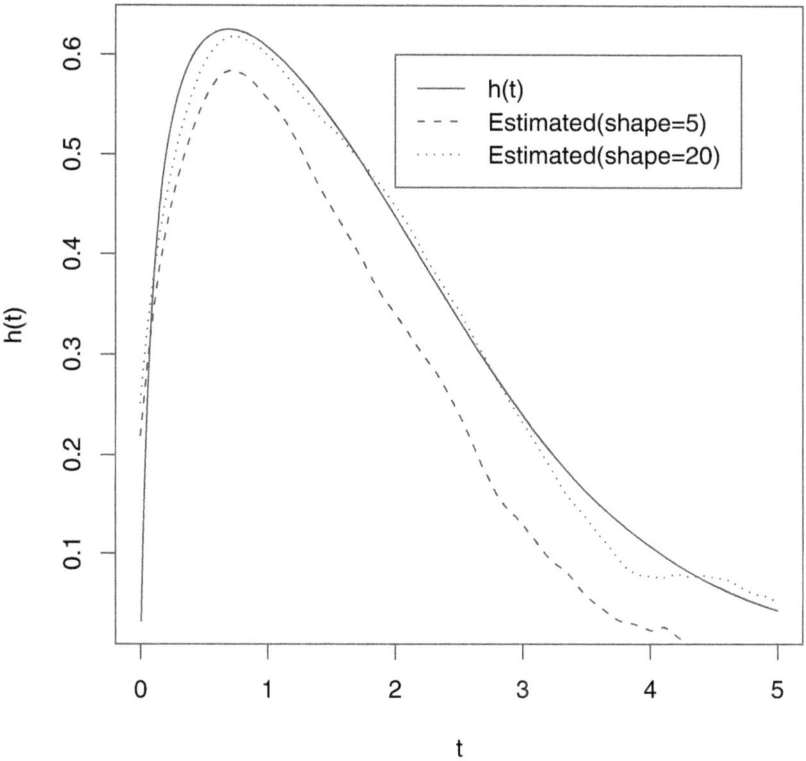

Figure 5.4
True and estimated exposure effects with placebo adjustment: constant baseline hazard with gamma frailty (shape = 5 and 20).

5.10 Random sample simulation from exposure-risk models

5.10.1 Basic simulation approaches for time-to-events

Time-to-event samples that follow some standard parametric distributions can be generated easily. If T_i has the distribution function $F(t)$, and $F^{-1}(u)$ can be easily calculated, a straightforward way to generate T_is is to generate a uniform distribution $U_i \sim U(0,1)$, the uniform distribution function within (0,1), then $T_i = F^{-1}(U_i) \sim F(t)$. One can also use the survival function $S(t)$ to generate $T_i = S^{-1}(U_i) \sim F(t)$, since $S^{-1}(u)$ and $F^{-1}(u)$ are symmetric on (0,1). Note that for the same U_i, $F^{-1}(U_i)$ and $S^{-1}(U_i)$ follow the same distribution and are also negatively correlated. This approach can be used to generate TTE data under time-constant exposures efficiently as long as the survival function under the exposure has an analytical inverse function.

Generating TTE samples from a Cox model with an underlying parametric distribution corresponding to the baseline risk needs more careful consideration. We start from Cox models with constant exposures and then turn to those with time-varying exposures. Consider the following Cox regression model

$$h(t, \boldsymbol{\beta}) = h_0(t) \exp(\mathbf{X}^T \boldsymbol{\beta}). \tag{5.66}$$

The survival function of this model is

$$S(t|\mathbf{X}) = \exp[-H_0(t) \exp(\mathbf{X}^T \boldsymbol{\beta})]. \tag{5.67}$$

When its inverse function can be found, a sample T following the Cox model can be generated in the way of Bender et al. [2005]

$$T = H_0^{-1}[-\log(U) \exp(-\mathbf{X}^T \boldsymbol{\beta})]. \tag{5.68}$$

One can choose from some standard parametric distributions for the baseline risk. For example, the Weibull distribution with scale and shape parameters s and γ, respectively, has

$$H_0^{-1}(t) = (s^{-1}t)^{1/\gamma}, \tag{5.69}$$

which can be inserted into (5.68) to generate a random sample of Ts following a Cox model with the baseline risk corresponding to the Weibull distribution.

For a Cox model with time-varying covariate

$$h(t, \boldsymbol{\beta}) = h_0(t) \exp(\mathbf{X}^T(t) \boldsymbol{\beta}), \tag{5.70}$$

simulation becomes much more complex. We can still write

$$S(t|\mathbf{X}) = \exp[-\int_0^t h_0(\tau) \exp(\mathbf{X}(\tau)^T \boldsymbol{\beta})]d\tau, \tag{5.71}$$

and, if the inverse of function $H(t) = \int_0^t h_0(\tau) \exp(\mathbf{X}(\tau)^T \boldsymbol{\beta}) d\tau$ can be calculated, we could still generate T from an equation similar to (5.68).

For special time-varying covariates, such as piecewise constants and linear functions of time, the simple approach in Austin [2012] based on $H^{-1}(u)$ can be used. For generating a piecewise exponential variable with risk λ_k in interval $(t_k, t_{k+1}), k = 1, ..., K, t_1 = 0$, the following is an algorithm adapted from Zhou [2001]. Start from $k = 1$ and $Y_0 \sim Exp(\lambda_1)$, then repeat the following steps

- If $Y \leq t_{k+1}$ then output Y and stop.
- Else $Y \leftarrow t_k + \lambda_k (Y - t_k)/\lambda_{k+1}$.
- $k \leftarrow k + 1$.

The following is a fully vectorized R program for implementing this algorithm, which generates a large number of samples simultaneously, and the loop in it runs over the K intervals regardless of whether an individual $Y < t_k + 1$. If it is programmed in software that does not support vectorized operations, the iteration should stop when an individual $Y \leq t_{k+1}$.

```
nsimu=10000
cut=1:10
rate=c(10/cut,11)
rate=rep(1,11)
yv=rexp(nsimu)/rate[1]
for (i in 1:length(cut)){
  ti=cut[i]
  yv=ifelse(yv<ti,yv,ti+(yv-ti)/rate[i+1]*rate[i])
}
```

Zhou [2001] suggested a monotone transformation to allow a time-varying baseline risk function within each interval in which the covariates are constant. If a transform $s = g(t)$ is used in t with a constant risk, then the baseline risk within an interval is proportional to $dg^{-1}(t)/dt$, and therefore the baseline risk can vary over time, yet the property of proportional risk still holds. This approach has recently been proposed by Hendry [2014]. The above code can also be used with transformation, but the intervals should also be transformed.

However, in most cases, a numerical calculation is needed to evaluate $H^{-1}(u)$ even when $H(t)$ has a simple analytical form. Consider the following simple case in which $h_0(t) = a$ (i.e., T_i follows an exponential distribution), $c(t) = 1 - \exp(-Kt)$, and $h(t) = h_0(t)c(t)$. The latter is a simple function that describes the process of exposure reaching steady state. Under these conditions, one can derive

$$\begin{aligned} h(t) &= a(1 - \exp(-Kt)) \\ H(t) &= \int_0^t a(1 - \exp(-K\tau))d\tau = a(t + (\exp(-Kt) - 1)/K) \\ S(t) &= \exp(-a(t + (\exp(-Kt) - 1)/K)). \end{aligned} \tag{5.72}$$

It is still not easy to sample directly from $S(t)$, as $H^{-1}(t)$ is not an explicit function. Although one can calculate it by numerically solving the implicit function

$$S(T_i) = U_i \tag{5.73}$$

to generate T_i for a given U_i, there are more efficient algorithms than this one, as we will show later. For general time-varying covariates, a permutation algorithm [Sylvestre and Abrahamowicz, 2008] can be used. However, it is inefficient to generate data with a large sample size.

5.10.2 Rejection-acceptance algorithms

The rejection-acceptance sampling technique is commonly used to generate samples from a distribution that is not easy to sample from. The idea is to generate samples from a distribution close to the target distribution, then reject those unlikely to follow the target distribution. Specifically, to sample from $f(t)$, we find $g(t)$ which is easy to sample from with $f(t) \leq Cg(t)$, where C is a constant, then we can:

- Generate $Y_i \sim g(t)$
- Generate $U_i \sim U(0, Cg(t))$
- If $U_i \leq f(Y_i)$ then accept Y_i, else regenerate Y_i and U_i

There is also an equivalent version in which one generates $U_i \sim U(0,1)$ then accepts Y_i if $U_i \leq C^{-1}f(Y_i)/g(t)$. Applying it to the example above, we note that

$$\begin{aligned} f(t) &= a(1-\exp(-Kt))\exp(-a(t+(\exp(-Kt)-1)/K)) \\ &\leq a(1-\exp(-Kt))\exp(-a(t-1/K)) \\ &\leq a\exp(-at)\exp(a/K) \end{aligned} \quad (5.74)$$

and we find that $g(t) = a\exp(-at)$ is the density function of the exponential distribution with parameter a, and $C = \exp(a/K)$. The following algorithm can be used to generate T:

- Generate $T_i^* \sim Exp(a)$
- Generate $U_i \sim U(0, a\exp(-aT^*)\exp(a/K))$
- If $U_i \leq f(T_i^*)$, then $T_i = T_i^*$; otherwise reject T_i^* and go back to the first step

Its efficiency depends on the ratio a/K. When the time to reach the steady state is comparable to the time to event or even longer than that, this algorithm may be quite inefficient. However, compared to the time needed for the model fitting, the lack of efficiency is acceptable in most practical situations.

This approach can also be used for some other $h(t)$s. Suppose that $h(t) = B(t)$ where $B(t)$ is the sum of spline functions, then

$$H(t) = \int_0^t B(\tau)d\tau, \quad (5.75)$$

which, in principle, can be derived analytically. When $S^{-1}(t)$ is difficult to calculate with this $H(t)$, the rejection method can be used. Since $f(t) = B(t)\exp(-H(t))$, if $N < B(t) < M$ then

$$f(t) \leq (M/N)N\exp(-tN), \quad (5.76)$$

and T can be generated with the rejection acceptance method based on an exponential distribution with parameter N. The efficiency of the generator depends on the ratio M/N. This approach is inefficient if the lower bound N is very low relative to the upper bound M.

5.10.3 Generating discrete event times

In clinical trials, it is often sufficient to record the event time in days; hence, using discrete time may allow considerable simplification of the simulation. In the following, we assume that $t = 1, 2, \ldots,$ so that we can write

$$h_i(t) = h_0(t)\exp(\mathbf{X}_i^T(t)\boldsymbol{\beta}) \tag{5.77}$$

as an approximation of the hazard on day t. A very general approach for discrete-time sample generation follows a similar idea to the conditional logistic regression model. That is, for a subject at risk at time t, the event at time t follows a binary distribution with probability $h(t)$. Here we assume that the day is a sufficiently small time unit so that $h(t) << 1$ for all t. Otherwise, a smaller unit may be used. With this approach, we can generate events from the hazard function directly hence it is straightforward even when the corresponding $f(t)$ and $S(t)$ have no analytical form and are difficult to calculate. $h(t)$ can be an analytical function or an empirical distribution, if the simulation is to mimic a specific practical scenario.

The following algorithm implements this approach (assuming that censoring is before the event occurrence at each time):

- for each subject set at-risk indicator $R_i = 1$
- do $t = 1, 2, ...J$:
  - while $R_i = 1$, generate $Y_i(t) \sim bin(h_i(t))$.
  - when $Y_i(t) = 1$ set event time to t and event indicator $\delta_i = 1$. Output subject i data.
  - when a censoring event occurs or when $Y_i(t) = 1$ set $R_i = 0$.
- next t
- If at $t = J$, $Y_i(t) = 0$ and $R_i = 0$, then set event time=J and event indicator $\delta_i = 0$. Output subject i data.
- repeat for all subjects.

Note that if a Cox model is to be fitted, only data at time points when an event occurs are needed. Dropping the other data may substantially reduce the size of the final dataset. On the other hand, one may want to keep all the records when a parametric model is used for analysis. A shortcoming of this algorithm is the lack of efficiency when the follow-up time is very long. In this case, the interval length may be increased to discretize the time. For example, in a trial with a 5-year follow-up period, the TTE may be sufficiently accurate if calculated in weeks.

Since this approach only needs the hazard function, it can be easily used for a complex model specified by $h_i(t)$. For example, to generate TTE from a frailty model with $h_i(t) = h_0(t)U_i \exp(\mathbf{X}_i^T \boldsymbol{\beta})$, we generate U_i from a desired distribution, then use the same algorithm. The same approach can also be used for a model $h_i(t) = h_0(t)U_i \exp(\beta_c C_i(t))$ with time-varying exposure $C_i(t)$.

This approach can be made more efficient for rare events simulation by simulating the number of events at each t for a set of subjects sharing the same covariates and exposure levels.

5.10.4 Simulation for recurrent and multiple events

Simulation for transition times based on a multi-state model seems complex, but it follows the same rules as for single TTE simulation. For example, in state k, suppose that the risk of having the event of moving to state k' is

$$h_{kk'}(t) = h_{0kk'}(t) \exp(\beta_{kk'} c(t)) \tag{5.78}$$

where $h_{0kk'}(t)$ is the specific baseline risk for the transition between the two states. Then, given a function $c(t)$, the transition time can be generated accordingly. Other state-dependent covariates can be added without additional difficulties. One special issue is whether one should restart the clock for $h_{0kk'}(t)$, i.e., using $h_{0kk'}(t - t_k)$ where t_k is the time to reach the state k. However, this is a model specification issue rather than a simulation issue, as the approaches stated here can cope with both situations.

The following algorithm generates recurrent events from a two-state (on and off events) model for piecewise-constant exposure within time intervals $t_j, t_{j+1}, j = 1, ..., J$. Let $\lambda_{kk'j}$ be the transition risk from k to k', calculated based on exposure in the interval j.

- Set state="off"
- For $j = 1, .., J$, do while $(T < t_{j+1})$
  - Set $T = t_j$.
  - if state="on" then generate $t \sim \exp(\lambda_{10j})$
    else generate $t \sim \exp(\lambda_{01j})$
  - Set $T = T + t$. If $T < t_{j+1}$ then switch to the state and return to the previous step, else let $T = t_{j+1}$ and go to the next j
- Collect all Ts and the state each time the state changes.

A SAS code implementing this algorithm can be found in the online Appendix.

A very simple algorithm can generate recurrent events on a discrete time scale, based on the dependence of current hazard on the history. Suppose that we denote if a patient is having an AE at day t by an indicator Y_t, $Y_t = 1$ for event occurrence and 0 otherwise. Then, between the days the event started and resolved, there is a series of "1"s. The continuation of the "1"s means when a patient is having an AE today, he is more likely to have the AE tomorrow than those having no event. Therefore, we may assume that

$$h(t, Y_{t-1}) = h_0(t) \exp(\beta_c c(t) + \beta_y Y_{t-1}), \tag{5.79}$$

where β_y controls the duration the patient stays in the "on" state. The term $\beta_y Y_{t-1}$ can be replaced by a more complex function of multiple lagged $y(t)$. One will find that this approach, in fact, uses a dynamic generalized linear model described in the next chapter. This algorithm can be easily implemented by adapting the algorithms in Section 5.10.3.

5.10.5 Simulation for TTE driven by complex dynamic systems

Often behind the TTE, there is a latent process, and the event occurs when the process hits a threshold. This assumption forms the first hit model (FHT) (Chapter 10, Aalen et al. [2008]) which provides simple hypothetical mechanisms for the TTE. The latent process may be abstract, but could also be real. The general latent health status can be considered an abstract process, which is 1 for prefect health and drops to 0 when a patient dies. There may also be real processes, such as CD4 cell counts in HIV / AIDS, that drive the TTE. An HIV patient is diagnosed with AIDS if the CD4 count is less than $200/\text{mm}^3$. Therefore, the time from HIV infection to AIDS may have the HIV dynamic as a latent process, and the event occurs when the CD4 count hits the limit $200/\text{mm}^3$. In oncology, disease progression (DP) for solid tumors is indicated if the increase in tumor size is greater than 20% and also greater than 5mm (RECIST V1.1). Hence, the time to DP is driven by a tumor dynamic model.

As an example, we consider the relationship between time-to-DP and tumor dynamics in cancer patients. Consider the tumor growth model [Claret et al., 2009] as the latent process,

$$\frac{dY(t)}{dt} = (K_L - K_D C(t))Y(t). \tag{5.80}$$

where $Y(t)$ and $C(t)$ are tumor size and exposure at time t, and K_L and K_D are constants. This model can be easily solved if the exposure is constant, but may only have numerical solutions for an arbitrary $C(t)$. Since we often only measure tumor size periodically at $t_j, j = 1, ...r$, e.g., by MRI or CT scans. For simplicity, we assume that the t_js are at equal distance Δ apart. At time t_j we observe Y_j which satisfies

$$\log(Y_j) = \int_0^{t_j} (K_L - K_D C(t))dt + \varepsilon_j \tag{5.81}$$

where ε_j is a measurement error. This leads to

$$\log(Y_j) - \log(Y_{j-1}) = \Delta K_L - \int_{t_j}^{t_{j-1}} K_D C(t)dt + \varepsilon_j. \tag{5.82}$$

Therefore, Y_j is a random walk on the log-scale with drift $\Delta K_L - \int_{t_j}^{t_{j-1}} K_D C(t)dt$. A random walk is a series of random variables that behaves like walking randomly. It has the form $x_{j+1} = x_j + K + e_j$, which goes from x_j to x_{j+1} by a random step e_j and a fixed step K, called draft. Let $Y_{min}(j) = \min(Y_1, ..., Y_j)$, the time to disease progression is the first t_j when $Y_j - Y_{min}(j) > 5$ and $Y_j/Y_{min}(j) > 1.2$ (20% increase) are observed. Therefore, generating the time to DP is essentially a generation of the latent process. The simulation provides a useful tool to evaluate empirical models when fitting to a TTE that has a clearly defined algorithm.

The time to AIDs for HIV infected patients may have a more complex mechanistic latent process, as the virus dynamic model is complex. Consider a dynamic model for a HIV study [Wu et al., 2008, 2010] where the amount of T-cells and drug exposure are described by models

$$\begin{aligned}
\frac{dT}{dt} &= \lambda - d_T T - (1-\gamma(t))kTV \\
\frac{dT^*}{dt} &= (1-\gamma(t))kTV - \delta T^* \\
\frac{dV}{dt} &= N\delta T^* - cV
\end{aligned} \tag{5.83}$$

and where T, T^* and V are the uninfected and infected T-cells and free virions, respectively, and $\gamma(t) = (1+\phi/(\sum_{k=1}^{K} w_k C_k A_k(t)/IC_{50}^k(t)))^{-1}$ represents treatment effect (described by an Emax model with $E_{max} = 1$). C_k, $A_k(t)$ and $IC_{50}^k(t)$ are the PK exposure, adherence and the exposure achieving 50% inhibition for the kth regimen at time t, respectively, all measured periodically during the study. To simulate TTE, we may use a numerical approach to solve the equations from time $t = 0$ to $T(t) < T_0$ for a given threshold T_0.

Using the mechanism, but without specifying a threshold, we can link the latent process in a normal way. We may assume that T-cells accounts $T(t)$ is associated with the risk of death and $h(t) = h_0(t)\exp(m(T(t), \boldsymbol{\beta}))$ represents the relationship between exposure, virus dynamics, and TTEs. However, even though we can solve $T(t)$ from the dynamic model and calculate $H(t)$ numerically, it is still not easy to sample from $S(t) = \exp(-H(t))$. Crowther and Lambert [2013] proposed using a Gaussian quadrature to calculate $H(t)$ and a numerical root finder to generate the event time $S^{-1}(u)$ in general situations. But applying this approach here is inefficient, as a large number of function evaluations are needed for generating a single TTE. A more efficient way is to use Gaussian quadrature in combination with a rejection-acceptance algorithm, with $H(t)$ calculated with a Gaussian quadrature. Since $H(t)$ is often bounded from below, it is easy to find an appropriate $g(t)$ that leads to a reasonably efficient rejection algorithm. For example, with an Emax model in $h(t)$: $h(t) = \exp(\beta_0 + E_{max}/(1 + EC_{50}/C(t)))$, and $N \leq h(t) \leq M$. With a positive E_{max}, $N = \exp(\beta_0)$ and $M = \exp(\beta_0 + E_{max})$ for any $C(t)$. Therefore, $f(t) \leq M \exp(-Nt) = N \exp(-Nt)(M/N)$, so we can use $g(t) = N \exp(-Nt)$. As $a = M/N = \exp(E_{max})$, when $E_{max} = 1$, $a \leq \exp(1) = 2.72$, that is, on average, a sample is generated by every 2.72 simulations.

As an example, suppose that T-cells accounts $T(t)$ is related to the risk of death by $h(t) = \exp(\beta_0 + m(T(t)))$, where $m(T(t))$ may be an Emax model. The rejection algorithm for the HIV dynamic model can be implemented as follows. Since $T(t)$ does not have a closed form, we need to solve the ODEs, which can be done together with the numerical integration for $H(t)$. To implement this approach, we add a dummy ODE:

$$\frac{dH}{dt} = \exp(\beta_0 + m(T(t))) \tag{5.84}$$

to the dynamic model (5.83). Then $f(t)$ is given as $f(t) = \exp(\beta_0 + m(T(t)))H(t)$, where $T(t)$ and $H(t)$ are the solutions to the 1st equation in (5.83) and equation (5.84). Then the same rejection-acceptance algorithms as discussed before, with N and M determined in the same way, can be implemented.

5.10.6 Example programs

The following R program simulates TTE data using the binary distribution with $c(t) = \exp(-t) - \exp(-2t)$. The censoring time is 5 and between 0 and 5, 1000 intervals of equal size are used. log(etime/ntime) converts log-baseline risk $h_0 = -1$ to that per interval.

```
etime=5
ntime=1000
ttime=(1:ntime)/ntime*etime
EC50=0.15
Emax=1
h0=-1
h0adj=h0+log(etime/ntime) #width=5year/1000
Yi=NULL
for(i in 1:5000){
 ct=(exp(-ttime))-exp(-2*ttime)
 hi=pmin(0.9999,exp(h0adj+Emax/(1+EC50/ct)))
ei=rbinom(ntime,1,hi)
tti=min(which(ei==1))
Yi=c(Yi,min(ntime+1,tti)) #min(NA)=Inf
}
Yi=Yi/1000*etime
```

This is a fully vectorized algorithm, which is efficient in R (but not necessarily in SAS) than using an additional loop for each individual to generate ei till ei=1 occurs.

The following R program uses the RA algorithm together with a numerical integration algorithm to generate TTE data with an Emax model and $c(t) = \exp(-t) - \exp(-2t)$

```
h0=-1
EC50=0.15
Emax=1
ht=function(t){
 ct=(exp(-t))-exp(-2*t)
 exp(h0+Emax/(1+EC50/ct))
}
M=exp(h0+Emax)
N=exp(h0)
nsimu=10000
  yv=rexp(nsimu,N)
  un=runif(nsimu,max=M*exp(-N*yv))
Yi=NULL
for(i in 1:nsimu){
  Ht=integrate(f=ht,lower=0, upper=yv[i])$value
  if (un[i]<exp(-Ht)*ht(yv[i])) Yi=c(Yi,yv[i])
}
```

where the R function intergate(.) calculates $H(t)$ and $f(t)$ in the RA algorithm.

Simulation algorithm for the HIV dynamic model:

```
parameters <- c(a =0.3, lmd=33,d=0.3,k=1,del=0.5,N=1,c=0.2,u=0.5)
 state <- c(T = 1, Ts = 0, V = 1,H=0)
gm=function(t) 0.5 #assume constant

h0=-1
EC50=1
Emax=1
#set upper and lower boundaries for h(t)
M=exp(h0+Emax)
N=exp(h0)

 HIV<-function(t, state, parameters) {
 with(as.list(c(state, parameters)),{
 # similar to $DES in NONMEM
 dT <- lmd - d*T-(1-gm(t))*k*T*V
 dTs <- (1-gm(t))*k*T*V -del*Ts
 dV= N*del*Ts-c*V
 dH= exp(h0+Emax*T/(T+EC50)) #h(t)
 list(c(dT, dTs, dV,dH))})
 }
 Yi=NULL
   yv=rexp(nsimu,N)
  un=runif(nsimu,max=M*exp(-N*yv))
for(i in 1:nsimu){
```

```
  out=ode(y = state, times = c(0,yv[i]), func = HIV,
     parms = parameters,method=''lsoda")
  T=out[2,2] #col2-5 are T, Ts, V and H
  h=exp(h0+Emax*T/(T+EC50))
  Ht=out[2,5]
  if (un[i]<exp(-Ht)*h) Yi=c(Yi,yv[i])
}
```

where $H(t)$ is also calculated by the ODE solver function ode(.), together with T, Ts and H.

5.10.7 Sample size estimation using simulations

As an application of the simulation approaches, here we use these simulation tools for sample size calculation to estimate the exposure effect, e.g., log-RR, when the exposure has a complex distribution. The sample size calculation for parametric models and Cox models for comparing two or more groups has been well developed; hence the reader is referred to a standard text such as Schoenfeld [1983]. In general, the sample size calculation for exposure-risk modeling is rather complex, since the information matrix for the model parameters cannot be easily calculated. The following simulation tools provide an easy way for applied statisticians and modelers. The basic idea is to use simulation in combination with model fitting to estimate the information matrix with a large sample simulation. Then the sample size needed to achieve a given precision (e.g., given by a target SE) can be determined accordingly. The approach described here can be applied almost directly to sample size calculation for other type of models.

We start from a simple situation of no covariates in a Cox model, which is often sufficient for the sample size calculation when the exposure $C_i(t)$ can be simulated. We would like to determine the sample size that gives SE_t, a target SE size, for $\hat{\beta}$, assuming a baseline hazard function. Although a trial-and-error approach using multiple simulations with different sample sizes can be used to determine the right sample size, a much more efficient way is to run a single simulation of a much larger sample size so that random variations in the SE estimate are almost eliminated. Suppose that we have run a simulation of the sample size n_l and obtained SE_l, from which we can calculate the information matrix (which is a scalar here) $I_l = SE_l^{-2}$ of sample size n_l. The contribution of one sample is then $I_u = I_l/n_l = SE_l^{-2}/n_l$. From I_u we can calculate that the SE of sample size n is $1/\sqrt{I_u n}$. Therefore, to obtain SE_t, the sample size needed is $n = n_l SE_l^2/SE_t^2$. As this n is based on asymptotic properties, we may still need to assess the small sample properties by running multiple simulations with the sample size n, and adjusting if necessary. However, the approach based on the asymptotic variances helps in determining the starting point for the multiple simulations. This formula can be derived directly based on the fact that the asymptotic SE^{-2} is proportional to the sample size. However, the derivation via the information matrix is a more general approach.

This basic approach can be extended to more complex situations. The following is a typical scenario in drug development when deciding exposure measures for later phase trials, where an active and a placebo arm are included. It is often needed to determine from how many patients in the active arm exposure measures should be taken. If the modeling strategy is to exclude the placebo arm, the previous approach can be used directly. However, if the placebo arm is included as having zero exposure, the approach has to be modified. In this case, the total information is

$$I = n_0 I_{u0} + n_1 I_{u1} \tag{5.85}$$

where n_k and I_{uk} are the sample sizes and the unit (of a single patient) information matrix in arms $k = 0$ (placebo) and $k = 1$ (active), respectively. We would like to decide the number of exposure measures in the active arm to obtain an estimate with a given SE_t value. For given $n_0 I_{u0}$ and I_{u1}, the sample size to obtain a given SE_t value is $n_1 = (SE_t^{-1} - n_0 I_{u0})/I_{u1}$. Therefore, the task becomes how to calculate $n_0 I_{u0}$ and I_{u1} based on simulations. This can be done by running two simulations with different sample sizes n_{1a} and n_{1b} for the active arm and obtaining SE_a and SE_b, respectively. Then $n_0 I_{u0}$ and I_{u1} can be solved from

$$\begin{aligned} n_0 I_{u0} + n_{1a} I_{u1} &= SE_a^{-2} \\ n_0 I_{u0} + n_{1b} I_{u1} &= SE_b^{-2} \end{aligned} \tag{5.86}$$

which leads to $I_{u1} = (SE_a^{-2} - SE_b^{-2})/(n_{1a} - n_{1b})$ and $n_0 I_{u0} = SE_b^{-2} - n_{1b} I_{u1}$. Note that we only need to estimate $n_0 I_{u0}$ as a single value.

Another extension of this approach is for multiple parameters to allow for time-varying effects or covariates in the model. These can be spline functions to increase model flexibility, which is important when the placebo arm is included in the analysis, or covariates must be adjusted for, particularly when the exposure is related to these covariates. The same approach can be applied to the information matrix of multiple parameters $\boldsymbol{\beta}$. The determinant of the information matrix is inversely proportional to the volume of the confidence region, hence is a general measure for the precision of multi-parameter estimates. Consider the situation with a placebo arm in the model; we can use the same approach of running two simulations with sample sizes n_{1a} and n_{1b}. Writing (5.86) in terms of the variance-covariance matrices

$$\begin{aligned} n_0 \mathbf{I}_{u0} + n_{1a} \mathbf{I}_{u1} &= \text{var}(\hat{\boldsymbol{\beta}}_a)^{-1} \\ n_0 \mathbf{I}_{u0} + n_{1b} \mathbf{I}_{u1} &= \text{var}(\hat{\boldsymbol{\beta}}_b)^{-1}, \end{aligned} \tag{5.87}$$

where $\text{var}(\hat{\boldsymbol{\beta}}_a)$ and $\text{var}(\hat{\boldsymbol{\beta}}_b)$ are the variance-covariance matrices from the two simulations, one can solve these equations to give $\mathbf{I}_{u1} = (\text{var}(\hat{\boldsymbol{\beta}}_a)^{-1} - \text{var}(\hat{\boldsymbol{\beta}}_b)^{-1})/(n_{1a} - n_{1b})$ and $n_0 \mathbf{I}_{u0} = \text{var}(\hat{\boldsymbol{\beta}}_b)^{-1} - n_{1b} \mathbf{I}_{u1}$. If the target is to make $|\text{var}(\hat{\boldsymbol{\beta}})| \leq K$, then the required sample size for the exposure measures can be solved from the equation

$$|n_0 \mathbf{I}_{u0} + n_1 \mathbf{I}_{u1}| = K^{-1} \tag{5.88}$$

numerically. Since there may not be any integer n_1 that satisfies equation (5.88), to do this efficiently, one can treat n_1 as a continuous variable and use a root finder to find the solution to (5.88) then round the value to the nearest integer. The following code defines an R function and calls a root finder:

```
obj=function(n1) det(n0*Iu0+n1*Iu1)-1/K
uniroot(f=obj, interval=c(lower,upper))
```

where we provide $n0$, $Iu0$ and $Iu1$ and K, as well as the lower and upper boundaries for the root search.

The approach is quite universal, as it can be used for almost any type of TTE models and model fitting procedures. When using a non-ML approach to estimate $\boldsymbol{\beta}$, one can still consider $(\text{var}(\hat{\boldsymbol{\beta}}))^{-1}$ as an information matrix and use the approach directly. This approach only uses the assumption that asymptotically $\text{var}(\beta) \propto 1/n$, which is satisfied by almost all estimates in this book. For multiple parameter models, there are a number of alternatives to the determinant of the information matrices to measure the precision of $\hat{\boldsymbol{\beta}}$, e.g., the trace and a linear combination of the information matrix. These measures can be found in standard texts for optimal experimental designs such as Atkinson et al. [2007].

5.11 Comments and bibliographic notes

There are several excellent books on TTE data analysis, among those the author has used extensively are Fleming and Harrington [2013], Kalbfleisch and Prentice [2002] Aalen et al. [2008]. Cook et al. [2007] (2007) is dedicated to recurrent events analysis. Putter et al. [2007] give a tutorial on competing risk and multi-state models. The use of parametric models for TTE data analysis has a long history, while a landmark in the semi-parametric approach is the Cox model [Cox, 1972; Therneau and Grambsch, 2000]. Afterward, numerous works have been published on the use of the Cox model for TTE data analysis, in particular, in biomedical fields.

Joint modeling is an active research area with a large number of publications. No attempt is made to review the literature. The reader is referred to Rizopoulos [2012] for methods and references.

6

Modeling dynamic dose-exposure-response relationship

Until now, we have assumed that the effect of dose and/or exposure on the response is instantaneous, with a few exceptions such as Section 2.1.1. This assumption is rarely true, although sometimes reasonable as an approximation. In pharmacometrics, in most cases, the response change lags behind the exposure change (PK) that caused it, a phenomenon known as hysteresis. In this case, it is important to investigate and model the temporal ER relationship. The same happens in the DR relationship. For example, the impact of warfarin dose adjustment on INR in the warfarin data [Avery et al., 2020] is lagged behind the adjustment. The dynamic (temporal) DER relationship is important in many situations, e.g., to predict the time of onset of an adverse event or the efficacy response to treatment, to optimize dosing schedule and dose adjustment. Csajka and Verotta [2006] give a comprehensive review of PKPD modeling, in particular, hysteresis in PKPD relationships. In PKPD modeling, there are mainly two ways to model the temporal DER relationship. One assumes that the response depends on a latent "exposure", which follows a dynamic model that links to the exposure we observe. The other is based on a dynamic response model that describes the natural course of the disease process, e.g., tumor growth. Exposure affects the disease process by changing its natural course. Similar approaches can also be used for DR relationships within and beyond pharmacometrics.

The modeling of the dynamic DER relationship may consist of three sub-dynamic systems DE, ER and DR relationships, and each is an integrated part of the dynamic system. Figure 6.1 shows the system with the three sub-dynamic systems, and among them the DE part has been discussed in Chapter 3. The two other sub-systems represent (i) exposure effect accumulation: the dynamic of drug effects, and (ii) disease processes: the dynamic of disease with or without exposure. The dynamic of exposure effect cumulation and disease process may not be separable.

The exposure dynamic may also be affected by the exposure and response via a feedback loop in, e.g., a trial with therapeutic dose monitoring. Dose adjustment can also be made according to clinical outcomes. These are exposure dynamics with mechanisms more complex than those under a fixed dosing scheme and will be discussed in Chapter 8.

DOI: 10.1201/9781003457008-6

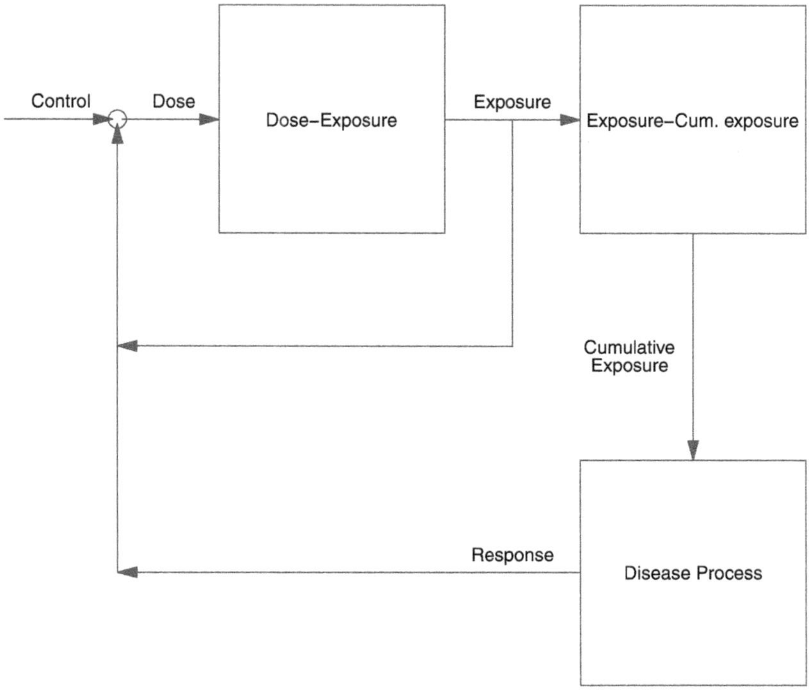

Figure 6.1
An illustration of the dynamic system between dose, exposure, cumulative exposure e.g., in an effect compartment, and disease process. The boxes represent dynamic sub-systems with a temporal relationship between the input and the output.

6.1 Effect compartment models

To introduce hysteresis in DER relationships, a widely accepted approach in PKPD modeling is to assume that the drug enters a hypothetic effect compartment, where the drug induces instantaneous effects. The hysteresis is due to the time it takes for the change in the central compartment to propagate to the effect compartment. The effect compartment model is an extension of well-developed PK compartment models, often supported by the pharmacological mechanism. A combination of an effect compartment model and an instantaneous response model such as the Emax model can describe nonlinear relationships with hysteresis. The effect compartment model approach has been widely used in practice. An example, among many others, is the modeling of PK/QT relationship [Minematsu et al., 2001].

First, we assume that the effect compartment is a linear system described by

$$C^*(t) = K_{in} \int_0^t \exp(-K\tau)C(t-\tau)d\tau \tag{6.1}$$

where $C^*(t)$ and $C(t)$ are the concentrations in the effect compartment and the central compartment in a population PK model, K_{in} and K are the rate constants of entry and elimination of the drug in and out of the effect compartment. Only for a few types of population PK models, (6.1) can be calculated analytically. One is the linear compartmental model with constant coefficients. A simple but typical model is the one-compartment model after an IV bolus injection, which gives

$$C(t) = C_0 \exp(-K_e t) \tag{6.2}$$

where C_0 is determined by dose and parameters such as volume of distribution and K_e is the elimination rate from the central compartment. Taking it into (6.1) we obtain

$$C^*(t) = \frac{C_0 K_{in}}{K - K_e}(\exp(-K_e t) - \exp(-Kt)). \tag{6.3}$$

In general, if the PK model is a linear compartmental model with constant parameters, the concentration $C(t)$ is a linear combination of exponential and polynomial functions, and hence the concentration in the effect compartment $C^*(t)$ always has an analytical form. However, the derivation of $C^*(t)$ is often complex. We recommend the use of software such as R to automatically derive it when the PK model is more complex than a one-compartment model with first-order absorption with oral doses or a two-compartment model with IV injection.

When repeated measurements are made for the exposure, we also need to use an NLMM for the effect compartment. Taking model (6.3) as an example, $C^*(t_{ij})$ for subject i can be written as

$$C^*_{ij} = \frac{C_0 K_{ini}}{K_i - K_{ei}}(\exp(-K_{ei}t) - \exp(-K_i t)) \tag{6.4}$$

where K_{ini}, K_{ei} and K_i are random parameters for subject i, as in the standard NLMM. However, in practice, the effect compartment is not observable, hence the unknown parameters can only be determined when fitting the PKPD model. Replacing C_{ij} in model (3.16) with C^*_{ij} we obtain

$$Y_{ij} = g(C^*_{ij}, \boldsymbol{\beta}_i) + e_{ij}. \tag{6.5}$$

Note that in addition to the parameters in (3.16), additional parameters are in C^*_{ij} and need to be estimated. The model (6.5) is nonlinear even when (3.16) is linear, hence it is more difficult to fit.

6.2 Indirect response models

The other type of model, the indirect response model [Csajka and Verotta, 2006] introduced as an example in Section 2.1.1, is based on another assumption that there is a baseline biomedical process and exposure acts to modify the baseline process by, e.g., inhibiting/promoting the input or elimination process. The PD process may be a biopharmaceutical process or a disease process such as tumor growth or glucose regulation. These models can be combined with non/semi-parametric approaches to reduce the dependence of model assumptions if appropriate.

Let $R(t)$ be the response at time t. The following are two simple but typical indirect response models to describe the dynamic relationship between exposure $C(t)$ and $R(t)$:

$$\begin{aligned} \frac{dR(t)}{dt} &= K_{in}(1 \pm g(C(t))) - K_{out}R(t) \\ \frac{dR(t)}{dt} &= K_{in} - K_{out}(1 \pm h(C(t)))R(t) \end{aligned} \tag{6.6}$$

where $g(C(t))$ and $h(C(t))$ are functions of exposure $C(t)$ with $g(0) = h(0) = 0$. The exposure effect can be inhibited (-) or stimulated (+) and can act on K_{in} or K_{out}. When $C(t) = 0$, model (6.6) degenerates to

$$\frac{dR(t)}{dt} = K_{in} - K_{out}R(t), \tag{6.7}$$

which describes the natural process without exposure. Note that if the system is stable without exposure, $R(t)$ will finally reach the level of K_{in}/K_{out}, derived by setting $dR(t)/dt = 0$. The same approach can be used on models (6.6) when $C(t)$ is constant or tends to a constant level. A common model for $g(C(t))$ and $h(C(t))$ is the Emax model (assuming $C(t) > 0$)

$$g(C(t)) = Emax/(EC_{50}/C(t) + 1) \tag{6.8}$$

on which random error and coefficients can be added. However, even when $C(t)$ is the output of a simple DE model such as (2.6), the model (6.6) may not have an analytical solution. Therefore, $R(t)$ has to be calculated via an ODE solver, which can be found in either NONMEM or R. The following R program calculates the solution of the above model with three parameter settings, using the deSolve(.) library.

```
yini <- c(y1 = 0, y2 = 1)
OneComp <- function(t,y,parms){
      with(as.list(c(parms,y)),{
      dy1 = 1 - Emax*y[2]/(EC50+y[2]) -kout*y[1] #response dynamic
      dy2 = - theta*y[2] #Central comp. with elimination rate ke=theta
```

```
list(c(dy1, dy2))
})
}
times <- seq(0, 10, by = 3/24)

out1 <- ode(func = OneComp, times = times,y = yini,
 parms = c(Emax=1.5,EC50=0.3,theta=0.3,kout=1), method = "ode45")
out2 <- ode(func = OneComp, times = times,y = yini,
 parms = c(Emax=1.5,EC50=0.6,theta=0.3,kout=1), method = "ode45")
out3 <- ode(func = OneComp, times = times,y = yini,
 parms = c(Emax=1.5,EC50=0.6,theta=0.9,kout=1), method = "ode45")
```

The solutions with the three parameter settings are plotted in Figure 6.2. There are only two $C(t)$ curves, as only K_e affects it. This program is for

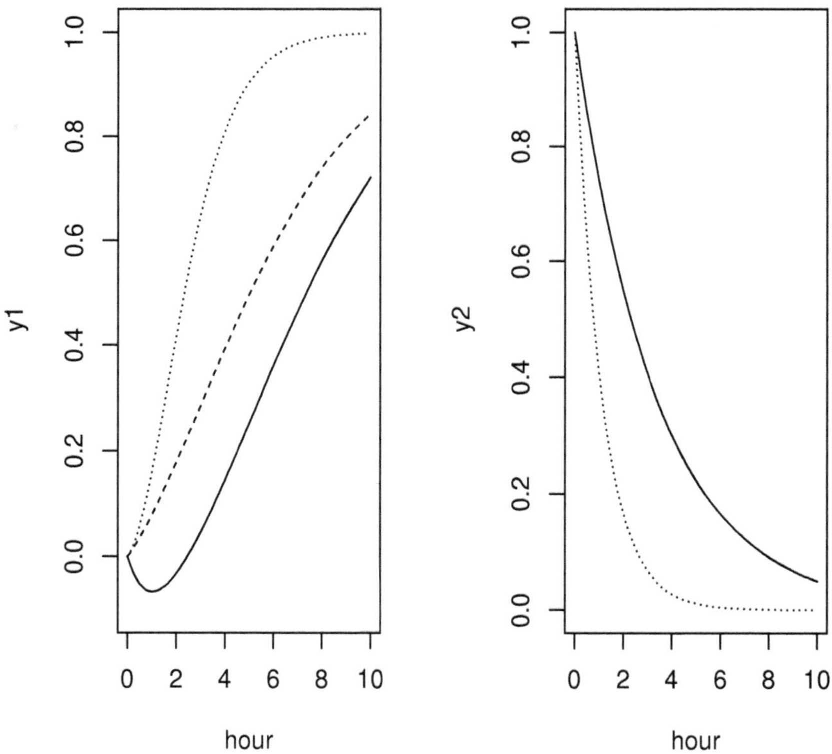

Figure 6.2
Solution to the system of ODEs consists of a central compartment, an indirect response model (6.6) and an Emax model for exposure effects, with $K_e = 0.3, EC_{50} = 0.3$ (solid line), $K_e = 0.6, EC_{50} = 0.3$ (dash line) and $K_e = 0.6, EC_{50} = 0.9$ (dot line) using the deSolve(.) library. Left panel: response; right panel: concentration in the central compartment.

the purpose of illustration of solving ODE systems with the R library. Since for this model, y[2] is not affected by y[1], a computationally more efficient approach is to solve y[2] analytically and only use deSolve(.) for y[1].

Using an ODE solver we can fit much more complex models than (6.5). For example, the natural course model (6.7) can be nonlinear; K_{in} and/or K_{out} may also be a time-varying function. However, although using complex models does not greatly increase programming complexity, it does increase computing intensity and reduce computational stability.

6.3 Disease process models

Disease process models follow a routine similar to indirect response models, but are more flexible. They form the basis for modeling exposure effects on disease processes following a complex time pattern with and without exposure, and they may also quantify the DER relationship. These models can be used in many situations in which a dynamic model dedicated to disease processes is needed. This section introduces a number of models for modeling different diseases.

6.3.1 Empirical models

Empirical models play an important role in the situation where mechanistic disease models are not available or difficult to use. These models describe the disease process by specifying the changes in measurements for disease outcomes, e.g., tumor sizes over time. Linear time trends with random coefficients, e.g.,

$$Y_i(t) = \beta_{0i} + \beta_{1i}t + e_i(t) \tag{6.9}$$

are frequently used. This model can be easily extended to use spline functions to increase flexibility. Fitting these models is easy with software for linear mixed models, as described in Chapter 3. It can also be combined with exponential functions, e.g., with

$$Y_i(t) = \beta_{0i} + \beta_{1i}t + \beta_{2i}\exp(-\beta_{3i}t) + e_i(t), \tag{6.10}$$

which offers a component that decays to zero naturally. A technical difficulty is that $Y_i(t)$ is not linear with respect to β_{3i}, hence the model (6.10) cannot be fitted with linear mixed model software.

Extending to other types of response is straightforward. For example, if $Y_i(t)$ is a binary indicator of a disease state, a logistic model can be used with the linear predictor (see Chapter 3) replaced by the right-hand side of (6.9). If $Y_i(t)$ is a count, e.g., of asthma attacks in the time interval t, a Poisson or negative binomial model can be adapted to include a time trend.

To use a disease model in DER modeling, we can link the model to, e.g., the exposure as the output of either the effect compartment or the indirect response model. It is obvious that the exposure can be directly added to the right-hand side of the two models as an additional term. But this setting leads to an instantaneous ER model. If the exposure has an impact on the rate of change, e.g.,

$$Y_i(t) = \beta_{0i} + \beta_{1i}t + \beta_{2i}\exp(-C_i(t)\beta_{3i}t) + e_i(t), \tag{6.11}$$

then the model is an empirical indirect response model specifying a dynamic relationship between $Y_i(t)$ and $C_i(t)$.

6.3.2 Slow and fast sub-systems

Although the combination of exposure and disease process systems is often complex, sometimes it can be simplified if one system (often the exposure dynamic) is much faster than the other. For example, suppose that the systems for the central and effect compartments are fast and slow systems, respectively:

$$\begin{aligned}\frac{dC(t)}{dt} &= h(C(t), C^*(t)) \\ \frac{dC^*(t)}{dt} &= \epsilon h^*(C(t), C^*(t))\end{aligned} \tag{6.12}$$

where $h(C(t), C^*(t))$ and $h^*(C(t), C^*(t))$ are functions of comparable value range, ϵ is a small number so that the second in model (6.12) is a slow system (i.e., with a much lower rate $dC^*(t)/dt$ than $dC(t)/dt$). Then, $C(t)$ changes much faster than $C^*(t)$ in the sense that it reaches steady state while $C^*(t)$ has almost not changed. Therefore, an approximation of the system solution can be obtained in two stages. First, when $t < t_0$ with a given t_0,

$$\lim_{\epsilon \to 0} C^*(t) = C^*(0) = 0, \tag{6.13}$$

where $C^*(0)$ may also be set to a non-zero value. Under this condition, the system is simplified to

$$\frac{dC(t)}{dt} = h(C(t), 0) \tag{6.14}$$

for which we assume that a solution $C(t) = \psi_0(t)$ exists. In the second stage, we replace $C(t)$ with $\psi_0(t)$ in the second system

$$\frac{dC^*(t)}{dt} = \epsilon h^*(\psi_0(t), C^*(t)), \tag{6.15}$$

then solve this system to obtain $C^*(t)$.

Now we consider a more specific system consisting of models for the central and effect compartments and the response:

$$\begin{aligned}
\frac{dC(t)}{dt} &= h(d(t), \gamma) \\
\frac{dC^*(t)}{dt} &= -KC^*(t) + K_{in}C(t) \\
Y(t) &= \beta_0 + E_{max}/(1 + EC_{50}/C^*(t))t
\end{aligned} \tag{6.16}$$

where the third is a linear disease process model with growth rate $E_{max}/(1 + EC_{50}/C^*(t))$ controlled by latent exposure $C^*(t)$. Note that since there is no $C^*(t)$ in the first sub-model, one can solve the system sequentially starting from the first one. However, we show that the system can be simplified as long as the first one is much faster than the rest.

We consider the above model with a single dose, but this approach also applies to a much complex model if it leads to solution $C(t) = \psi_0(t)$ that decays to 0 much quicker than $C^*(t)$ Since

$$\begin{aligned}
C^*(t) &= \int_0^t \exp(-K(t-\tau))K_{in}\psi_0(\tau)d\tau \\
&= K_{in}\exp(-Kt)\int_0^t \exp(K\tau)\psi_0(\tau)d\tau,
\end{aligned} \tag{6.17}$$

as long as the $C(t)$ dynamic is much faster than the elimination rate K, there exists a t_0 such that

$$\begin{aligned}
\exp(K\tau) \approx 1 &\qquad \tau \leq t_0 \\
\exp(K\tau)\psi_0(\tau) \approx 0 &\qquad \tau > t_0.
\end{aligned} \tag{6.18}$$

Using these approximations, we can write

$$\int_0^t \exp(K\tau)\psi_0(\tau)d\tau \approx \begin{cases} U(t_0) & t > t_0 \\ U(t) & t < t_0 \end{cases} \tag{6.19}$$

where $U(t) = \int_0^t \psi_0(\tau)d\tau$ is the AUC of $C(t)$, which may be calculated analytically for a simple system, or non-parametrically for a complex system. Note that as $\psi_0(t) \to 0$ quickly, $U(t) \approx U$, a constant when $t > t_0$, for not small t_0 (relative to the $C(t)$ dynamic), hence

$$C^*(t) \approx K_{in}\exp(-Kt)U \tag{6.20}$$

is a good approximation to (6.17). Taking $C^*(t)$ into the third equation of (6.16) leads to

$$Y(t) = \beta_0 + E_{max}/(1 + EC_{50}/(\exp(-Kt)U))t, \tag{6.21}$$

where we omitted K_{in}, as it is absorbed in EC_{50}. This simplification supports a simple approach to using the PK parameter AUC as a summary exposure in the effect-compartment model when the $C(t)$ sub-system is a much faster system, as used in the HIV dynamic models [Wu et al., 2008]. Further improvement to the simple approximation is possible by using the perturbation method to dynamic systems that consist of fast and slow subsystems. Due to the complexity of these approaches, the reader interested in the development in this area is referred to texts such as O'malley et al. [1991].

6.3.3 Semi-mechanistic models

Some models may be considered semi-mechanistic since there is no clear pharmacological mechanism to support them but may consist of hypothetical compartments to represent important quantities of measurement. For example, the Positive and Negative Syndrome Scale (PANSS) is a common measure for the symptoms of schizophrenia, a severe mental illness. To model the disease process of schizophrenia, the following model has been used [Reddy et al., 2013]

$$d\text{PANSS}(t)/dt = K_{in} - K_{out}(1 + \beta C_e)\text{PANSS}(t), \tag{6.22}$$

where C_e is a constant exposure or dose ($C_e = 0$ for placebo). The model assumes that the treatment affects the elimination rate of PANSS. The model also assumes the existence of $d\text{PANSS}(t)/dt$, although PANSS is, in fact, on a discrete scale. However, this assumption allows for the fitting of the practical model using the solution $\text{PANSS}(t) = \text{PANSS}(0)\exp((K_{in} - K_{out}(1+\beta C_e))t)$. A similar approach was used to model the Unified Parkinson's Disease Rating Scale (UPDRS) scores.

6.3.4 Modeling tumor growth and drug effects

A number of empirical models have been used to model tumor growth and treatment effects on it. Wang et al. [2009] used the following model for non-small cell lung cancer (NSCLC). Let $Y(t)$ be the tumor size at time t, and the model assumes a linear growth and an exponential decay:

$$Y(t) = Y(0)\exp(-St) + Kt \tag{6.23}$$

where S and K are decay and growth parameters. Another model [Claret et al., 2009] incorporated treatment effects of dose D:

$$\begin{aligned} dY(t)/dt &= K_g Y(t) + K_d D\exp(-\lambda t)Y(t) \\ &= (K_g + K_d D\exp(-\lambda t))Y(t). \end{aligned} \tag{6.24}$$

In this model, $D\exp(-\lambda t)$ can be considered as a solution to an exposure kinetic model.

Houk et al.'s model [Houk et al., 2010] replaces the dose in model (6.24) with concentration $C(t)$:

$$dY(t)/dt \quad = \quad (K_g + K_d C(t)\exp(-\lambda t))Y(t). \tag{6.25}$$

This model is an indirect response model with exposure that affects the rate of tumor decay. The solution to (6.25) can be written as

$$Y(t) = Y(0)\exp(K_g t + K_d \int_0^t C(\tau)\exp(-\lambda\tau)d\tau). \tag{6.26}$$

When $C(t)$ is considered piecewise constant, e.g., $C(t) = C_j, t \in (t_j, t_{j+1})$, the solution can be written as

$$Y(t_{j+1}) = Y(t_j)\exp(K_g\Delta_j + K_d C_j[\exp(-\lambda t_j) - \exp(-\lambda t_{j+1})]/\lambda). \tag{6.27}$$

where $\Delta_j = t_{j+1} - t_j$. Taking the log-transformation on both sides, we obtain on the log-scale

$$\begin{aligned} \log(Y_{j+1}) &= \log(Y_j) + K_g\Delta_j + K_d C_j[\exp(-\lambda t_j) - \exp(-\lambda t_{j+1})]/\lambda \\ &= \log(Y_j) + K_g\Delta_j + K_d C_j \exp(-\lambda t_j)(1 - \exp(-\lambda\Delta_j))/\lambda. \end{aligned} \tag{6.28}$$

Hence the tumor growth rate has a constant and an exposure-dependent component, and the latter decays at a rate λ.

Tumor growth treatment effect modeling is a fast-growing area with many recent works. See Yin et al. [2019] for a review of recent developments.

6.4 Fitting dynamic models for longitudinal data

We have described a number of dynamic systems. To fit longitudinal data to these models, for those with an analytical solution, the approaches given in Chapter 3 can be applied directly. For complex models without an analytical solution, one has to combine the algorithm for fitting NLMM with an ODE solver to solve the dynamic system numerically. Both NONMEM and R provide options to implement them in a straightforward manner. The implementation in R uses an ODE solver interface to the NLMM model fitting library nlme. NONMEM uses the same solver and a similar model specification as in R. For example, to fit the following models:

$$\begin{aligned} \frac{dR(t)}{dt} &= E_{maxi}/(EC_{50}/(C(t)) + 1) - K_{out}R(t) \\ \frac{C(t)}{dt} &= -\theta C(t) \end{aligned} \tag{6.29}$$

where $E_{maxi} \sim N(E_{max} + U_i, \sigma_e^2)$ is the only random coefficient in the models, the following program, similar to that in Chapter 3, can be used.

```
bdata=bdata[order(bdata$Subject,bdata$Time),]
gdata=groupedData(conc~Time|Subject,bdata)

OneComp <- list(DiffEq=list(
      dy1dt = ~ Emax*y2/(EC50+y2) -kout*y1 ,    #Absoprtion dynamic
      dy2dt = ~ - theta*y2, #Central comp. with elimination rate ke
  ObsEq=list(
      c1 = ~ y1,          #No measure for absorption
      c2 = ~ y2,  #Observe concentration c2=amount y2/volume
  Parms=c("Emax","EC50","theta"),
  States=c("y1","y2"),
  Init=list(0,0))  #Initial states for the ODE

moximodel=nlmeODE(OneComp,gdata) #generate function for nlme() call

jk=nlme(conc~moximodel(ka,ke,Cl,Time,Subject)  ,fixed=ka+ke+CL~1,
   random=pdDiag(Cl~1), start=c(Emax=1,EC50=0.5,theta=1), data=gdata,
   control=list(returnObject=TRUE,msVerbose=TRUE),
   verbose=TRUE)
```

The call to the R function nlme(.) follows the same way as shown in Chapter 3, except the model specification is via the moximodel, which calls the ODE solver.

6.5 Semi-parametric and non-parametric approaches

6.5.1 Effect compartment model with non-parametric exposure estimates

So far we have considered parametric dynamic DER models. To reduce dependence of model assumptions, a part of the model may be set non-parametric. For example, when the PK model is not well established, we may prefer to use a non-parametric method to describe concentration time profile in the dynamic system. A simple approach is to use linear interpolation to approximate $C(t)$ within $t_{j+1} \le t \le t_j$ as

$$\begin{aligned} C(t) &= C_j + \frac{C_{i+1} - C_j}{\Delta_j}(t - t_j) \\ &\equiv a_j + b_j t \end{aligned} \tag{6.30}$$

where $\Delta_j = t_{j+1} - t_j, b_j = (C_{j+1} - C_j)/\Delta_j$, $a_j = C_j - t_j b_j$, and C_j is the concentration measured at t_j. Taking (6.30) into the effect compartment model (6.1) and using the well-known formula for integration by parts, $\int x \exp(ax)dx = \exp(ax)(ax - 1)/a^2$, we obtain for $0 < t \le t_1$ with $C(0) = 0$,

$$C^*(t) = K_{in} K^{-2}[Kt - 1 + \exp(-Kt)]. \tag{6.31}$$

$C(t)$ in other intervals can be calculated consecutively. See Wang [2005] for details. When sampling times are well designed, a moderate number of PK samples provides a good approximation to a moderately complex PK profile [Wang, 2001]. Since $C(t)$ is a piecewise linear function in (6.30), it is possible to calculate the effect-compartment concentration analytically. The class of approximation tools for PK profiles allowing analytical effect-compartment concentrations includes spline functions and polynomials. This algorithm can be implemented in SAS proc NLMIXED with some simple programming [Wang, 2005]. Although the calculation is elementary, it is recommended to use R or other software to derive them and generate programming codes automatically, particularly when high-order polynomials are involved.

6.5.2 Non-parametric dynamic models and lagged covariates

In this section we explore the relationship between the dynamic model approach and the non-parametric lagged covariate method [Diggle, 2002] to model delayed exposure effects. Let Y_{ij} and C_{ij} be the response and exposure of subject i at time t_j, respectively. A linear model with the exposure as lagged covariates can be written as

$$Y_{ij} = \beta_0 C_{ij} + \sum_{r=1}^{R} \beta_r C_{ij-r} + U_i + \varepsilon_{ij}, \tag{6.32}$$

where we have omitted other covariates for simplicity. The coefficients $\beta_r, r = 1, ..., R$, represent the contribution of the delayed exposure effect (hysteresis) to the present response, hence the existence of hysteresis can be tested by the null hypothesis $H_0 : \cap_{r=1}^{R} \beta_r = 0$. This model is easy to fit as long as all necessary data are observed, for example, from a longitudinal study with repeated measures at fixed intervals at equal distances. Note that the test for the null hypothesis may not work in some situations. An example is when hysteresis is short and the time intervals between t_js are wide. Specifically, the method may not detect a constant delay with $C^*(t) = C(t-\delta)$ if the time intervals are larger than δ.

The lagged covariate model can be considered as a discrete approximation to a model based on the effect compartment model (6.1). With sufficiently dense time intervals $t_1, ..., t_R$, (6.1) can be approximated as

$$C^*(t) = K_{in} \int_0^t \exp(-K\tau) C(t-\tau) d\tau \approx K_{in} \sum_{r=1}^{R} \exp(-Kt_r) C(t-t_r). \tag{6.33}$$

It is clear that β_r is an estimate of $\exp(-Kt_r)$. In fact, the lagged covariate model can be considered as a non-parametric approximation to a linear model in combination with a more general linear system.

$$C^*(t) = K_{in} \int_0^t h(\tau) C(t-\tau) d\tau, \tag{6.34}$$

for the effect compartment without assuming a constant rate K. In this case, β_r is an estimate of $h(t_r)$.

Next we apply the lagged covariate approach to the moxifloxacin data. To this end, we use the fitted popPK model as described in Section 3.3.2. The prediction of PK profiles based on the fitted model can also be found there. To create lagged concentrations as covariates for each response, we predict the PK profiles with a number of different time lags as the covariates. For this example, we have used unequal lag intervals (0.5, 1, 3, 6, 10) to cover a large range of time intervals with a relatively small number of lag times. Some earlier QT measures may have some lagged concentrations set to zero. The lagged concentrations were included in a LMM with random effects on all their coefficients. The fitted model is summarized below.

```
       AIC      BIC    logLik
  3779.202 3933.431 -1853.601

Random effects:
 Formula: ~PHKRSL1N + pk05 + pk1 + pk3 + pk6 + pk10 | id
 Structure: General positive-definite, Log-Cholesky parametrization
            StdDev       Corr
(Intercept) 4.276355e+00 (Intr) PHKRSL pk05   pk1    pk3    pk6
PHKRSL1N    2.498573e-03 -0.226
pk05        1.381401e-03  0.051  0.048
pk1         1.614406e-03 -0.035 -0.620 -0.645
pk3         7.838476e-07 -0.071 -0.112 -0.682  0.584
pk6         1.773276e-03 -0.173  0.209  0.117 -0.285 -0.281
pk10        2.191611e-03  0.092  0.027 -0.025  0.078  0.170 -0.544
Residual    6.323127e+00

Fixed effects: dd_tavg ~ PHKRSL1N + pk05 + pk1 + pk3 + pk6 + pk10
                 Value Std.Error  DF   t-value p-value
(Intercept)  2.3008091 1.2376942 470  1.858948  0.0637
PHKRSL1N     0.0029934 0.0005968 470  5.015411  0.0000
pk05         0.0004095 0.0005101 470  0.802786  0.4225
pk1          0.0006924 0.0004593 470  1.507614  0.1323
pk3         -0.0000001 0.0000002 470 -0.451544  0.6518
pk6          0.0004219 0.0004832 470  0.873148  0.3830
pk10         0.0007972 0.0005246 470  1.519473  0.1293
 Correlation:
         (Intr) PHKRSL pk05   pk1    pk3    pk6
PHKRSL1N -0.625
pk05     -0.127 -0.226
pk1       0.013 -0.179 -0.636
pk3       0.041 -0.068 -0.145  0.353
pk6      -0.368  0.302  0.083 -0.218 -0.222
pk10     -0.334  0.260  0.057  0.012  0.018 -0.329

Standardized Within-Group Residuals:
        Min          Q1         Med          Q3         Max
-3.76389458 -0.52315789  0.00844584  0.52550998  3.76154683
```

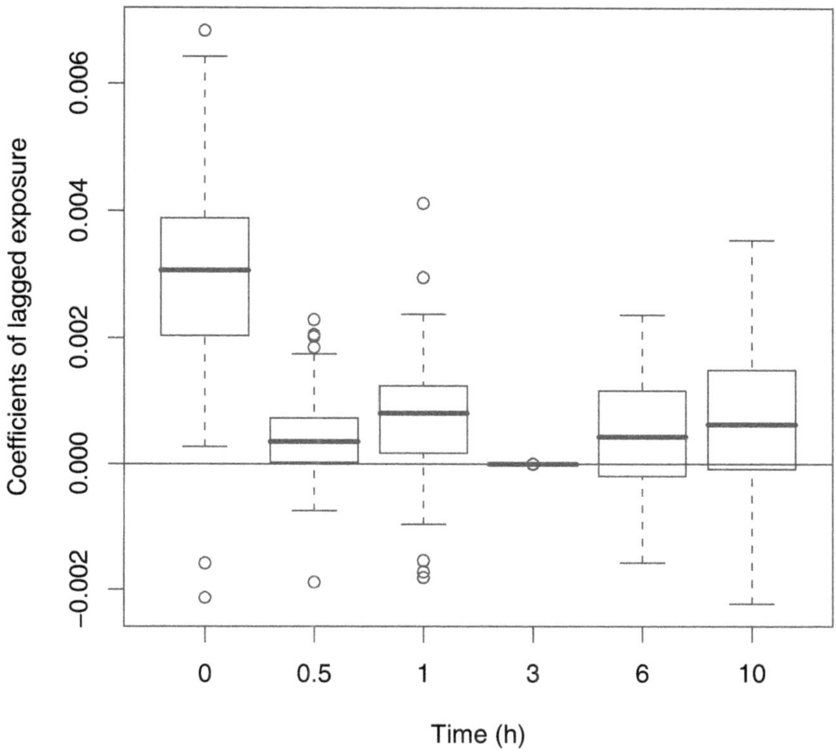

Figure 6.3
Distribution of predicted coefficients of lagged moxifloxacin exposures in the linear mixed model with lagged exposures for QTcF change from baseline.

```
Number of Observations: 536
Number of Groups: 60
```

The distribution of the individual predicted coefficients of the model can be found in Figure 6.3. Note that if the linear effect compartment model holds, the coefficients should follow the shape of $\exp(-Kt)$. However, for the QTcF data this seemed not the case, as there was no exponential decay in the exposure effects. This suggests that the temporal relationship between moxifloxacin concentration and its QT effect may be more complex than a linear effect compartment model with constant rate can describe.

6.6 Dynamic linear and generalized linear mixed models

The effect compartment and indirect response models are based on ODE that describe the response dynamic and its relationship to exposure. The model fitting heavily relies on solving the ODE, either analytically or numerically. In some situations where repeated measures of response, for example tumor size or biomarker value, are taken at equally spaced time intervals $t_1, ..., t_J$, with $t_j - t_{j-1} = \Delta, j = 1, ..., J$, some simple models can also be used to describe the dynamic relationship. The dynamic linear model (DLM) is among the simplest and yet has a wide range of applications. Let Y_{ij} be the jth, $j = 1, ..., J$, response measure of subject $i, i = 1, ..., n$, we assume that

$$Y_{ij} = \beta_y Y_{ij-1} + \beta_c C_{ij} + U_i + \varepsilon_{ij} \tag{6.35}$$

where parameter β_y controls the dependence of Y_{ij} on Y_{ij-1}, the other parts are the same as in a simple repeated measurement model without random coefficient. Models like this with lagged responses as covariates are known as autoregression models and are widely used in time series analysis. Their correlation structures have also been used for the residual error term. However, these models can also describe complex dynamic DER relationships as the ODE does. In fact, they are known as difference equations, a discrete-time version of ODEs. We will show their applications to modeling dynamic DER relationship with dose adjustment.

Apparently, fitting this model could be done by the LS method, treating U_i as fixed parameters. However, with fixed (and often small) J, the LS estimates are inconsistent when $n \to \infty$. With U_i as a random effect, the MLEs for all the model parameters are consistent with small J. However, to do so, we need to correctly specify the distribution of U_i. In addition, sometimes Y_{i0} is not observed, which is an important issue when J is small. See Hsiao [2022] for more details.

When U_i is ignored, this model can be written as a marginal model

$$Y_{ij} = \beta_y^j Y_{i0} + \beta_c \sum_{j'=1}^{j} \beta_y^{j-j'} C_{ij'} + \varepsilon_{ij}^* \tag{6.36}$$

depending on the entire exposure history. The first term represents the marginal time profile of the system dynamic without exposure, and the second is a sum of cumulative exposure effects in the past. Model (6.36) is not linear with respect to β_y and the error term ε_{it}^* is variance heterogeneous and correlated within subjects, making the fitting of this model more difficult than fitting model (6.35).

The dependence on the history may also occur on ε_{ij}, e.g., through a model:

$$\varepsilon_{ij} = \rho\varepsilon_{ij-1} + \varepsilon_{ij}^* \tag{6.37}$$

where ε_{ij}^* are independent, but ε_{ij} and ε_{ij-1} are correlated via ρ. This is a model for the AR(1) error introduced in Chapter 3, given here to illustrate the similarity to the model (6.35). However, there is a fundamental difference between the two models, as this AR(1) model does not introduce dynamics into the mean response.

The model (6.35) without random terms U_i and ε_{ij} is, in fact, an approximation to an ODE. To see this, we write the model as

$$(Y_{ij} - Y_{ij-1})/\Delta = [(\beta_y - 1)Y_{ij-1} + \beta_c C_{ij}]/\Delta. \tag{6.38}$$

Let $\Delta \to 0$, this model becomes ordinary differential equation

$$\frac{dY_i(t)}{dt} = \eta Y_i(t) + \beta^* C_i(t) \tag{6.39}$$

where $\eta = \lim_{\Delta\to 0}(\beta_y - 1)/\Delta$ and $\beta^* = \lim_{\Delta\to 0}\beta_c/\Delta$. These limits exist when $Y_i(t)$ (without random components) is sufficiently smooth. Ignoring random terms avoids the technical complexity of introducing a stochastic differential equation [Oksendal, 2013].

A more general DLM contains a hidden dynamic part

$$\begin{aligned} \xi_{ij} &= \beta_\xi \xi_{ij-1} + \beta_c C_{ij} + U_i \\ Y_{ij} &= \xi_{ij} + \varepsilon_{ij} \end{aligned} \tag{6.40}$$

in which the first is a dynamic model and the second is an observation model, in which ξ_{ij} can only be observed through Y_{ij}. DLMs have been used for prediction in engineering for a long time, and the most significant method using these models is the Kalman filter. But model (6.40) is much more difficult to fit than model (6.35). One may be tempted to write the former into the form of the latter by replacing ξ_{ij} in the first one in (6.40) with $Y_{ij} - \varepsilon_{ij}$ and getting

$$\begin{aligned} Y_{ij} &= \beta_\xi Y_{ij-1} - \beta_\xi \varepsilon_{ij} + \beta_c C_{ij} + U_i + \varepsilon_{ij} \\ &= \beta_\xi Y_{ij-1} + \beta_c C_{ij} + U_i + \varepsilon^*_{ij} \end{aligned} \tag{6.41}$$

where $\varepsilon^*_{ij} = \beta_\xi \varepsilon_{ij-1} + \varepsilon_{ij}$. Although this model looks like model (6.35), it cannot be fitted with lagged Y_{ij}, as ε^*_{ij} and Y_{ij} are correlated. This issue can also be looked at from the measurement error aspect, as (6.40) can be considered as a measurement error model in which we only observe ξ_{ij} via Y_{ij} with measurement error ε_{ij}. The measurement error of ξ_{ij} does not cause bias, but that of ξ_{ij-1} does. Recent developments in the fitting of these models have focused on Bayesian approaches, since, unlike model (6.35), model (6.40) cannot be fitted with linear mixed model software, and the performance of the MLE is unsatisfactory [Hsiao, 2022].

Another useful extension of the DLM is introducing time-varying coefficients, yet still keeping the linear structure. For example, if the exposure effect β_y is time-varying, then it can be described by a dynamic system of its own

$$\beta_{yj} = \gamma\beta_{yj-1} + b \tag{6.42}$$

where γ and b are parameters to be estimated. Subject effects can also be introduced to these parameters. When $|\gamma| < 1$, β_{yj} tends to its asymptote

$b/(1-\gamma)$. One may choose to write β_{yj} as an explicit function in model (6.35) without the DLM (6.42). But the model is no longer linear with respect to β_{yj}.

As an application, a linear dynamic model can be a simple alternative to the model (6.28) for tumor size per cycle and has non-zero asymptotes. Let $Z_k = \log(Y_k)$ be the log-size at the end of the treatment cycle k

$$Z_k = \beta_z Z_{k-1} + K - g(C_k) \tag{6.43}$$

where $g(C_k)$ represents exposure effect, $\beta_z \geq 0$, K is a constant and C_k is the cumulative treatment effect in cycle k. This model is more general than (6.28) as in which $\beta_z = 1$. With constant treatment $C_k = C$ and $|\beta_z| < 1$, $Z_k \to (K - g(C))/(1 - \beta_z)$, i.e., tumor size $Y_k \to \exp((K - g(C))/(1 - \beta_z))$ when the equilibrium between nature growth and treatment effects is reached. Therefore, β_z plays a key role in determining the long-term outcome. This is derived by assuming $Z_k = Z_{k-1} = Z$ in the model, which becomes $Z = \beta_z Z + K - g(C_k)$, then solving Z from it, a similar approach to finding equilibrium from an ODE by setting the derivatives to zero. Note that these approaches only work when Z_k tends to a constant, that is, the system is stable under the condition $|\beta_z| < 1$. When $\beta_z = 1$, it is a random walk on the log scale again, while $\beta_z > 1$ leads to unstable growth, both have no equilibrium states.

As another example, we consider a crossover clinical trial that compares FEV1 in patients after receiving two active treatments (a) and (c) and a placebo (p) with a crossover design. FEV1 was measured hourly for eight hours after each treatment, and a baseline measure was also taken 11 hours before the application of the treatment to 24 patients. The dataset has been used in multiple publications. Figure 6.4 gives individual curves of the FEV1 measures for all subjects, together with their means. There is a small placebo effect, as the placebo curve increases slightly after treatment. Both active treatments show a significant initial increase in the first hour, then the effects of the treatment gradually reduce. Therefore, treatment effects may be measured by the initial increase and also the rate of reduction. From the individual curves, one can also find patterns of correlation between consecutive measures.

We first fit a model to FEV1, i.e., Y_{ijk} from patient i under treatment k at hour j on the log-scale:

$$\log(Y_{ijk}) = \beta_y \log(Y_{ij-1k}) + \beta_k I(j = 1) + U_i + \varepsilon_{ijk} \tag{6.44}$$

where β_k is the effect of treatment k at 1 hour after the treated is given at 0 hour. Note that using $\log(Y_{i0k})$ as the lagged dependent variable for $\log(Y_{i1k})$ is not restrictively correct, due to the much longer than one hour interval the post treatment measures have, but we use this model for illustration. This setting assumes a direct effect on the first observation of this dynamic system. Direct effects on later hours can be tested by adding, e.g., $\beta_{2k} I(j = 2)$. the model is fitted with codes, where logy and loglag are $\log(Y_{ijk})$ and $\log(Y_{ij-1k})$ respectively,

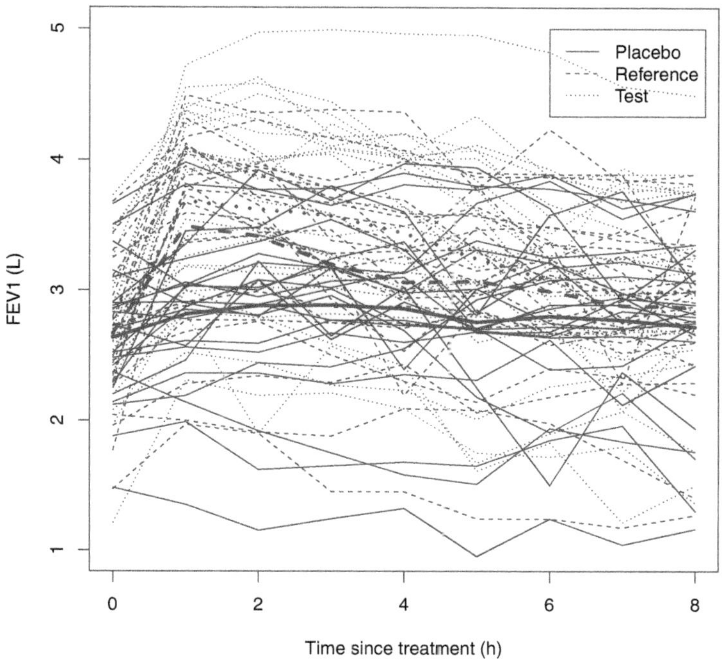

Figure 6.4
Mean (bold lines) and individual time profile of FEV1 measures after three treatments.

```
proc mixed data=fev1;
 class drug hour1 hour2 patient;
 model logy=loglag drug*hour1/solution;
 random patient;
 estimate 'a vs p' drug*hour1 -1 1 0 0 -1 1;
 estimate 'c vs p' drug*hour1 -0 0 -1 1 -1 1;
run;
```

which results in fixed effect estimates and comparisons of the two active treatments with placebo.

Effect	DRUG	hour1	Estimate	Standard Error	t Value
Intercept			0.3738	0.03966	9.43
loglag			0.6722	0.03051	22.03
DRUG*hour1	a	0	-0.03488	0.02289	-1.52
DRUG*hour1	a	1	0.2065	0.02948	7.00
DRUG*hour1	c	0	-0.01760	0.02340	-0.75
DRUG*hour1	c	1	0.2736	0.02948	9.28
DRUG*hour1	p	0	-0.05162	0.02235	-2.31
DRUG*hour1	p	1	0		

```
                          Standard
Label        Estimate        Error        DF      t Value      Pr > |t|

a vs p         0.1897      0.03168       546         5.99        <.0001
c vs p         0.2396      0.03198       546         7.49        <.0001
```

Both active treatments showed significant effects at 1 hour. There is also a strong dependency on the previous measure.

One may suspect if treatments also have effects on the time course (represented by β_{yi}), e.g., lowering the rate of decay. This can be tested by adding treatment effect on loglag in the code.

```
*effect on rate change;

proc mixed data=fev1;
 class drug hour1 patient;
 model logy=loglag loglag*drug drug*hour1 /solution;
 random patient;
run;
```

The results show no effect on it (the term loglag*DRUG).

```
          Type 3 Tests of Fixed Effects

                   Num      Den
 Effect             DF       DF     F Value     Pr > F

 loglag              1      544      476.68     <.0001
 loglag*DRUG         2      544        0.79     0.4552
 DRUG*hour1          5      544       53.81     <.0001.
```

One can also test whether there is a random effect on β_{yi} by adding loglag in the random statement:

```
*random dynamic?;

proc mixed data=fev1;
 class drug hour1 patient;
 model logy=loglag loglag*drug drug*hour1 /solution;
  random intercept loglag/subject=patient;
run;
```

But the results also did not show any random effect.

```
 Covariance Parameter Estimates

Cov Parm       Subject     Estimate

Intercept      PATIENT     0.007296
loglag         PATIENT            0
Residual                    0.01043
```

Finally, we add a term to represent direct effects at 2 hours

```
*drug effect later (hour2);
proc mixed data=fev1;
 class drug hour1 hour2 patient;
 model logy=loglag drug*hour1 drug*hour2/solution;
 random patient;
  estimate 'a vs p' drug*hour1 -1 1 0 0 1 -1;
 estimate 'c vs p' drug*hour1  0 0 -1 1 1 -1;
 estimate 'a vs p 2h' drug*hour2 -1 1 0 0 1 -1;
 estimate 'c vs p 2h' drug*hour2 0 0 -1 1 1 -1;
run;
```

However, although the effects are overall significant, there is no significant difference between the actives and the placebo.

Effect	Num DF	Den DF	F Value	Pr > F
loglag	1	543	413.52	<.0001
DRUG*hour1	3	543	86.51	<.0001
DRUG*hour2	3	543	3.92	0.0087

Estimates

Label	Estimate	Standard Error	DF	t Value	Pr > |t|
a vs p	0.1899	0.03162	543	6.01	<.0001
c vs p	0.2367	0.03190	543	7.42	<.0001
a vs p 2h	0.02590	0.03169	543	0.82	0.4140
c vs p 2h	0.02159	0.03168	543	0.68	0.4958

In general, it seems the first model we fit is reasonable.

6.7 Testing hysteresis

Since hysteresis indicates the need to use dynamic models, a proper assessment of hysteresis is advisable before fitting a complex dynamical model to deal with hysteresis. Even when hysteresis is statistically significant, it can sometimes not affect the ER modeling significantly enough to warrant modeling it in the ER model. When repeated measures are taken at several time points for both PK and PD, a pharmacometrics approach to identify hysteresis is plotting the PKPD data and linking the points in the order of observation times [Csajka and Verotta, 2006]. Hysteresis is indicated by an anti-clockwise loop, showing different responses at the same concentration level in the ascending and descending PK phases. The anti-clockwise curves provide an initial view on hysteresis. However, a formal test may also be useful.

As the effect compartment (6.1) is the source of hysteresis, a natural approach to testing the existence of hysteresis is to test if this compartment is necessary. Intuitively, the larger the K (here we assume $K_{in} = K$) the less the hysteresis, since with a sufficiently large K, the effect compartment becomes almost instantaneous. This suggests testing hysteresis with hypotheses

$$\begin{aligned} H_0 &: C^*(t) = C(t) \\ H_a &: C^*(t) = K\int_0^t \exp(-K\tau)C(t-\tau)d\tau, \end{aligned} \tag{6.45}$$

where $K < \infty$. It can be verified that if $C(t)$ is absolutely continuous, then $C^*(t) \to C(t)$ when $K \to \infty$. Therefore, we reject H_0 by showing $K < \infty$ with an appropriate statistical test procedure. To this end, a natural approach is the likelihood ratio test. This test compares the values of the likelihood function evaluated at H_0 and at H_a, therefore fitting a model for $C(t)$ together with (6.1) is needed.

The profile likelihood approach can be used to test the hypothesis (6.45). The procedure is very simple, but we should often concentrate on one or two parameters only in the effect compartment. The key parameter for hysteresis is K, therefore the first stage is, for a number of values K, to calculate the profile likelihood curve for statistical inference on K (see Appendix 10.2.2).

In the following, instead of using the effect compartment model, we propose using a very simple model as an instrument to perform the score test for hysteresis. Note that to control the type I error of the test, it is sufficient that the model under H_0 is correct. We can consider the simplest model :

$$C^*(t) = C(t-\delta), \tag{6.46}$$

where δ represents a constant delay between exposure changes in the central and effect compartments. Therefore, we can test hysteresis by testing $H_0 : \delta = 0$ vs $H_a : \delta > 0$. A more general instrumental model can also be introduced as

$$C_i^*(t) = C_i(t-\delta_i), \tag{6.47}$$

where $C_i^*(t)$ and $C_i(t)$ are concentrations of subject i, and $\delta_i = \delta_0 \exp(s_i)$ is the hysteresis of the i th subject with a fixed component δ_0 and a random component $\exp(s_i)$. However, since it is more difficult to test both together, we will only use (6.46). This model is rarely true, but as an instrumental model, it yields a simple score statistic for δ. It is easy to find $\partial C^*(t)/\partial\delta|_{\delta=0^-} = \dot{C}^-(t)$, the left derivative of $C(t)$ at time t.

We illustrate the approach with a simple ER model

$$Y_j = g(C^*(t_j), \boldsymbol{\beta}) + \varepsilon_j. \tag{6.48}$$

The score statistic can be written as

$$S(\boldsymbol{\beta}) = \sum_{j=1}^{J} \dot{C}^{-}(t_j) \frac{\partial g}{\partial C}(C(t_j), \boldsymbol{\beta})(Y_j - g(C(t_j - \delta), \boldsymbol{\beta}))|_{\delta=0}. \tag{6.49}$$

Under some technical conditions, $S(\boldsymbol{\beta})$ follows a normal distribution asymptotically with a zero mean and a variance that can be derived [Wang and Li, 2014]. The score test based on the instrumental model does not need to fit the model with an effect compartment, but still requires additional programming for the calculation of $S(\boldsymbol{\beta})$ and its variance.

The score statistic for a mixed model can also be derived, but the calculation is complex. To further simplify it, we propose using an approximation for the instrumental model:

$$C^*(t) = C(t - \delta) \approx C(t) - \delta \dot{C}^{-}(t). \tag{6.50}$$

Note that H_0 is equivalent to $\delta = 0$, so the approximation does not affect the type I error. To illustrate the implementation, we take the linear longitudinal model

$$Y_{ij} = C^*_{ij}\beta_i + U_i + \varepsilon_{ij}, \tag{6.51}$$

with $\beta_i = \beta + U_i$ as an example. To test H_0, we fit the model

$$Y_{ij} = C_{ij}\beta_i + \eta\dot{C}^{-}_{ij} + \mathbf{Z}^T_{ij}\gamma_i + w_i + \varepsilon_{ij}, \tag{6.52}$$

where $\dot{C}^{-}_{ij} = \dot{C}^{-}(t_{ij})$ and $w_i = -U_i\delta\dot{C}^{-}_{ij}$, that is to add $\dot{C}^{-}_{ij}$ in the model as a covariate. Then H_0 is tested by testing $H^*_0 : \eta \equiv -\beta\delta = 0$. Although H^*_0 is equivalent to H_0 only when $\beta \neq 0$, this restriction does not limit practical use of the test since it is only when $\beta \neq 0$ that the test for hysteresis is meaningful. The power may depend on how good is the approximation in (6.50). In practice, $\dot{C}^{-}_{ij}$ may be derived from a compartmental PK model. For example, with model (2.6), $\dot{C}^{-}_{ij}$ is proportional to $(-K_e \exp(-K_e t) + K_a \exp(-K_a t))|_{t=t_{ij}}$. Alternatively, it can also be estimated by a linear interpolation approach. The major advantage of this test over the others is the easiness in implementation using common statistical software. This test can also be applied to other models. For example, we can test $H_{0a} : \eta = 0$ for hysteresis in a logistic or beta regression model

$$\text{logit}(E(Y_{ij})) = C_{ij}\boldsymbol{\beta}_i + \dot{C}^{-}_{ij}\eta + \mathbf{Z}^T_{ij}\gamma_i. \tag{6.53}$$

Alternatively, the same approach can be used for GEE approaches. The details are very similar to that using GLMM, hence are omitted here.

We apply the score test procedure to the moxifloxacin and QT example described in the introduction, using both analytical derivatives and one using the finite difference approximation. For the approximation, the slope of linear interpolation is used to the left of each time point. To calculate the analytical one, the concentration data from each subject are fitted to the open one-compartment model with first-order absorption (6.2). The derivative of concentration at each time point is calculated from the fitted PK model for each individual. Then we fit a mixed linear model to repeated measures Δ QTcF with the corresponding concentrations and their analytical or approximate derivatives as fixed effects and subject as random effect. Hysteresis is tested using the coefficient of $\dot{C}_{ij}^{-}$. With the analytical derivatives, the χ^2 statistic (with 1 degree of freedom) is 16.19 and with the approximate one it is 12.45, both indicate a very significant hysteresis. The profile likelihood test can also be used and yields a χ^2 of 9.0, consistent with the other two tests. Therefore, all three tests suggest the existence of hysteresis between the PK and PD measures.

The test based on instrumental models is closely related to the lagged covariates model. Hysteresis can be tested based on this model since the contribution of lagged covariates represents the hysteresis. It has been shown Wang and Li [2014] that in some special situations the score test for a lagged covariate is equivalent to the instrumental model-based test using an approximate of $\dot{C}_{ij}^{-}$. However, in general cases, the instrumental model-based test is more powerful.

6.8 Comments and bibliographic notes

Many real examples for how dynamic models play a central role in ER modeling can be found from papers in *Journal of Pharmacokinetics and Pharmacodynamics*, as well as in Bonate [2006] and Ette and Williams [2007]. As typical disease process models, tumor growth models with different levels of complexity vary from empirical models to those derived from biological and pharmacological mechanisms. Bonate [2011] gives a nice summary and can serve as a starting point. Collaboration with clinical and pharmacological experts is the key to the successful dynamic modeling of the ER relationship.

Discrete-time dynamic models have been used in statistics as empirical models for longitudinal and time series data. As ways of describing a dynamic system with a simple model, they seem underused in general. A statistical introduction can be found in Fitzmaurice et al. [2008]. For more technical details, the reader is referred to Hsiao [2022], and their application in dose adjustment will be discussed in detail in Chapter 9.

7

Bayesian dose-exposure-response modeling

This chapter deals with Bayesian modeling for DER relationships, but most parts will take DR modeling as an example. The same principle and methods apply to DE and ER modeling or a combination of them. We will mainly consider parametric models, but we will also include the use of other Bayesian approaches with fewer model and prior specification. As there are several excellent books on Bayesian modeling and inference, e.g., Bernardo and Smith [2009]; Gelman et al. [1995]; Robert et al. [2007], we will mainly consider specific topics in DER modeling, especially prior specification, Bayesian modeling with a misspecified model, and approximate Bayesian inference using Bayesian bootstrap.

7.1 Bayesian modeling of dose-response relationship

7.1.1 Bayesian inference and information update

In recent years, we have seen rapid development in Bayesian modeling and inference, as well as their applications, in many areas, including modeling the DER relationship. Rather different from frequentist approaches that we have discussed so far, the Bayesian inference framework considers model parameters θ as random variables about which we may have prior information, and we update our information after observing data relating to them. This process of information update is presented by the Bayesian formula for the posterior density (or distribution) of $\boldsymbol{\theta}$:

$$p(\boldsymbol{\theta}|Y) = \frac{p(Y|\boldsymbol{\theta})\pi_0(\boldsymbol{\theta})}{p(Y)}, \tag{7.1}$$

where we use Y to represent the data we observed, $\pi_0(\boldsymbol{\theta})$ is the prior reflecting our prior knowledge of $\boldsymbol{\theta}$. The posterior distribution represents the updated information on $\boldsymbol{\theta}$ and is the key to Bayesian inference. $p(Y|\boldsymbol{\theta})$ is the density of Y given $\boldsymbol{\theta}$, which may include a DER model, and $p(Y)$ is the marginal density. Since $p(Y)$ is not a function of $\boldsymbol{\theta}$, we may write (7.1) as

$$p(\boldsymbol{\theta}|Y) \propto p(Y|\boldsymbol{\theta})\pi_0(\boldsymbol{\theta}) \tag{7.2}$$

DOI: 10.1201/9781003457008-7

An interesting point is that, if we have observed data Y^1, Y^2 sequentially, then we may write $p(\boldsymbol{\theta}|Y^1, Y^2) \propto p(Y^2|\boldsymbol{\theta})p(\boldsymbol{\theta}|Y^1)$, where $p(\boldsymbol{\theta}|Y^1)$ is the posterior of $\boldsymbol{\theta}$ after observing Y^1. This formula shows a sequential information update. However, we can also write $p(\boldsymbol{\theta}|Y^1, Y^2) \propto p(Y^1|\boldsymbol{\theta})p(\boldsymbol{\theta}|Y^2)$, therefore, the update after having observed the data Y^1, Y^2 does not depend on the time order of Y^1, Y^2.

7.1.2 Bayesian regression models

This section introduces the models for $p(Y|\boldsymbol{\theta})$ in (7.1) using the model we have introduced in previous chapters and shows the form of $p(\boldsymbol{\theta}|Y)$ for some common priors for $\pi_0(\boldsymbol{\theta})$. How to calculate $p(\boldsymbol{\theta}|Y)$, or sample from it, is left to the later sections. We will denote a vector that includes the dose and an intercept as X_i, which may also include covariates and Y_i here is the response in the DER relationship.

7.1.2.1 Linear models

For linear models

$$Y_i = X_i^T \boldsymbol{\beta} + \varepsilon_i \tag{7.3}$$

the following priors

$$\begin{aligned} \boldsymbol{\beta}|\sigma^2 &\sim N(\boldsymbol{\beta}_0, \sigma^2 \boldsymbol{\Sigma}) \\ \sigma^2 &\sim IG(a, b), \end{aligned} \tag{7.4}$$

where $x|y \sim F$ means that x conditional on y follows distribution F, leads to a posterior distribution in closed form. Note that the prior for$\boldsymbol{\beta}$ is specified as a distribution condition on σ. Let $S_x = \sum_{i=1}^n \mathbf{X}_i^T \mathbf{X}_i$, $\hat{\boldsymbol{\beta}}$ be the LS estimate for $\boldsymbol{\beta}$, $\boldsymbol{\Sigma}^* = (S_x + \boldsymbol{\Sigma})^{-1}$, and s^2 be the residual sum squares, the posterior distributions are

$$\begin{aligned} \boldsymbol{\beta}|\sigma^2 &\sim N(\Sigma^*(S_x \hat{\boldsymbol{\beta}} + \boldsymbol{\Sigma}^{-1}\boldsymbol{\beta}_0), \sigma^2 \boldsymbol{\Sigma}^*) \\ \sigma^2 &\sim IG(a + n/2, b + (s^2 + (\hat{\boldsymbol{\beta}} - \boldsymbol{\beta}_0)^T \boldsymbol{\Sigma}^* (\hat{\boldsymbol{\beta}} - \boldsymbol{\beta}_0))/2). \end{aligned} \tag{7.5}$$

They have the same form as their priors. With these posteriors, one can easily generate posterior samples by first taking samples for σ^2, then samples for $\boldsymbol{\beta}$, plugging the σ^2 sample as a parameter in the $\boldsymbol{\beta}$ distribution. Although we cannot use the conditional posterior distribution directly, the MCMC approach with Gibbs sampling can take advantage of this form [Gelman et al., 1995; Robert et al., 2007].

If we replace the prior for $\boldsymbol{\beta}$ by Zellner prior[Zellner, 1986]

$$\boldsymbol{\beta}|\sigma^2 \sim N(\boldsymbol{\beta}_0, \sigma S_x / n_0), \tag{7.6}$$

the posterior distributions has a simpler form:

$$\begin{aligned} \boldsymbol{\beta}|\sigma^2 &\sim N((\hat{\boldsymbol{\beta}} + n_0\boldsymbol{\beta}_0)/(n_0+1), \sigma^2 S_x/(n_0+1)) \\ \sigma^2 &\sim IG(a+(n-p)/2, b+(s^2+n_0(\hat{\boldsymbol{\beta}}-\boldsymbol{\beta}_0)^T S_x(\hat{\boldsymbol{\beta}}-\boldsymbol{\beta}_0)/(n_0+1))/2). \end{aligned} \tag{7.7}$$

where p is the dimension of $\boldsymbol{\beta}$. This prior has a simple relationship with the effect sample size (ESS) [Morita et al., 2008], as it means that the prior information on $\boldsymbol{\beta}$ is equivalent to n_0 "copies" of the observed data. This is reflected in the posterior distribution, as its mean is the weighted average of the LS and prior mean based on the observed and "pseudo" sample sizes, and the inverse variances are proportional to the total sample size. One may specify a weak prior by specifying a prior equivalent to, say, 1 copy of the observed information.

7.1.2.2 Generalized linear and nonlinear models

For GLM models, such as the logistic model, we can also use a multivariate normal prior $\boldsymbol{\beta} \sim N(\boldsymbol{\beta}_0, \boldsymbol{\Sigma})$ for the parameters of the linear predictor $\mathbf{X}_i^T\boldsymbol{\beta}$. The major difference is that not all parameters have an explicit conditional distribution as we have for linear models. To take a posterior sample, we will need another approach.

For nonlinear models with multiple parameters, we can also use the same form of priors, although often a transformation is needed for some parameters with range restrictions, such as ED50.

7.1.2.3 Mixed models

With linear mixed model

$$\begin{aligned} Y_{ij} &= \mathbf{X}_i^T\boldsymbol{\beta}_i + \epsilon_{ij} \\ \boldsymbol{\beta}_i &\sim N(\boldsymbol{\beta}, \boldsymbol{\Sigma}) \end{aligned} \tag{7.8}$$

the only new set of parameters is $\boldsymbol{\Sigma}$. A commonly used prior for it is the inverse Wishart prior. Therefore, for linear mixed models we may use priors

$$\begin{aligned} \boldsymbol{\beta} &\sim N(\boldsymbol{\beta}_0, \boldsymbol{\Sigma}) \\ \sigma^2 &\sim IG(a,b) \\ \boldsymbol{\Sigma} &\sim IW(\rho, \mathbf{R}) \end{aligned} \tag{7.9}$$

where $IW(\rho, \mathbf{R})$ is the inverse Wishart distribution with degree of freedom ρ and variance-covariance matrix $\mathbf{R}$. These priors are commonly used for technical convenience, but there are several alternatives.

Extending the model-prior combination to GLMM is also straightforward. Suppose that

$$g^{-1}(Y_{ij}) = \boldsymbol{\beta}_i^T\mathbf{X}_i \tag{7.10}$$

with $\boldsymbol{\beta}_i \sim N(\boldsymbol{\beta}, \boldsymbol{\Sigma})$, we can use

$$\begin{aligned} \boldsymbol{\beta} &\sim N(\boldsymbol{\beta}_0, \boldsymbol{\Sigma}) \\ \boldsymbol{\Sigma} &\sim IW(\rho, \mathbf{R}). \end{aligned} \tag{7.11}$$

Sometimes there may be additional parameters in the conditional distribution for Y_{ij}, for example, the over-dispersion parameter. In general, for a parameter that represents the magnitude of variation, a prior for variance σ^2 such as the inverse-gamma distribution can be used.

For NLMM

$$Y_{ij} = g(D_{ij}, \boldsymbol{\beta}_i) + \varepsilon_{ij} \tag{7.12}$$

with $\boldsymbol{\beta}_i \sim N(\boldsymbol{\beta}, \boldsymbol{\Sigma})$, we use a similar set of priors, together with that for ε_{ij}.

```
prior sigu ~ igamma(0.01,scale=0.01);
prior sig ~ igamma(0.01,scale=0.01);
 prior var_y ~ igamma(0.01, scale=0.01);
 parms  theta0 {-5 -2} beta {20 5 5} sig {1} Sigma var_y {4} sigu {1};
cl=exp(theta1);
v=exp(theta2);
pk=(dose/cl)*(1-exp(-cl*t2/v))*exp(-cl*(1-t1)*(time-tinf)/v);
var=(sig**2)*(pk**(2*0.22));
if ind=1 then pred=pk;
else if ind=0 then do;
   emaxi=exp(emax+u1);
   ec50i=exp(ec50);
   pred=E0+(emaxi-E0)*pk/(pk+ec50i);
   var=var_y;
end;
  random u1 ~ normal(0,var=sigu) subject=subject;
  random theta ~mvn(theta0,Sigma) subject=subject;
model resp ~ normal(pred,var=var);
run;
```

The summary of posterior distribution for the parameters are as follows.

Posterior Summaries

Parameter	Mean	Standard Deviation	Percentiles 25%	50%	75%
theta01	-5.4194	0.0723	-5.4642	-5.4183	-5.3734
theta02	-1.9020	0.0470	-1.9334	-1.9040	-1.8735
emax	9.1851	0.0569	9.1463	9.1765	9.2121
ec50	6.6917	0.1381	6.6074	6.7166	6.7978
e0	30.0969	0.5443	29.6991	30.0835	30.4841
sig	22.9332	0.7897	22.3485	22.9465	23.4893
Sigma1	0.1741	0.0427	0.1429	0.1661	0.1972
Sigma2	0.00937	0.0206	-0.00422	0.00849	0.0215
Sigma3	0.00937	0.0206	-0.00422	0.00849	0.0215

```
Sigma4        0.0631     0.0187    0.0504    0.0594    0.0721
var_y        16.5058     1.9074   15.1683   16.2539   17.6840
sigu         22.8149     5.4977   18.9758   21.6388   26.1234
```

However, diagnostic plots (not shown here) suggested that not all Markov chains converged properly. Nevertheless, comparing the Bayesian posterior means of the parameters with the estimates using proc NLMIXED, there is no substantial difference. The time for the proc MCMC run with the above setting took about ten times the CPU time as that for the proc NLMIXED run. Hence, one may ask what the added value is of the Bayesian approach. In terms of statistical inference, the most substantial one is that the Bayesian approach does not require asymptotic assumptions, which is essential for inference based on fitted models using proc NLMIXED. The distribution of posterior samples.

7.1.2.4 Time-to-event models

For a parametric survival model, the prior specification is similar to that for GLM or a nonlinear model. However, for a Cox model, additional consideration is needed for its unspecified baseline function $h_0(t)$. In the Bayesian framework, the baseline function does not cancel out. Therefore, one has to specify a prior distribution for $h_0(t)$ then calculate the likelihood from

$$S(t) = \exp(-H_0(t)\exp(\boldsymbol{\beta}\mathbf{X}_i)) \tag{7.13}$$

and $f(t) = -dS(t)/dt$ for Bayesian analysis. The main difficulty is that $h_0(t)$ is a functional and needs a more complex prior. A common choice is a piecewise increment prior for $H_0(t)$ within the intervals formed by the failure times, which is equivalent to piecewise constant priors for $h_0(t)$. Piecewise constant priors can be implemented in SAS proc PHREG [SAS Institute Inc., 2011], with the following command as a simple example:

```
BAYES CPRIOR=UNIFORM PIECEWISE=(NINTERVAL=10 PRIOR = UNIFORM);
```

where CPRIOR specifies the prior for the coefficient $\boldsymbol{\beta}$ and PIECEWISE=(NINTERVAL=10 PRIOR = UNIFORM) asks using a piecewise constant baseline function with 10 intervals and a uniform prior for the log-hazards for each interval, that is, we assume that $h_0(t) = h_k, k = 1, ..., K$ when t is in the kth interval and $h_k \propto C$. Several other options are available.

An alternative Bayesian approach to the above for fitting a Cox model is to treat the partial likelihood as an ordinary likelihood and derive the posterior distribution for $\boldsymbol{\beta}$ as

$$p(\boldsymbol{\beta}|\mathbf{Y}) \propto L_p(\mathbf{Y}|\boldsymbol{\beta})\pi_0(\boldsymbol{\beta}) \tag{7.14}$$

where $L_p(\mathbf{Y}|\boldsymbol{\beta})$ is the partial likelihood (5.6) and $\pi_0(\boldsymbol{\beta})$ is the prior distribution for $\boldsymbol{\beta}$. Note that the prior for the baseline risk is not needed as it does not exist in $L_p(\mathbf{Y}|\boldsymbol{\beta})$. Although this approach seems very simple, its implementation is not easy, as the calculation of $L_p(\mathbf{Y}|\boldsymbol{\beta})$ (5.6) requires identification of the risk set at each failure time. An example for implementing this approach can be found in examples for SAS proc MCMC.

7.1.2.5 Semiparametric Bayesian models

Recall that the model with a parametric part and a non-parametric part such as

$$Y_i = \beta_d D_i + \boldsymbol{\beta}^T B(D_i) + \epsilon_i \tag{7.15}$$

where $\boldsymbol{\beta}^T B(D_i)$, although seemed a part of the linear model, is to model an arbitrary, but smooth function of D_i. One may ask why bother having the linear part if the other part aims to capture all smooth curves. The rationale is that if the parametric part is correct, the semiparametric model can be more efficient than a non-parametric one. However, if it is not, the non-parametric part can capture the incorrect part.

A semiparametric model can also be constructed by adding a non-parametric term to the parametric part. The Emax model is flexible, but may still not enough to cover some types of DER curve, e.g., those with non-monotone patterns. For DR models with limited dose levels, one remedy is to add an extra flexible term:

$$Y_i = E_0 + E_{max}/(1 + EC_{50}/D_i) + U_{D_i} + \varepsilon_i. \tag{7.16}$$

where $U_{D_i} \sim N(0, \sigma_u^2)$ and $\sigma_u^2 \sim IG(a, b)$ [Gajewski et al., 2019]. When the model fits the data well, the posterior of σ_u^2 is small and the model behaves like an Emax model. But when the model is severely misspecified, the posterior mean of σ_u^2 is high and (7.16) becomes essentially a non-parametric model. This flexibility comes with costs: When misspecification occurs at, e.g., the high dose end, the whole model breaks down to non-parametric. Also, this approach does not work for the ER model with continuous exposure.

We use a logistic model to illustrate implementation of the semiparametric model approach and compare it with the simple logistic model. We take the probability of toxicity in scenarios 1 and 5 of Lee et al. [2015], for the latter, the logistic model is clearly misspecified. The model with random dose effect has wider quantiles, particularly when the model is misspecified, as a cost of its flexibility. The following code implements

```
library(brms)
yi=rbinom(5,100,Tox5)
doseb=1:5
dosef=as.factor(dose) #Dose as a factor for the radom effect
mdata=data.frame(yi=yi,ni=rep(100,5),doseb=doseb,dosef=dosef)
fit20 <- brm(yi| trials(ni) ~doseb ,  data=mdata,family = binomial())
fit21 <- brm(yi| trials(ni) ~doseb  + (1|dosef),  data=mdata,family = binomial())
pred0=predict(fit20)
pred1=predict(fit21)
```

```
> pred0
     Estimate Est.Error   Q2.5 Q97.5
[1,] 44.62950  6.328249 32.975    57
[2,] 61.72325  5.532297 51.000    72
[3,] 76.29025  4.770607 67.000    85
[4,] 86.51100  3.972194 78.000    94
[5,] 92.71100  3.018154 86.000    98
```

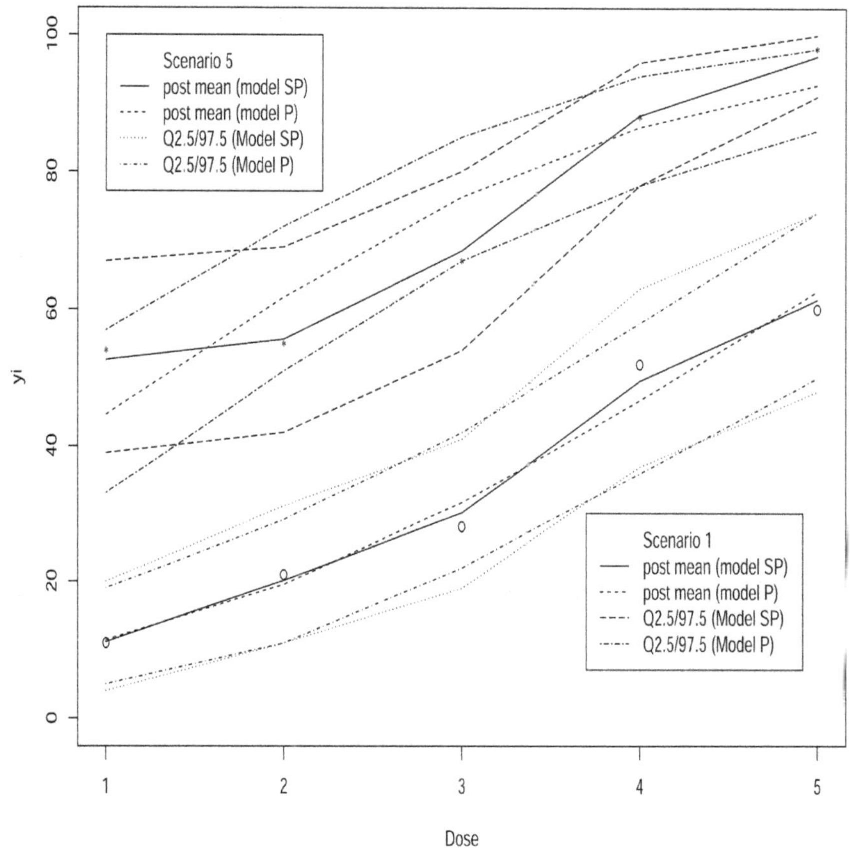

Figure 7.1
Posterior means and 0.025%, 0.975% quantiles of predicted posterior distribution using simple logistic regression (model P) and the logistic model with a random effect Model SP at dose level, for scenarios 1 and 5 in Lee et al. [2015], 100 subjects per dose.

An alternative that also works for ER models is to replace U_{D_i} with a realization of a Gaussian process. We assume that the ER curve is a sum of a parametric part and a non-parametric part with $U_{c_i} \sim N(0, \sigma_u^2)$ and $cov(U_{c_i}, U_{c_j})$ is a function depending on $d = |c_i - c_j|$, e.g., the Ornstein–Uhlenbeck covariance function $cov(U_{c_i}, U_{c_j}) = \exp(-d/C_d)$ with parameter C_d. Then we need to specify the prior distributions of both σ_u^2 and C_d, hence it is more complex than U_{D_i} as a non-parametric term.

The following Stan code implements the semiparametric model with Gaussian-process driven non-parametric term, with data generated as in the code:

```
  N=5
ni=100
dose=1:5
bdose=dose
prob=c(1,3,6,8,6)/10 #logistic model misspecified
#prob=1/(1+exp(3-dose))  # logisitc model
yi=rbinom(5,100,prob)

N1=5
ndose=seq(from=1,to=5,by=0.25)
ldose=c(dose,ndose)
N=length(ldose)
dat=list(z1=yi,N1=N1,N=N,ni=ni,x1=dose,x=ldose,bx=ldose,bdose=dose)

gpcode <- "
data {
  int<lower=1> N1;
    int<lower=1> N;
    int<lower=1> ni;
  array[N1] int<lower=0> z1;
    vector[N1] bdose;
  array[N] real x;
      vector[N] bx;
}
transformed data {
  real delta = 1e-9;
  int<lower=1> N2=N-N1;

}
parameters {
  real<lower=0> rho;
  real alpha;
  real beta;
  real a;
  vector[N] eta;
}
transformed parameters {
  vector[N] f;
  {
    matrix[N, N] L_K;
    matrix[N, N] K = gp_exp_quad_cov(x, alpha, rho);

    // diagonal elements
    for (n in 1:N) {
      K[n, n] = K[n, n] + delta;
    }

    L_K = cholesky_decompose(K);
    f = L_K * eta;
  }
}
model {
  rho ~ inv_gamma(5, 5);
```

```
  alpha ~ std_normal();
  beta ~ std_normal();
  a ~ std_normal();
  eta ~ normal(0, 10);
  z1 ~ binomial_logit(ni,a +beta*bdose+ f[1:N1]);
}
generated quantities {
  array[N2] int z2;
  array[N2] real p2;
  for (n2 in 1:N2) {
  z2[n2] = binomial_rng(ni,inv_logit(a +beta*bx[N1 + n2]+ f[N1 + n2]));
    p2[n2] = inv_logit(a +beta*bx[N1 + n2]+ f[N1 + n2]);
  }
}
"


fit <- stan(model_code = gpcode, model_name = "example",
          data = dat, warmup =5000, iter = 7000, chains = 3, verbose = F)

predz=summary(fit,pars="z2")$summary

par(mfrow=c(1,2),mar=c(5,4,2,1))
plot(dose,yi,ylim=c(0,100),xlab="Dose",ylab="Number of responses")
lines(ndose,predz[,1])
lines(ndose,predz[,4],lty=2)
lines(ndose,predz[,8],lty=2)
lines(ndose,predz[,5],lty=3)
lines(ndose,predz[,7],lty=3)

legend(x=1,y=100,legend=c("Posterior Mean",
      "2.5/97.5% quantiles","25/75% quantiles"),lty=1:3)
```

The posterior means and 0.025/0.975%, 25/75% quantiles of predicted number of events by the semi-parametric logistic model when the data are generated with and without model misspecification are plotted in Figure 7.2. The posterior distributions are much narrower when there is no model misspecification, while when misspecification occurs at the high-dose end, the posterior distribution is generally wider, especially in the region when the misspecification occurs.

7.2 Prior specification

The first key step in Bayesian modeling is to specify the prior distribution $\pi_0(\boldsymbol{\theta})$ for the model parameters. $\pi_0(\boldsymbol{\theta})$ should reflect our prior information (or lack of it) about $\boldsymbol{\theta}$. The prior distribution is often specified in a parametric form $\pi_0(\boldsymbol{\theta}|\boldsymbol{\theta}_0)$, with hyper-parameters $\boldsymbol{\theta}_0$. Therefore, the task of prior

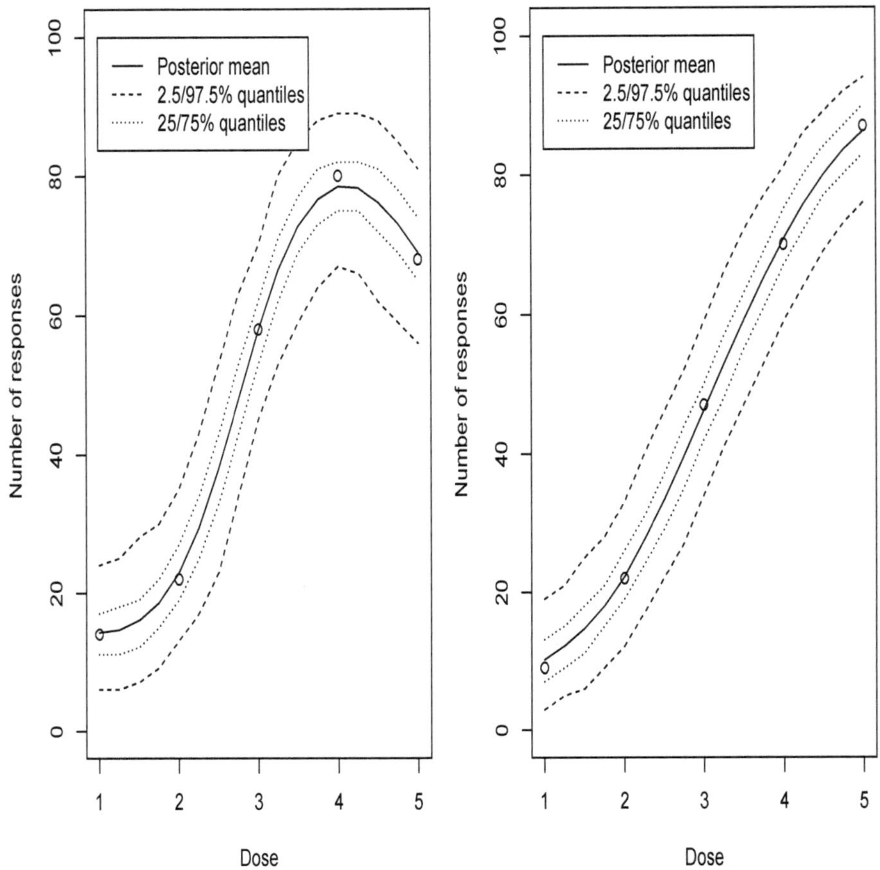

Figure 7.2
Posterior means and 0.025/0.975%, 25/75% quantiles of predicted number of events by the semi-parametric logistic model with a Gaussian process prior. Left panel: data generated with probabilities (0.1, 0.3, 0.6, 0.8, 0.6) for dose levels (1, 2, 3, 4, 5); right panel: data generated by a logistic model, 100 subjects per dose.

specification can be simplified to determine the hyperparameter values after the function $\pi_0(\boldsymbol{\theta}|\boldsymbol{\theta}_0)$ is determined.

The posterior distribution depends on both the prior and the model (or data) parts. The data part will dominate with increasing sample sizes. However, for sparse data, the prior can be a crucial factor in the posterior. To show the impact of the prior, we take the scenario in Neuenschwander et al. [2008] as an example, in which five doses (1,2.5, 5, 10, 25) are tested in (3, 4, 5, 4, 2) subjects, respectively. Only two subjects at dose=25 had dose-limiting

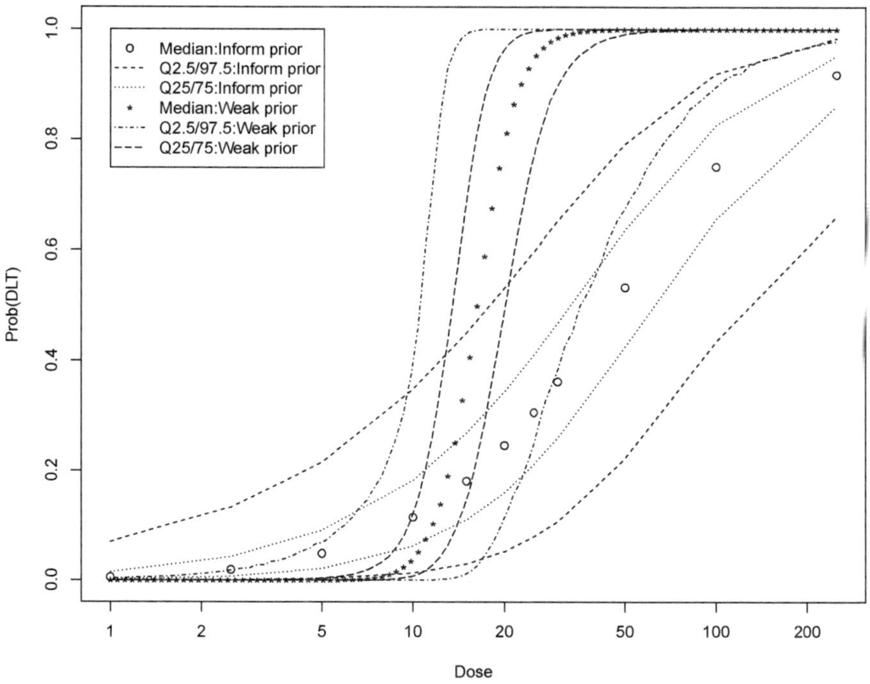

Figure 7.3
Predicted posterior 2.5, 25, 50, 97.5% quantiles of probability of DLT by fitted logistic regression models with weakly informative prior and a strongly informative prior.

toxicity, the response of interest. Hence, we cannot fit a logistic model, as this is known as a separated case, and the coefficient of dose cannot be estimated.

With informative priors, the Bayesian approach can fit the model, although the fitted model heavily depends on the prior. Using the weakly informative prior of Cauchy(0, 2.5) [Gelman et al., 2008], we can fit a logistic model. However, the predicted posterior probability of DLT, as shown by the median and quantiles, has a rapid jump in the middle of the dose range, as the data suggested. With a strong informative prior as elicited in Neuenschwander et al. [2008], the fitted logistic model gives a rather different posterior probability pattern. Figure 7.3 shows the difference in the fitted models with these two priors.

The following are codes for fitting the logistic model with weakly informative prior (which can be implemented by calling the function brm in R-library brms. However, using the prior given in Neuenschwander et al. [2008], in which the coefficient of dose is exponentially transformed to enforce monotonicity, but not for the intercept, requires some programming. The following code calls rstan (with the Stan code) for its implementation. The code for implementing the weakly informative prior is also included, but the other parts (sample extraction and plotting) are omitted.

```
    DoseRef=250 # Ref dose
dose=log(c(1,2.5, 5, 10, 25)/DoseRef) #log dose (tested) normalized
dname=c(1, 2.5, 5, 10, 15, 20, 25, 30,50,100,250) #dose levels for prediction
alldose=log(c(1, 2.5, 5, 10, 15, 20, 25, 30,50,100,250)/DoseRef)
nlong=length(alldose)
ni=c(3, 4, 5, 4, 2) #Number of subjects
yi=c(0,0,0,0,2)  #Number of DLTs
N=length(yi)
data1=data.frame(dose=dose,ni=ni,yi=yi)

# Weakly informative prior
prior=c(set_prior("normal(0,10)", class ="Intercept"),set_prior("cauchy(0, 2.5)"
          , class = "b", coef = "dose"))
fit00 <- brm(yi| trials(ni) ~dose , iter=4000, thin=2, data=data1
            ,family = binomial(),prior=prior)
# Prior in Neuenschwander et al (2008)
Sig=matrix(c(0.84,0.2,0.2,0.8),2,2)
mu=c(2.15,0.52)

gpcode <- "
data {
  int<lower=1> N;
  array[N] int ni;
    int<lower=1> nlong;
  vector[N]   dose;
  vector[nlong] alldose;
    vector[2] mu;
    matrix[2,2] Sig;
  array[N] int<upper=100> yi;
}

parameters {
  vector[2] beta;
}

model {

   beta ~ multi_normal(mu, Sig);
  yi ~ binomial_logit(ni, beta[1] + exp(beta[2])*dose);
}
generated quantities{
  vector[nlong] predp;
     predp=inv_logit(beta[1] + exp(beta[2])*alldose);
}
"
dat=list(yi=yi,N=N,ni=ni,dose=dose,mu=mu, Sig=Sig,nlong=nlong
                                                ,alldose=alldose)
fit<-stan(model_code = gpcode, model_name = "Neuenschwander et al (2008)",
            data = dat, warmup =3000, iter = 5000, chains = 3, verbose = F)
predp=summary(fit,pars="predp")$summary

plot(dname,predp[,6],ylim=c(0,1),xlab="Dose", ylab="Prob(DLT)",log="x")
lines(dname,predp[,4],lty=2)
lines(dname,predp[,8],lty=2)
lines(dname,predp[,5],lty=3)
lines(dname,predp[,7],lty=3)
```

Although there are many choices in terms of prior distribution, the most commonly used are conjugate priors, which makes the posterior distribution belong to the same family. See the example in the linear model cases. Conjugate priors are also available for some other type of outcomes. For example, if $Y \sim Bin(n,p)$ with prior p following $Beta(a,b)$ prior, then $p(p|y) \sim Beta(a+y, b+n)$ after having observed $Y = y$. Other model-conjugate prior combinations are the Poisson-gamma and multinomial-Dirichlet pairs. One practical advantage of using a conjugate prior is that, for some simple situations, the posterior distribution can be derived analytically. This advantage is not as important as in the past, since for many DER models it is not easy to specify a conjugate prior, and widely used Bayesian software in combination with modern computer power can easily calculate the posterior distribution without conjugate priors. However, the use of conjugate priors has some other advantage, e.g., to determine ESS[Morita et al., 2008].

Sometimes, we also need a non-parametric prior when the model or a part of it is non-parametric, e.g., a non-parametric ER curve or the baseline risk in Cox regression. Another example of using a non-parametric prior is the Bayesian bootstrap [Rubin, 1981], as described in the Appendix 10.5.

Ideally, the prior distribution should reflect the information and knowledge before observing the data in the analysis. Priors of this nature are called informative priors. However, often non-informative priors that carry no information are preferred. One reason is to make analyses as objective as possible; hence, the analysis uses the Bayesian framework but is not influenced by prior information or knowledge. Another reason is that there is often no prior knowledge or information, or they are too vague to be quantified.

Often it is not easy to specify noninformative priors, as it may not be clear if a prior is truly non-informative or not, even in some very simple cases. For example, a prior of equal probability for any possible parameter value (uniform prior) seems to be non-informative. However, if the parameter is transformed on log-scale, then this prior on the log-scale is no longer uniform, hence its non-informativeness is not transformation invariant. This uniform prior is improper (i.e., it does not have a density function) if the parameter range is not finite. This might not be a problem for Bayesian inference, as long as the resulting posterior distribution is proper. Nevertheless, improper priors do cause issues in some situations such as model selection.

There are priors derived for a model that minimize the information it carries into the posterior distribution, known as reference priors. The most commonly used is Jeffrey's prior,

$$f(\boldsymbol{\xi}) \sim |\mathbf{I}(\boldsymbol{\theta})|^{1/2} \tag{7.17}$$

where $|I(\boldsymbol{\theta})|$ denotes the determinant of the information matrix $I(\boldsymbol{\theta})$. It can be easily checked that this prior is transformation invariant, so it does not have the problem of uniform priors. Details about reference priors and Bayesian analysis based on these priors involve some technical complexity. They can be found in, e.g., Robert et al. [2007]. In practice, standard software such as SAS and R has an option to use Jeffreys prior, hence its implementation is an easy task.

To avoid the problem of improper uniform priors, one may specify a prior distribution that carries a very small amount of information but is also easy to handle. For example, $f(\boldsymbol{\beta}) \sim N(1,1)$ is a strong prior suggesting that β is around 1. However, $f(\beta) \sim N(1,10000)$, contains almost no information, although it is still centered around 1. An apparently informative prior, but with huge variability, is known as a diffused prior and has been widely used in practice. However, a highly variable prior may make the model fitting unstable, particularly when the sample size is small.

Informative priors are useful as they represent the expert's best knowledge on the ER relationship, which is invaluable for decision making when data are sparse. The process of transferring knowledge (or belief) to the prior is called prior elicitation. A common way to elicit prior is to let the expert specify some statistics and then to use a parametric distribution to approximate them. For example, if a coefficient is believed to have a mean = 2 and 90% chance to be within the range of 1 and 3, then a normal prior distribution with this property should have a mean 2 and SD=$\Phi^{-1}(0.95) = 0.61$. Note that in this case the form of prior distribution, i.e., normality, is also a part of prior, which is often suggested by the data analyst rather than the expert. Other distributions can also be specified to meet the same criteria, and they may behave quite differently when putting into a model. The issue is that although the mean and range are specified correctly, different distributions extrapolate them into different global specifications, which may not reflect the expert's knowledge. Therefore, using informative priors carries considerable risk, especially when the sample size is small.

For DR models, the prior information elicited can be presented as the range of possible DR curves by dose level. To use this prior in a parametric model, we can approximate it with a prior for the model parameters. The following code shows how to convert a hypothetical prior given by the quantiles 5% and 95% at multiple dose levels.

```
    # Find optimal normal prior
dose=log(c(1,2,5,10,20))
q1=c(0,0,0.1,0.15,0.2) #Q5
q2=c(0.3,0.4,0.6,0.8,0.9) #Q95

obj=function(beta){
  mu=beta[1]+dose*beta[2]
  sig=sqrt(beta[3]+2*beta[4]*sqrt(beta[3]*beta[5])*dose+dose^2*beta[5])
  p1=qnorm(0.05,mu,sig)
  p2=qnorm(0.95,mu,sig)
  mean((c(q1,q2)-1/(1+exp(-c(p1,p2))))^2)
}
beta=optim(par=c(-1,0.5,1,-0.5,1),fn=obj,method="L-BFGS-B",
            lower=c(-9,-9,0,-1,0),upper=c(9,9,9,1,9))$par
```

```
mu=beta[1]+dose*beta[2]
sig=sqrt(beta[3]+2*beta[4]*sqrt(beta[3]*beta[5])*dose+dose^2*beta[5])
p1=1/(1+exp(-qnorm(0.05,mu,sig)))
p2=1/(1+exp(-qnorm(0.95,mu,sig)))
plot(dose,p1,type="l",ylim=c(0,1),ylab="Quantile",xlab="log-dose")
lines(dose,p2,lty=2)
lines(dose,q1,lty=3)
lines(dose,q2,lty=4)
legend(x=0,y=1,legend=c("Elicited Q5","Elicited Q95","Fitted Q5",
                                   "Fitted Q95"),lty=1:4)
```

The generated plot (Figure 7.4) shows the difference between the elicited quantiles and model quantiles with the fitted multivariate normal prior.

A Bayesian approach should be robust to prior mis-specification in the sense that when the sample size becomes large, the impact of the prior distribution becomes weak and finally diminishes. However, when using a Bayesian approach in practice, we are more interested in its small sample properties, in which the prior may have a considerable impact. A measure of the impact of prior on the modeling is ESS [Morita et al., 2008]. To show how ESS is defined, consider the situation of using a vague or non-informative prior and observing data of sample size k. Suppose that one can derive the posterior distribution based on the vague prior and the data. If an informative prior gives the same amount of information, e.g., in terms of the posterior variance-covariance matrix of parameters, then k can be considered as the ESS of the informative prior. ESS can be found easily for some specific situations, in particular, for conjugate priors. For example, for $Y_i \sim N(\mu, 1)$ with prior $\mu \sim N(\mu_0, \sigma^2)$, the

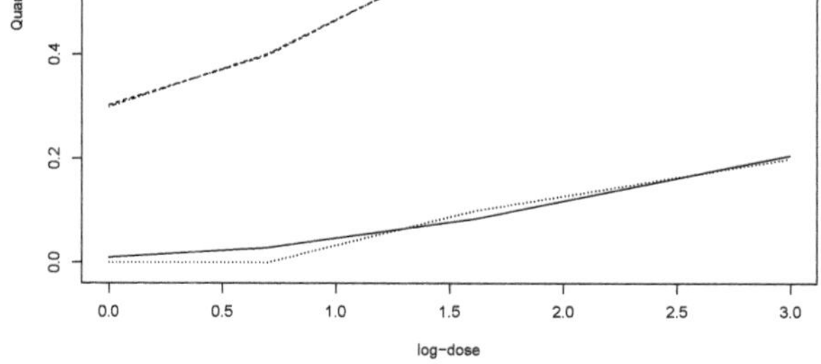

Figure 7.4
Fitted multivariate normal prior for logistic regression models to elicited prior quantiles.

ESS is $1/\sigma^2$. In many cases, e.g., when the prior-model are not conjugate, there may be no exact equivalence between the prior and a dataset of certain size, but the ESS can be defined as the sample size that minimize the determinant of the difference between the information matrices of the posterior distribution from the data and vague prior, and of the informative prior distribution. Different definitions of distance may lead to different ESS in non-conjugate situations.

For DER modeling, the definition of ESS is more complex, since it also depends on at which doses the samples are taken. If the dose distribution is known, we can average over it. An interesting point is that the ESS of a prior is the lowest if the doses are assigned according to an optimal design. In some sittings, such as a linear model in matrix form: $Y = X^T\boldsymbol{\beta} + \epsilon$ with n subjects, where X includes dose and intercept, the g prior for $\boldsymbol{\beta}$ has a multivariate normal distribution $\boldsymbol{\beta} \sim N(\boldsymbol{\beta}_0, g\sigma(X^TX)^{-1})$, where σ^2 is the variance of the error term. In terms of posterior variance var($\boldsymbol{\beta}$), this prior is equivalent to having observed $g^{-1}n$ subjects with mean $\boldsymbol{\beta}_0$, hence $ESS = g^{-1}n$.

Closely related to ESS is the pseudo-data prior [Whitehead and Williamson, 1998], which is in the form of data, but may reflect prior knowledge about model parameters. Sometimes, this comes naturally from a prior elicitation process. For example, a physician may have treated 3 patients with a treatment and believe that if the 3 patients are given 1mg dose, it is likely that two-thirds of them may have an AE. Then a record in the pseudo-data prior will be 2 events from 3 trials with 1mg dose. Approximately the ESS of this pseudo-data prior is 3 from a binary distribution with $p = 2/3$. The whole pseudo-data set may consist of multiple records at different dose levels. To use pseudo-prior we simply fit the prior data together with the current data to the model. The resulting parameter estimates are for the posterior modes, hence this approach may be a good choice if one only needs the posterior mode, e.g., for a simulation study to assess dose escalation algorithms, as it is simple and more efficient than using prior distributions in combination with a MCMC approach to obtain the posterior distribution. The pseudo data may not correctly reflect the uncertainty of prior information. For example, to specify a complex prior, one may need 10 records in the pseudo data, but the expert feels that the amount of information, after taking uncertainty into account, should be equivalent to ESS=3. A practical way to adjust it is to weight the records properly so that the contribution of the prior relative to the real data reflects the uncertainty. In the example above, the weight for the prior data should be 3/10, while observed data have weight 1.

For regression models such as a DR model, where X contains dose and intercept, the ESS of a pseudo-prior data also depends on the distributions of both pseudo and real data. Suppose that the real data has determinant of information $\sigma^2|X^TX|$ with sample size k and that of the pseudo data $\sigma^2|X_p^TX_p|$, then

$$ESS = k\frac{\sigma^2|X_p^TX_p|}{\sigma_p^2|X^TX|}. \tag{7.18}$$

The prior specification is closely related to the model structure. Taking the Emax model

$$Y_i = E_0 + E_{max}/(1 + EC_{50}/D_i) + \varepsilon_i. \tag{7.19}$$

as an example. Here, the parameters are E_0, E_{max}, EC_{50} and $\text{var}(\varepsilon_i) = \sigma^2$. For convenience, we denote $\boldsymbol{\beta} = (E_0, E_{max}, EC_{50})$. Note that one needs to specify the prior distribution for all parameters, including σ^2, to find the posterior distribution (7.2). In general, for model

$$Y_i = g(c_i, \boldsymbol{\beta}) + \varepsilon_i \tag{7.20}$$

we often use the following priors:

$$\begin{aligned} \boldsymbol{\beta} &\sim N(\boldsymbol{\beta}_0, \boldsymbol{\Sigma}) \\ \boldsymbol{\Sigma}^2 &\sim IG(a, b), \end{aligned} \tag{7.21}$$

where $IG(a, b)$ is an inverse gamma distribution, in which parameters $\boldsymbol{\beta}_0, \boldsymbol{\Sigma}$, a and b are hyper-parameters we have to supply as a part of the prior distributions. To reduce the impacts of the prior selection, often the hyper-parameters are selected to make the distribution as wide as possible to diffuse the prior.

7.2.1 Argatroban example by Bayesian analysis

Here we revisit the argatroban example to fit the same models with Bayesian approaches. To start with, we used the sequential approach to fit the Emax model for the relationship between aPTT and predicted concentration. For simplicity, we reuse the frequentist concentration prediction to focus on ER modeling. The following proc MCMC program is adapted from the proc NLMIXED program in Section 4.2.3.

```
proc mcmc data=pred nbi=5000 nmc=3000 outpost=postout seed=23 init=random;
ods select Parameters REParameters PostSummaries;
array theta[3] emax ec50 e0;
array mu0[3] (0 0 0);
array Sig0[3,3] (1000 0 0 0 1000 0 0 0 1000);
prior theta ~ mvn(mu0, Sig0);
prior sigu ~ igamma(0.01,scale=0.01);
 prior var_y ~ igamma(0.01, scale=0.01);
 parms  theta {20 5 5} var_y {4} sigu {1};
   emaxi=exp(emax+u1);
   ec50i=exp(ec50);
   pred=E0+(emaxi-E0)*conc/(conc+ec50i);
  random u1 ~ normal(0,var=sigu) subject=subject;
model pd ~ normal(pred, var=var_y);
run;
```

In the program diffused priors are used for all the parameters, and the MCMC starting values for some parameters are based on the fitted model by the frequentist approach. The following show summary statistics of the posterior samples. The means are similar to those of the frequentist estimate, but some SDs are considerably different from the SEs of the frequentist ones.

Parameter	Mean	Standard Deviation
emax	4.8384	0.1205
ec50	7.6948	0.1220
e0	30.7843	0.0888
var_y	21.3648	2.4320
sigu	0.0925	0.0317

However, this fitting, as shown, did not converge properly. The following program fits a model with a slightly different parameterization and with additional random effects on the baseline.

```
proc mcmc data=pred nbi=10000 nmc=3000 outpost=postout seed=23 init=random;
ods select Parameters REParameters PostSummaries;
array theta[3] emax ec50 e0;
array mu0[3] (0 0 0);
array Sig0[3,3] (1000 0 0 0 1000 0 0 0 1000);
prior theta ~ mvn(mu0, Sig0);
prior sigu ~ igamma(0.01,scale=0.01);
 prior var_y ~ igamma(0.01, scale=0.01);
 parms  theta {20 5 5} var_y {4} sigu {1};
   emaxi=exp(emax+u1);
   ec50i=exp(ec50);
   pred=E0+(emaxi-E0)*conc/(conc+ec50i);
  random u1 ~ normal(0,var=sigu) subject=subject;
model pd ~ normal(pred, var=var_y);
run;
```

The posterior samples for the model parameters are summarized as follows.

Posterior Summaries

Parameter	Mean	Standard Deviation	Percentiles 25%	50%	75%
emax	4.8846	0.1188	4.8038	4.8787	4.9665
ec50	7.7193	0.1185	7.6394	7.7106	7.7984
e0	30.6840	0.0932	30.6036	30.6947	30.7614
var_y	21.5298	2.4275	19.8539	21.3968	23.0193
sigu	0.0851	0.0291	0.0646	0.0805	0.1001

The proc NLMIXED program for joint modeling can be adapted to fit the joint models with proc MCMC. Again we use the results from proc NLMIXED to determine the initial parameter values here.

```
proc mcmc data=arg nbi=20000 nmc=3000 thin=5 outpost=postout
     seed=123 init=random PROPCOV=QUANEW;
ods select Parameters REParameters PostSummaries;
array beta[3] emax ec50 e0;
array theta[2] theta1 theta2;
array mu0[3] (0 0 0);
array S[2,2] (1 0 0 1);
array theta0[2];
array Sigma[2,2];
array theta00[2] (0 0);
array Sig0[3,3] (1000 0 0 0 1000 0 0 0 1000);
array Sigb[2,2] (1000 0 0 1000);
prior beta ~ mvn(mu0, Sig0);
prior theta0 ~ mvn(theta00, Sigb);
prior Sigma ~ iwish(4, S);
prior sigu ~ igamma(0.01,scale=0.01);
prior sig ~ igamma(0.01,scale=0.01);
 prior var_y ~ igamma(0.01, scale=0.01);
 parms  theta0 {-5 -2} beta {20 5 5} sig {1} Sigma var_y {4} sigu {1};
cl=exp(theta1);
v=exp(theta2);
pk=(dose/cl)*(1-exp(-cl*t2/v))*exp(-cl*(1-t1)*(time-tinf)/v);
var=(sig**2)*(pk**(2*0.22));
if ind=1 then pred=pk;
else if ind=0 then do;
   emaxi=exp(emax+u1);
   ec50i=exp(ec50);
   pred=E0+(emaxi-E0)*pk/(pk+ec50i);
   var=var_y;
end;
  random u1 ~ normal(0,var=sigu) subject=subject;
  random theta ~mvn(theta0,Sigma) subject=subject;
model resp ~ normal(pred,var=var);
run;
```

The summary of posterior distribution for the parameters are as follows.

Posterior Summaries

Parameter	Mean	Standard Deviation	Percentiles 25%	50%	75%
theta01	-5.4194	0.0723	-5.4642	-5.4183	-5.3734
theta02	-1.9020	0.0470	-1.9334	-1.9040	-1.8735
emax	9.1851	0.0569	9.1463	9.1765	9.2121
ec50	6.6917	0.1381	6.6074	6.7166	6.7978
e0	30.0969	0.5443	29.6991	30.0835	30.4841
sig	22.9332	0.7897	22.3485	22.9465	23.4893
Sigma1	0.1741	0.0427	0.1429	0.1661	0.1972
Sigma2	0.00937	0.0206	-0.00422	0.00849	0.0215

Sigma3	0.00937	0.0206	-0.00422	0.00849	0.0215
Sigma4	0.0631	0.0187	0.0504	0.0594	0.0721
var_y	16.5058	1.9074	15.1683	16.2539	17.6840
sigu	22.8149	5.4977	18.9758	21.6388	26.1234

However, diagnostic plots (not shown here) suggested that not all Markov chains converged properly. Nevertheless, comparing the Bayesian posterior means of the parameters with the estimates using proc NLMIXED, there is no substantial difference. The time for the proc MCMC run with the above setting took about ten times the CPU time as that for the proc NLMIXED run. Hence, one may ask what the added value is for the Bayesian approach. In terms of statistical inference, the most substantial one is that the Bayesian approach does not require asymptotic assumptions, which is essential for inference based on fitted models using proc NLMIXED. The distribution of posterior samples is ready to use for estimation of credible intervals, hypothesis testing, and decision analysis that we will introduce later.

7.2.2 Bayesian inference based on posterior distribution or sample

Bayesian inference for model parameters of interest can be mainly based on the posterior distribution. After obtaining $p(\boldsymbol{\theta}|Y)$ with observed data Y, inference for $\boldsymbol{\theta}$ is straightforward. For example, we can calculate $P(\theta > \theta_0|Y)$, or the 95% credible interval defined as the narrowest interval (C_1, C_2) that satisfies $P(C_1 \leq \theta \leq C_2|Y) = 0.95$. One may also test hypothesis $H_0 : \theta < \theta_0$ according to $P(\theta < \theta_0|Y)$ and reject H_0 if $P(\theta < \theta_0|Y) < \alpha$. This approach is similar to the frequentist test procedure. But an important difference is that the type I error of the frequentist test refers to the rejection rate of repeating the experiment under H_0, while $P(\theta < \theta_0|Y)$ is simply the probability that H_0 is true, given the data and model. Similarly, $P(C_1 \leq \theta \leq C_2|Y)$ is the probability of $C_1 \leq \theta \leq C_2$, given the data and the model. Therefore, the Bayesian framework leads to a more intuitive interpretation of the modeling results.

Bayesian point estimate for $\boldsymbol{\theta}$ can also be derived from the posterior distribution. Note that $\boldsymbol{\theta}$ is a random vector, but its posterior mean, median, and mode can be estimated. If a criterion for point estimate can be specified, an optimal one can be found too. For example, the posterior mean is the optimal estimate that minimizes the posterior mean squared error of the prediction, in the sense of Bayesian decision analysis, as discussed later.

In the frequentist framework, although one can predict further outcomes with estimated parameters, it is often difficult to quantify the uncertainty and variability of the prediction, as they typically depend on true parameter values. Bayesian prediction can be based on the posterior distribution. Let Y_f be the response in the future; after observing Y, its distribution can be written as

$$p(Y_f|Y) = \int p(Y_f|\boldsymbol{\beta})p(\boldsymbol{\beta}|Y)d\boldsymbol{\beta}. \tag{7.22}$$

As the Markov chain Monte Carlo (MCMC) approach (described in the next section) gives the posterior samples $\boldsymbol{\beta}_1, .\boldsymbol{\beta}_s.., \boldsymbol{\beta}_S$, rather than $p(\boldsymbol{\beta}|Y)$, we can calculate (7.22) by

$$\hat{p}(Y_f|Y) = \sum_{s=1}^{S} p(Y_f|\boldsymbol{\beta}_s). \tag{7.23}$$

7.2.3 Bayesian computing: from prior to posterior distributions

Bayesian inference is based on the posterior distribution, hence its calculation has been the key issue in the implementation of Bayesian approaches. Today, this calculation can be done much easier and quicker, even for quite complex models, than twenty years ago, thanks to the development of efficient MCMC algorithms and powerful modern computers. Although $p(\boldsymbol{\theta}|Y)$ has no closed form for most of the model-prior combinations, sampling from $p(\boldsymbol{\theta}|Y)$ with MCMC is still an efficient approach to Bayesian inference.

MCMC uses Markov chains in simulations to obtain posterior samples from posterior distributions that are difficult or impossible to sample directly, including distributions with no analytical form. Two samplers have been used for MCMC for a long time and are implemented in common statistical software. When sampling from a multi-dimension distribution is not feasible, the Gibbs sampler is a standard tool to use, if the distribution of an individual element, conditional on the others is easy to sample from. For example, if we would like to sample $\mathbf{Y} = (Y_1, ..., Y_k)$ from $p(Y_1, ..., Y_k)$, using the Gibbs sampler, we first sample Y_1^* from $p(Y_1|Y_2, ..., Y_k)$ where $Y_2, ..., Y_k$ are initial values, then Y_2 from $p(Y_2|Y_1^*, Y_3, ..., Y_k)$. After obtaining $(Y_1^*, ..., Y_k^*)$, we repeat these steps again. After a large number of cycles (known as burn-in in MCMC), under some technical conditions on $p(Y_1, ..., Y_k)$, the samples $(Y_1^*, ..., Y_k^*)$ approximately follow the distribution $p(Y_1, ..., Y_k)$. To use the Gibbs sampler, the conditional distributions should be in a simple form.

In some situations, even a conditional distribution may not be easy to sample from. The Metropolis-Hastings (MH) algorithm provides a feasible way to sample from a wide range of distributions. Suppose that we would like to sample from a posterior distribution $p(\boldsymbol{\theta})$, the algorithm starts from an initial value, which may be the estimate of a fitted model using a non-Bayesian approach, such as the MLE. The algorithm iteratively samples from a "proposal" distribution $q(\boldsymbol{\theta}^*|\boldsymbol{\theta})$. In step k after obtaining the sample $\boldsymbol{\theta}^{(k)}$, $\boldsymbol{\theta}^*$ is sampled from the proposal distribution $q(\boldsymbol{\theta}^*|\boldsymbol{\theta}^{(k)})$. Then

$$r = \frac{p(\boldsymbol{\theta}^*)q(\boldsymbol{\theta}^{(k)}|\boldsymbol{\theta}^*)}{p(\boldsymbol{\theta}^{(k)})q(\boldsymbol{\theta}^*|\boldsymbol{\theta}^{(k)})} \tag{7.24}$$

is calculated and $\boldsymbol{\theta}^*$ is taken as $\boldsymbol{\theta}^{(k+1)}$ with probability $\min(1, r)$, and $\boldsymbol{\theta}^{(k+1)} = \boldsymbol{\theta}^{(k)}$ with probability $1-\min(1, r)$. It can be shown that with a large number of iterations, $\boldsymbol{\theta}^{(k)}$ is approximately $p(\boldsymbol{\theta})$ distributed. The proposal distribution should satisfy some technical conditions to avoid the algorithm running in cycles in a region and to ensure that $\boldsymbol{\theta}^k$ explores all the parameter space. The proposal distribution might be symmetric, i.e., $q(\boldsymbol{\theta}^*|\boldsymbol{\theta}^{(k)}) = q(\boldsymbol{\theta}^{(k)}|\boldsymbol{\theta}^*)$. For example, the normal proposal distribution $\boldsymbol{\theta}^* \sim N(\boldsymbol{\theta}^{(k)}, \boldsymbol{\Sigma})$ is symmetric. An algorithm using a symmetric proposal distribution is known as a random-walk Metropolis algorithm.

Although with MCMC Bayesian computing is feasible to program, in practice, using readily made software is much more convenient. For some specific models such as GLM or survival models, the MCMC procedure has been integrated into proc GENMOD, LIFEREG and PHREG, so the user only needs to specify options for the prior and the MCMC algorithm. There are other MCMC packages such as WinBugs with an R-interface. One practical advantage of SAS proc MCMC is that it has a similar structure for random effects as in proc NLMIXED, hence it is easier to program mixed models than in other software. The proc MCMC has the same random statement to specify random effects in the same way as in the proc NLMIXED. The PRIOR statement specifies the prior distribution for the parameters. The PARMS statement declares model parameters (except the hyper-parameters, for which values are specified directly in the distribution function) and assigns initial values. See Section 7.2.1 for details. NONMEM can also be used for Bayesian analysis, with fewer options than SAS and R.

A major development in Bayesian computing is the Hamilton Monte Carlo and the no-U-turn sampler, which are more efficient and stable than the Gibbs sampler above. Although the mechanism is more involved, Stan [Stan Development Team, 2023] is an implementation of these algorithms, with an easy-to-use interface in R. For its use in PK and PK/PD modeling, see Margossian et al. [2022].

7.2.4 Bayesian model selection and averaging

Bayesian approaches that we have introduced so far are all based on correctly specified models, including distributional assumptions. However, this assumption is often questionable in practice. An obvious approach to avoid using a wrong model is to fit multiple models and select the one most likely to be correct. Bayesian model selection can be based on the posterior probability that a model is correct. Suppose that there are two possible models M_1 and M_2 and their prior probability are $P(M_1)$ and $P(M_2)$, and under model M_k the response Y has distribution $p(Y|\boldsymbol{\theta}_k, M_k)$ one can calculate the odds that the model M_1 is true

$$\frac{P(M_1|Y)}{P(M_2|Y)} = \frac{p(Y|M_1)}{p(Y|M_2)} \frac{P(M_1)}{P(M_2)} \tag{7.25}$$

where $p(Y|M_1)/p(Y|M_2)$ is known as the Bayesian factor, and, e.g., $p(Y|M_1)$ can be calculated as $p(Y|M_1) = \int p(Y|\boldsymbol{\theta}_1, M_1)p(\boldsymbol{\theta}_1|M_1)d\boldsymbol{\theta}_1$. Note that the approach applies when the models M_1 and M_2 are completely different, as are the parameters. In contrast, the likelihood ratio test for model selection requires nested models, i.e., M_1 is included in M_2, or vice versa. Therefore, the Bayesian approach also has an advantage for model selection. This approach obviously only works when one of the candidate models is correct.

Since a common Bayesian inference, in particular with DER modeling, is to predict the response at a given dose, although this can be done with the selected model, there are better alternatives for prediction. Instead of selecting one model, an approach, known as Bayesian model averaging [Hoeting et al., 1999], uses all fitted models and averages posterior prediction with weights that can be determined in several ways. This is a better approach than the single model prediction, particularly the case of the so-called M-open settings in which none of M_ks is the true model [Bernardo and Smith, 2009].

For model averaging, the Occam window is a powerful tool that excludes all models with $P(M_k|Y)$ smaller than a smaller fraction of $\max_k P(M_k|Y)$. This way may substantially reduce the number of models for averaging.

7.3 Bayesian inference with misspecified models and approximate Bayesian

We start with the famous quote by George Box: All models are wrong, but some are useful. This is true in both the frequentist and Bayesian senses. For the latter, theoretical results have been developed relatively recently.

7.3.1 Bayesian inference with misspecified DR models

In the Bayesian formula, we have assumed that

$$p(\boldsymbol{\theta}|Y, D) \propto p(Y|\boldsymbol{\theta}, D)\pi_0(\boldsymbol{\theta}) \tag{7.26}$$

where $p(Y|\boldsymbol{\theta}, D)$ is the density of the response Y, given $\boldsymbol{\theta}$ and the dose D, which also contains a regression model for the DR relationship, e.g., $Y \sim N(\beta_0 + \beta_d D, 1)$, and $\boldsymbol{\theta}$ contains β_0, β_d and other parameters. When $p(Y|\boldsymbol{\theta}, D)$ is correctly specified, we can obtain the posterior distribution, or a sample taken from it. By a correctly specified model for Y, we mean that there exists a $\boldsymbol{\theta}^0$ with $\pi(\boldsymbol{\theta}^0) > 0$ such that $Y \sim p(Y|D, \boldsymbol{\theta}^0)$ [Bernardo and Smith, 2009]. It is obviously violated when the true DR relationship is nonlinear, while we specify $p(Y|\boldsymbol{\theta}, D)$ by a linear DR model. A less obvious one is that we specify a Poisson model for Y, while the true $p(Y|\boldsymbol{\theta}, D)$ has overdispersion (e.g., a negative-binomial model).

What $p(Y|\boldsymbol{\theta}, D)\pi_0(\boldsymbol{\theta})$ represents if the model is misspecified? As a simple example, we consider a model with an additive error term:

$$Y_i = g(D_i, \boldsymbol{\beta}) + \epsilon_i \tag{7.27}$$

where we assume that $\epsilon_i \sim N(0,1)$, but the true model is $g^0(D_i)$, an unknown function. The model is misspecified if there is no such $\boldsymbol{\beta}$ to make $g(\boldsymbol{\beta}, d) = g^0(d)$. A relevant topic is the behavior of frequentist approaches under misspecified models. This topic has been investigated for a long time by the classical work of White [1981, 1982]. Applying his result to the above example, we can claim that the MLE (or LS) estimate $\hat{\boldsymbol{\beta}} \to \boldsymbol{\beta}^*$, where

$$\boldsymbol{\beta}^* = \text{argmin}_{\boldsymbol{\beta}} \sum_{i=1}^{n} (g(D_i, \boldsymbol{\beta}) - g^0(D_i))^2, \tag{7.28}$$

and $\hat{\boldsymbol{\beta}}$ follows an asymptotic normal distribution with $\sqrt{n}(\hat{\boldsymbol{\beta}} - \boldsymbol{\beta}^*) \sim_a N(0, \boldsymbol{\Sigma})$. Here we consider $D_i, i = 1, ..., n$ fixed.

Generally, if $\hat{\boldsymbol{\theta}}$ is the MLE based on $p(Y|\boldsymbol{\theta}, D)$, then when $n \to \infty$, $\hat{\boldsymbol{\theta}} \to \boldsymbol{\theta}^*$ which minimizes the Kullback-Leibler (KL) divergence of the model $P(Y|D, \boldsymbol{\theta})$ from the true $P_0(Y|D)$

$$\boldsymbol{\theta}^* = \text{argmin}_{\boldsymbol{\theta}} KL(P(Y|D, \boldsymbol{\theta}), P_0(Y|D)), \tag{7.29}$$

where $KL(P, P^0) = \int \log(dP_0/dP)dP^0$. It is easy to verify that for the regression example above, the KL divergence is the sum of squares on the right-hand side of (7.28).

Intuitively, there might be a similar large-sample property for Bayesian approaches with misspecified DER models. Indeed, for our example, we have $\sqrt{n}(\boldsymbol{\beta} - \boldsymbol{\beta}^*) \sim_a N(0, \boldsymbol{\Sigma}_b)$ with a proper prior $\pi_0(\boldsymbol{\beta})$. This property follows the Bayesian framework as $\boldsymbol{\beta}$ here is a random variable. Note that we have $\hat{\boldsymbol{\beta}} \to \boldsymbol{\beta}^*$ and $\sqrt{n}(\boldsymbol{\beta} - \hat{\boldsymbol{\beta}}) \sim_a N(0, \boldsymbol{\Sigma}_b)$ also hold [Kleijn and Van der Vaart, 2012; Lyddon et al., 2019].

In the example, we have assumed fixed doses; hence, the KL distance is in the form of a sum of squares. In general, if we consider the dose as random $D_i \sim F(d)$, then the right-hand side of (7.28) can be written as $E_d((g(D_i, \boldsymbol{\beta}) - g(D_i))^2)$. Hence, $\boldsymbol{\beta}^*$ also depends on $F(d)$. The importance of this property is that, with model misspecification, the fitted model and parameter estimates all depend on the distribution of the dose in both frequentist and Bayesian frameworks.

7.3.2 Approximate Bayesian DR modeling

A fast-developing area in Bayesian analysis is approximate Bayesian analysis. There are multiple motivations: The classical Bayesian approaches are based on correctly specified models and priors, which may be difficult to specify and fit, and are often subject to large uncertainty. In particular, prior selection is often driven by computing feasibility; hence, conjugate priors are often selected, which may not necessarily reflect prior information. Even these can be correctly specified, with an increasingly large sample size of current data and database, The computation needed to calculate the posterior distribution may become infeasible.

One simple approach to approximate Bayesian is to replace the likelihood function by a quasi-one, which is simple but still captures the essential of model fitting. A general Bayesian knowledge update framework from the prior $\pi_0(\boldsymbol{\theta})$ can be based on a loss function rather than likelihood [Bissiri et al., 2016],

$$p(\boldsymbol{\theta}|Y, D) \propto \prod_{i=1}^{n} \exp(-wl(Y_i|D_i, \boldsymbol{\theta}))\pi_0(\boldsymbol{\theta}), \tag{7.30}$$

where $l(Y, \boldsymbol{\theta})$ is a loss function, e.g., a normal quasi log likelihood with variance equal to $1, l(Y, \boldsymbol{\theta}) = (Y - g(D, \boldsymbol{\theta}))^2/2$ which is known as the quasi-normal likelihood, w is a weight, often referred to as a learning rate for updating knowledge on $\boldsymbol{\theta}$ from the data. This approach is known as a general Bayesian (GB) update.

Recall that for given data $Y_i, D_i, i = 1, ..., n$, the likelihood of $\boldsymbol{\theta}$ can be written as

$$L(\boldsymbol{\theta}|D) = \prod_{i=1}^{n} f(Y_i|D_i, \boldsymbol{\theta}), \tag{7.31}$$

where $f(Y|D, \boldsymbol{\theta})$ is the density function of Y_i, the MLE $\hat{\boldsymbol{\theta}}$ has an asymptotically normal distribution: $\sqrt{n}(\hat{\boldsymbol{\theta}} - \boldsymbol{\theta}) \sim N(0, \boldsymbol{\Sigma}_\theta)$, where $\boldsymbol{\theta}$ is the true value if the model is correctly specified. With a proper prior $\pi_0(\boldsymbol{\theta})$, the asymptotic posterior distribution of $\boldsymbol{\theta}$ satisfies $\sqrt{n}(\boldsymbol{\theta} - \hat{\boldsymbol{\theta}}) \sim N(0, \boldsymbol{\Sigma}_b)$, where $\boldsymbol{\Sigma}_\theta, \boldsymbol{\Sigma}_b$ are unknown variance-covariance matrices. The same property holds when $f(Y|D, \boldsymbol{\theta})$ is replaced by $\exp(-l(Y|D, \boldsymbol{\theta}))$, where $l(Y|D, \boldsymbol{\theta})$ is a loss function, e.g., a normal quasi-log-likelihood $l(Y, \boldsymbol{\theta}) = (Y - g(D, \boldsymbol{\theta}))^2$. A quasi-likelihood based on loss function $l(.\boldsymbol{\theta})$ can be written as

$$L^q(\boldsymbol{\theta}|D) = \prod_{i=1}^{n} \exp(-wl(Y_i|\boldsymbol{\theta})). \tag{7.32}$$

The maximum quasi-likelihood estimate, in that w does not play a role, also follows an asymptotic normal distribution: $\sqrt{n}(\hat{\boldsymbol{\theta}} - \boldsymbol{\theta}) \sim N(0, \boldsymbol{\Sigma}_q)$, but in general $\boldsymbol{\Sigma}_q \geq \boldsymbol{\Sigma}_b$. Using this loss function for an approximate Bayesian analysis with Bayesian knowledge update (7.30), in which w becomes important, the asymptotic posterior distribution of $\boldsymbol{\theta}$ satisfies $\sqrt{n}(\boldsymbol{\theta} - \hat{\boldsymbol{\theta}}) \sim N(0, \boldsymbol{\Sigma}^2_{bq})$.

An important step in using the general Bayesian update is to determine w. For example, if Y_i is generated by $Y_i = g(D_i, \boldsymbol{\beta}) + \epsilon_i$ with $\text{var}(\epsilon_i) = 2$ while $l(Y, \boldsymbol{\theta}) = 0.5(Y - g(D, \boldsymbol{\theta}))^2$, which corresponds to $\text{var}(\epsilon_i) = 1$, is specified in Eq (7.30), that is, the variance in the model is misspecified. Then Eq (7.30) will underestimate the variability of the posterior distribution of $\boldsymbol{\theta}$. Several approaches to the determination of w, known as posterior recalibration, have been proposed. Here we introduce only some simple ones. With the above example, an intuitive approach would be to set $w = 1/2$, which makes the loss function a correct log-likelihood, hence (7.30) becomes exactly the posterior distribution.

Recall that some GLMs may be misspecified if Y_i has overdispersion, that is, its variance is higher than that specified in the GLM. Two common models taking overdispersion into account are the overdispersed Poisson and binomial models. Recall that if the overdispersion parameter is ψ for an overdispersed Poisson model, then the variance of MLE $\hat{\boldsymbol{\theta}}$ is

$$Var(\hat{\boldsymbol{\theta}}) = \psi \sum_{i=1}^{n} D_i^T \mathrm{diag}(\mu_i) D_i \tag{7.33}$$

where D_i includes an intercept and $\mu_i = E(Y_i|D_i)$. Therefore, since ψ can be estimated, we can calibrate $Var(\hat{\boldsymbol{\theta}})$ by replacing ψ with the estimated one. This idea can be used in approximate Bayesian analyses by recalibrating the posterior with weight w so that the posterior variance is equal to the empirical one. The following R and Stan codes generate Y_i from a negative binomial distribution, and then a Poisson model is fitted to estimate the overdispersion parameter "disp". Then it is used to calibrate in the GB as $w = 1/disp$.

```
di=rep(1:3,10)
nsub=length(di)
pi=0.5 #Make Y_i overdispersed.
yi=rnbinom(nsub,size=exp(di-1.5),prob=pi)
fitp=glm(yi~di,family=poisson())
disp=sum((fitp$weights * fitp$residuals^2)[fitp$weights > 0])/fitp$df.residual
> disp
[1] 2.071181
#disp=1
dat=list(y=yi,dose=di,p=2,N=nsub,disp=disp,ldose=ldose,nlong=nlong)
gpcode <- "
data {
  int<lower=0> N;
    int<lower=0> p;
  vector[N] dose;
  vector[N] y;
  real<lower=0> disp;
}
parameters {
  vector[p] beta;
}
transformed parameters {
  vector[N] mu;
  vector[N] eta;
  eta=beta[1]+beta[2]*dose; //beta[1]=inertcept; beta[2]=dose
  mu=exp(eta);
}
model {
  for (i in 1:N) {
    target += (y[i]*eta[i]-mu[i])/disp;
```

```
  }
}
"
fit <- stan(model_code = gpcode, model_name = "Overdispersed Poisson",
      data = dat, warmup =1000, iter = 2000, chains = 3, verbose = F)
summary(fit, pars="beta")$summary
               mean    se_mean         sd       2.5%        25%        50%
beta[1] -1.1407223 0.02997278 0.6654802 -2.5314267 -1.5723510 -1.1224990
beta[2]  0.8823657 0.01138360 0.2535547  0.4079696  0.7077209  0.8774962

# Fitting a Poisson model
summary(glm(y~dose,family = poisson(),data=dat))
glm(formula = y ~ dose, family = poisson(), data = dat)
Coefficients:
             Estimate Std. Error z value Pr(>|z|)
(Intercept)  -1.0560     0.4407  -2.396   0.0166 *
dose          0.8624     0.1691   5.100  3.4e-07 ***
```

With the Poisson model, the SE of the estimated coefficient for dose is under estimated (0.17), while the SD of the same parameter (beta[2]) in the GB model is 0.25; and the variance ratio $(.25/.17)^2 = 2.16$ is similar to the value of the overdispersion parameter, showing that the recalibration has corrected for the issue of under-estimated variability in the Poisson model. For simplicity, we used the glm(.) function to estimate ψ. GB without recalibration results in posterior variances similar to those glm(.) gives. The reader can set disp=1 (a line commented out in the code) and rerun the code to verify.

7.3.3 Bayesian bootstrap for approximate Bayesian inference

Bayesian bootstrap is a simple way to sample the posterior distribution with non-parametric priors [Rubin, 1981]. Without going into the details of non-parametric Bayesian, we directly describe how BB works. Let $\prod_{i=1}^n f(Y_i|\boldsymbol{\theta})$ be the likelihood function and assume a uniform Dirichlet prior $Dir(1, ..., 1)$ for each subject, a posterior sample of $\boldsymbol{\theta}$, given the data, can be generated by a weighted MLE:

$$\hat{\boldsymbol{\theta}}^b = \text{argmax}_\theta \prod_{i=1}^n f(Y_i|\boldsymbol{\theta})^{\xi_i^b} \tag{7.34}$$

with weights generated from the uniform Dirichlet $\xi_i^b \sim Dir(1, ..., 1)$. Then, with MLE $\hat{\boldsymbol{\theta}}$, $\sqrt{n_0}(\hat{\boldsymbol{\theta}}^b - \hat{\boldsymbol{\theta}})$ and $\sqrt{n_0}(\boldsymbol{\theta} - \hat{\boldsymbol{\theta}})$ have the same asymptotic posterior distribution [Newton and Raftery, 1994], hence the BB posterior sample can be used for Bayesian inference. Therefore, BB is very easy to implement and does not need an MCMC.

Similar properties hold when $f(Y_i|\boldsymbol{\theta})$ in (7.34) is replaced by $\exp(-l(Y_i, \boldsymbol{\theta}))$ [Lyddon et al., 2019]. Although the properties are derived based on minimizing the loss function, under some technical conditions, this approach is equivalent to solving a set of estimating equations corresponding to (7.34) either with $f(Y_i|\boldsymbol{\theta})$ or with $\exp(-l(Y_i, \boldsymbol{\theta}))$ [Van der Vaart, 2000]. Furthermore, the weighted likelihood or negative loss function leads to weighted estimating equations. Therefore, using BB for DER modeling is straightforward. For example, to obtain a posterior sample of coefficients in a Poisson regression, we generate multiple copies of $\xi_i^b \sim Dir(1, ..., 1), b = 1, ..., B$ and fit a weighted EE

$$\sum_{i=1}^{n} \xi_i^b (1, D_i)^T (Y_i - \text{expit}(\beta_0 + \beta_d D_i)) = 0 \tag{7.35}$$

to obtain $\hat{\beta}_0^b, \hat{\beta}_d^b, b = 1, ..., B$. Note that we do not specify any prior for the parameters. Suppose that Y_i are generated from a negative binomial model (hence it is over-dispersed relative to Poisson distribution). Although one may estimate the over-dispersion parameter and adjust for it in the inference for β_d, the BB approach automatically takes this into account.

The following is R-code for a small simulation to examine the SE of the BB estimate for an over-dispersion model similar to the previous one. At the end of the code we give the SEs of the naive estimate based on the Poisson distribution, the empirical estimate by 1000 simulation runs, and the BB estimate, which shows that the SE of BB is quite close to the empirical one, while the naive estimate is much lower. However, this similarity is based on the large sample properties of BB, and a smaller sample size and/or a higher over-dispersion can result in a significant difference between them.

```
  di=rep(1:3,100)
nsub=length(di)
nsimu=1000
nboot=60
Pout=NULL
for (s in 1:nsimu){
    pi=0.7
    yi=rnbinom(nsub,size=exp(di-1),prob=pi)
  fitp=glm(yi~di,family=poisson())
  estp=fitp$coef[2]
  sep=summary(fitp)$coef[2,2]
  bvar=NULL
  for (b in 1:nboot){
    wei=rexp(nsub)
    wei=wei/mean(wei)
    fit=glm(yi~di,family=poisson(),weights=wei)$coef[2]
    bvar=c(bvar,fit)
  }
  Pout=rbind(Pout,c(estp,sep^2,var(bvar)))
}
SEs=sqrt(c(apply(Pout,2,mean)[2:3],apply(Pout,2,var)[1]))
names(SEs)=c("Poisson","Emprircal","Bayesyan boot.")
round(SEs,4)
      Poisson      Emprircal Bayesyan boot.
        0.0708           0.0827          0.0849
```

Compared to the Bayesian approach with full model specification, the BB approach lacks a guarantee of small sample properties. It is closely related to normal bootstrap, which is equivalent to sampling binary weights ξ_i^b. Therefore, BB can be considered a smoothed version of the Bayesian bootstrap, but it provides Bayesian justification and can be used for (approximate) Bayesian inference with minimum model/ distribution specification.

BB is very scalable, since it only needs to fit a model like (7.35) (we may also add a large number of covariates) repeatedly. It does not have problems of convergence of the MCMC algorithms, although the HMC and no-U-turn sampler have made much improvement on their convergence. BB may not be efficient if a large posterior sample, e.g., of sample size 5000, is needed, which can be generated by the MCMC algorithms easily after it reaches convergence. However, for small to moderate BB sample size B but large n and p, the advantage of BB is significant. An extreme situation in which BB is very efficient is the use of Thompson sampling to allocate doses to one or a few subjects in dose-finding studies (Section 9.3), since we only need a posterior sample of a very small size, but the MCMC approach needs a large number of warm-up runs before taking any sample.

BB can also be used to recalibrate GB. The following code is for calibration of the GB code in Section 7.3.2 with the same dataset

```
   # BB estimate disp
nb=500
Pout=NULL
for (j in 1:nb){
  wei=rexp(nsub)
  jk=summary(glm(yi~di,family = poisson(),weights=wei))$coef
  Pout=rbind(Pout,c(jk[,1],jk[,2]^2)) # Estimate and SE^2
}

J=apply(Pout,2,mean)[3:4]  # Mean variance
IJI=apply(Pout,2,var)[1:2]  # Var of estimates
sum(IJI)/sum(J) #Pooled psi estimate
[1] 1.614226
mean(IJI/J)  #mean psi2 of the two paras.
[1] 1.662117
```

Both estimates underestimated ψ (2.07), perhaps due to the small sample size. Note that the sample size in the simulation to verify the BB variance in this section is ten times larger than the data set for GB.

Prior information can also be included in BB [Pompe, 2021]. The prior can be either a distribution or data that represent the information. For the latter, one can simply include the data and apply BB weights on them. For the former, it can be included as an additional term in the loss function, or using the approach for the latter by generating pseudo data from the prior distribution. The prior information should be properly weighted, as discussed above.

Suppose that a previous study fitted a logistic model with mean $\text{expit}(\boldsymbol{\beta}^T\mathbf{Z}_i)$, where $\mathbf{Z}_i = (1, D_i, \mathbf{X}_i)$ includes the intercept, dose and covariates, and resulted in MLE $\hat{\boldsymbol{\beta}}$ with variance-covariance matrix $\boldsymbol{\Sigma}_\beta$. The pseudo-sample approach then generates n_0 samples with $Y_j \sim Bin(\text{expit}(\tilde{\boldsymbol{\beta}}_j^T \tilde{\mathbf{Z}}_j))$, where $\tilde{\boldsymbol{\beta}}_j \sim N(\hat{\boldsymbol{\beta}}, \boldsymbol{\Sigma}_\beta)$ and $\tilde{\mathbf{Z}}_j \sim F_n(Z), j = 1, ..., n_0$ is a sample from the current data. The

$$\sum_{j=1}^{n_0} w_0 \xi_j^b D_j (Y_j - \text{expit}(\boldsymbol{\beta}^T \tilde{\mathbf{Z}}_j)) + \sum_{i=1}^{n} \xi_i^b D_i (Y_i - \text{expit}(\boldsymbol{\beta}^T \mathbf{Z}_i)) = 0 \quad (7.36)$$

where ξ_j^b are generated in the same way as ξ_i^b and w_0 is to mitigate the impact of the n_0 samples so that we have $ESS = n_0 w_0$ small enough to make it a weak informative prior. However, when the distributions of $\tilde{\mathbf{Z}}_j$ and $\mathbf{Z}_i$ are different, the ESS will depend on what to estimate. When the information on all parameters is the measure, the formula (7.18) for ESS can be used. Sometimes the prior comes from real data, e.g., when we have access to individual data from a previous study. Then $Y_j, \tilde{\mathbf{Z}}_j$ in (7.36) can be replaced by real data, and the weight w_0 is set to controls the impact of the prior data on the analysis.

7.4 Bayesian sequential modeling and Bayesian bootstrap

The classical Bayesian approach to DER modeling is to fit the DE and ER models jointly, the same as the frequentist joint modeling approaches. It is an efficient approach when all model specifications are correct; however, it has the same drawback as its frequentist counterpart, since a wrongly specified ER model can affect the fitting of the DE model (known as a feedback effect). In addition, it is more difficult to fit a joint model, due to the complexity of the joint model and more parameters to be estimated. This is particularly important for Bayesian approaches when MCMC is needed. Although in view of frequentist approach, sequential modeling is an obvious solution to avoid the "feedback" problem and is easy to implement, Bayesian sequential modeling is conceptually more controversial and practically difficult to implement.

A solution to "cut the feedback" [McCandless et al., 2010] from the ER part to the DE part is relatively easy when using a Gibbs sampler, since it samples from the conditional distribution of each parameter conditional on the others. Therefore, we can leave out terms in the ER part of the joint model when forming the full conditional posterior density for parameters in the DE model. A cut(.) function in Jags (an R package for MCMC) for this purpose implements this idea,

A Bayesian approach to "cut the feedback" follows a similar route as the frequentist sequential modeling, with the following steps, including those for response prediction with a given dose:

1. Fit the DE model using a Bayesian approach and generate posterior samples of DE parameters.
2. Fitting a distribution to the posterior sample as prior for each posterior sample, predict the exposure and any quantity that is required in the ER model
3. Fit the ER model with a Bayesian approach and generate a posterior sample of ER parameters
4. For a given dose, generate posterior sample of mean response by combining the DE and ER models, with the posterior samples their model parameters.

This approach is known as a modular approach in which the DE and ER models are in separate modules and the interaction between modules is properly controlled for, e.g., cutting the feedback.

The BB for DE and ER modeling can be easily arranged as a modular approach, hence naturally cutting the feedback [Pompe and Jacob, 2021]. The approaches can be summarized by the following algorithm.

1. Take $w_i^b \sim Exp(1), i - 1, ..., n$ as BB weights, and repeat steps 3 and 4 B times
2. $\hat{\boldsymbol{\theta}}_1^b = \text{argmax}_{\theta_1} \sum_{i=1}^n w_i^b \log(f_1(C_{ij}, \boldsymbol{\theta}_1)$
3. $\hat{\boldsymbol{\theta}}_2^b = \text{argmax}_{\theta_2} \sum_{i=1}^n w_i^b \log(f_2(Y_i, h(C_i, \hat{\boldsymbol{\theta}}_1^b), \boldsymbol{\theta}_2)$

where $f_1(.), f_2(.)$ are likelihoods or $\exp(-l_1(.)), \exp(-l_2(.))$ with loss functions $l)1(.), l_2(.)$ for the DE and ER models. The weight $w_i^b \sim Exp(1)$ proposed in Pompe and Jacob [2021] is equivalent to the weights $w_i^b \sim Dir(1, ..., 1)$ in the last section. $\hat{\boldsymbol{\theta}}_1^b$ and $\hat{\boldsymbol{\theta}}_2^b$ are the posterior samples of the DE and ER models, respectively. Then, a posterior sample of the response at a given dose can be obtained by combining the DE and ER models, with the BB posterior samples of the model parameters. Obviously, due to the sequential nature, the properties of $\hat{\boldsymbol{\theta}}_1^b$ do not depend on the specification of $f_2(.)$

7.5 Bayesian decision analysis

The purpose of decision analysis (DA) is to find the best action based on available information to optimize some criteria that reflect the objective of the decision maker. For example, optimal dose selection based on a phase II trial is to maximize the probability of success in a phase III trial. This example is typical of using DA for drug development. Individual patient dose adjustment to balance their benefits and risk of the drug can also benefit from DA. Bayesian DA (BDA) [Parmigiani and Inoue, 2009] benefits from the

Bayesian framework that allows one to calculate the posterior risk (or benefit) based on data and prior information to optimize the criterion related to the objective.

Formally, DA consists of three elements:

- the action to be determined,
- the criterion for optimization,
- the outcome determined by the model and action.

Specifying the optimization criterion based on the task and the model is a key step, as is fitting the model to predict the outcome of taking an action. We will show how these elements link to a specific task later.

7.5.1 Decision analysis and dose selection

We start from a simple logistic DR model for safety endpoints:

$$Y_i \sim Binomial(n_i, p(D_i, \boldsymbol{\beta})), \;\; p(D_i, \boldsymbol{\beta}) = \text{expit}(\beta_0 - \beta_d D_i). \tag{7.37}$$

where $Y_i = 1$ indicates the occurrence of a DLT, and $\boldsymbol{\beta} = (\beta_0, \beta_d)$ are parameters. Suppose that our target response level is $E(Y_i) = y^0$ and the goal is to find a dose as close to y^0 as possible. Therefore, we need a measure of the distance between the response rate $p(d, \boldsymbol{\beta})$ and y^0, here we choose $L(d) \equiv (y^0 - p(d, \boldsymbol{\beta}))^2$, which is known as the loss function (but not that of approximate Bayesian), and our criterion is to find the dose d that minimizes $L(d)$. When β_0, β_d are known, this dose is the one that leads to $y^0 = p(d, \boldsymbol{\beta})$. When they are unknown, one approach is to replace them with their estimates, which has been widely used in practice. Taking the logistic model as an example, the calibrated dose based on the fitted model is $\hat{d} = (\log(y0/(1 - y0)) - \hat{\beta}_0)/\hat{\beta}_d$. How variation of these estimates affects dose selection remains a question.

Now we put this practical question into the BDA framework, assuming that $\boldsymbol{\beta}$ are random variables but that their posterior distribution can be found using data and priors. The action in this context is obviously the dose. Let $\pi(\boldsymbol{\beta}|D)$ be the posterior density of $\boldsymbol{\beta}$ given data D, with the loss function $L(d, \boldsymbol{\beta})$ (which is not the loss function in the approximate Bayesian analysis), we can average random variations out, given the posterior distribution of $\boldsymbol{\beta}$

$$R(d) = \int_{\beta} L(d, \boldsymbol{\beta}) \pi(\boldsymbol{\beta}|D) d\boldsymbol{\beta} = \int_{\beta} (y^0 - p(d, \boldsymbol{\beta}))^2 \pi(\boldsymbol{\beta}|D) d\boldsymbol{\beta}. \tag{7.38}$$

It is called a risk function and will be the criterion to minimize in BDA. Hence, a BDA is to minimize $R(d)$ by taking the optimal action (here is the dose).

Even for this simple task, since $p(d, \boldsymbol{\beta})$ is a nonlinear function with respect to d, there is no analytical solution to the optimal dose. However, as long as the right-hand-side can be calculated numerically, we can find the optimal dose $\hat{d}^* = \text{argmin}_d \hat{R}(d)$ with a numerical minimize such as optimize( ) in R. The following code implements this approach and compares the optimal dose with the calibration based on the fitted model at three target mean responses with a hypothetical dataset.

```
   dose=1:4
yi=c(0,1,1,2)
ni=rep(3,4)
Beta=NULL
for (b in 1:3000){
  wei=rexp(4)
  beta=glm(cbind(yi,ni)~dose,family = "binomial",weights = wei)$coef
  Beta=rbind(Beta,beta)
}
sq=function(dose,y0){
  mean((y0-1/(1+exp(-Beta[,1]-dose*Beta[,2])))^2)
}
beta0=glm(cbind(yi,ni)~dose,family = "binomial")$coef

y0=0.1  #Target mean response
> (log(y0/(1-y0))-beta0[1])/beta0[2] #Calibration using fitted model
(Intercept)
   1.322265
>
> optimize(sq,c(1,7),y0=y0)$min #Optimal Bayesian dose
[1] 1.166849
> y0=0.3  #Target mean response
> (log(y0/(1-y0))-beta0[1])/beta0[2] #Calibration using fitted model
(Intercept)
   3.255447
> optimize(sq,c(1,7),y0=y0)$min #Optimal Bayesian dose
[1] 3.232522
>
> y0=0.7  #Target mean response
> (log(y0/(1-y0))-beta0[1])/beta0[2] #Calibration using fitted model
(Intercept)
   5.682216
> optimize(sq,c(1,7),y0=y0)$min #Optimal Bayesian dose
[1] 5.505128
```

The results show that when the optimal dose is in the middle of the DR curve $y^0 = 0.3$, the simple calculation $\hat{d} = (\log(y0/(1-y0)) - \hat{\beta}_0)/\hat{\beta}_d$ works quite well. However, some moderate differences between the Bayesian optimal dose and the simple one occur at each end of the curve when $y^0 = 0.1$ and $y^0 = 0.7$. This is mainly due to the higher variability of $p(d, \hat{\boldsymbol{\beta}})$ when d is at the end of the curve.

The optimal dose may also need to satisfy certain constraints, the most common is to control the probability of overdose, e.g., to ensure for a selected dose d, the probability of an AE is lower than a limit:

$$P(p(d,\boldsymbol{\beta}) > U|D) < \Delta. \tag{7.39}$$

for given U and $\Delta > 0$. Note that $p(d,\boldsymbol{\beta}) > U$ is a random variable and $P(p(d,\boldsymbol{\beta}) > U|D)$ can be estimated if the posterior distribution of $\boldsymbol{\beta}$ can be calculated. This constraint can be combined with the quadratic loss function and

$$\begin{aligned} &\min_d \int_\beta (y^0 - p(d,\boldsymbol{\beta}))^2 \pi(\boldsymbol{\beta}|D) d\boldsymbol{\beta} \\ &\text{subj. } P(p(d,\boldsymbol{\beta}) < U|D) < \Delta \end{aligned} \tag{7.40}$$

Again, BB is an easy way to calculate the constraint. With the posterior sample $\hat{\boldsymbol{\beta}}^1, ..., \hat{\boldsymbol{\beta}}_B$, $P(p(d,\boldsymbol{\beta}) > U|D)$ can be calculated as

$$\hat{P}(d) = B^{-1} \sum_{b=1}^{B} I(p(d,\hat{\boldsymbol{\beta}}_b) > U) \tag{7.41}$$

This problem is a nonlinear optimization with a nonlinear constraint. Common optimization software may not have an option to solve this problem. An easy approximation is to make the constraint a "soft boundary". With this approach, we solve

$$\min_d \int_\beta (y^0 - p(d,\boldsymbol{\beta}))^2 \pi(\boldsymbol{\beta}|D) + K\text{expit}(\lambda(\hat{P}(d) - \Delta)) \tag{7.42}$$

where the last term is a "soft-switch" between 0 and K when λ is large enough. The above algorithm can be easily adapted to include the second term in Eq (7.42). The choice of the two parameters λ and K depends on the data, but more details are beyond the scope of the book.

Suppose that instead of achieving a specific response level we would like the response to be within a certain range (L, U), hence we select d to maximize $P(L < Y < U)$, then the criterion

$$\begin{aligned} P(L < Y < U|d,\boldsymbol{\beta}) &= P(L < g(d,\boldsymbol{\beta}) + \varepsilon < U) \\ &= P(L - g(d,\boldsymbol{\beta}) < \varepsilon < U - g(d,\boldsymbol{\beta})) \end{aligned} \tag{7.43}$$

not only depends on $g(d,\boldsymbol{\beta})$, but also on the variability of $\boldsymbol{\beta}$. In the same way as in the previous example, we can define a loss function as $l(d,\boldsymbol{\beta}) = P(L < Y < U|d,\boldsymbol{\beta})$ and the corresponding risk function is obtained by averaging $\boldsymbol{\beta}$ on its posterior distribution in the same way as (7.38).

We have focused so far on BDA using DR models. The same approaches can also be used if the DR relationship can be predicted by a DE model and an ER model. In this case, we can write $p(d,\boldsymbol{\beta},\gamma)$ and, if the BB approach is used, the BB samples for $\boldsymbol{\beta}$ and γ should use the same BB weights to reflect that each individual dose, exposure and response measures are from the same subject.

There are many other types of loss function, and the selection of the loss function is a task of multiple disciplines and should involve, e.g., clinicians and pharmacologists, for the example we consider. For example, if treatment is to control the response within a normal range (L, U), the loss function may be the probability of the response within this range. Outside of this range, the distance between the limits and the response may also be taken into account. A loss function for this purpose may be written as

$$l(d, \boldsymbol{\beta}) = \begin{cases} \int_{\boldsymbol{\beta}}(g(d, \boldsymbol{\beta}) - U)^2 & g(d, \boldsymbol{\beta}) > U \\ 0 & L \leq g(d, \boldsymbol{\beta}) \leq U \\ \int_{\boldsymbol{\beta}}(g(d, \boldsymbol{\beta}) - L)^2 & g(d, \boldsymbol{\beta}) < L \end{cases} \tag{7.44}$$

This loss function is a combination of the squared loss function and (7.43). Its risk function can be calculated by averaging $\boldsymbol{\beta}$ over the posterior distribution. Also, using BB, the integrals can be approximated by a sum of $l(d, \hat{\boldsymbol{\beta}}^b)$, where $\hat{\boldsymbol{\beta}}^b, b = 1, ..., B$ is a posterior sample.

Although BDA uses a quite different approach from the frequentist one, it is more general, hence the Bayesian decision has some desirable frequentist properties as well. For example, a decision in the frequentist framework is admissible if no other decision is better than it for some $\boldsymbol{\beta}$, and not worse than it for any $\boldsymbol{\beta}$ value. Since in the frequentist framework, one cannot find a uniformly optimal decision, an admissible decision is often the best one can find, in general. However, it can be shown that every Bayesian decision with a proper prior is admissible, and furthermore, for every admissible decision, there is a prior (which might be improper) that makes the decision a Bayesian decision. This result is a reassurance that BDA is not worse and often better than frequentist decisions for the same problem.

7.5.2 Utility, preference, and uncertainty

We introduced BDA using the loss function and Bayesian risk previously, assuming that the outcome of the decision can be measured by the loss function, whose definition is often pragmatic. However, in many cases, the evaluation of the outcome is a difficult task, as a pragmatic loss function often does not reflect the true benefit and risk. This section gives a brief introduction to the concept of utility and preference of outcomes from practical points of view. The reader is referred to Parmigiani and Inoue [2009] for technical details.

The key concept in utility theory is that there exists a utility function $U(Y)$, a function of the response Y, whose value reflects the decision maker's (DM's) preference. Under some assumptions reflecting rationale preference, if DM prefers $Y = A$ over $Y = B$ then $U(A) > U(B)$. The rationale for the preference is reflected in the properties of $U(.)$. These include that if $U(A) > U(B)$ and $U(B) > U(C)$, then $U(A) > U(C)$, and if $U(A) \leq U(B)$ and $U(B) \geq U(A)$ then $U(A) = U(B)$, and that $U(Y)$ is defined for all possible Ys so the utility of any response can be compared. As the response y

is often random, $U(Y)$ is a random variable. The foundation of classical DA is the principle of expected utility (EU), and the BDA problem becomes finding the optimal decision A to maximize the EU: $E(U(Y))$. Here we assume that the action affects $U(.)$ only through the response Y for simplicity.

Sometimes, the DM's preference seems obvious. For example, a larger tumor shrinkage is preferred over a smaller one; lower blood pressure (within a certain range) is better than higher blood pressure for hypertension patients. However, one major issue in ranking responses and defining $U(.)$ is the uncertainty of response, which may contain uncertainty in nature, or in the model and model parameter. Therefore, the utility should take the DM's attitude toward uncertainty into account. One common approach to elicit utility under uncertainty is called a standard gamble. For example, to determine the utility of the current state of health, this approach gives the DM a hypothetical scenario with options between living in the current state of health Y_0 and taking a gamble with probability p of having $U = 1$ (perfect health) and $1-p$ of having $U = 0$ (death). The p value that makes the DM indifference between the two choices is the value of $U(Y_0)$, as it makes the EUs of both choices equal. Taking the gamble, the utility is $1 \times p + 0 \times (1-p) = p$, which is the same as $U(Y_0)$ as Y_0 is certain. However, often the elicited $U(Y)$ is a concave function, since normal people are risk averse, that is, they tend to avoid uncertainty. The concept of risk averse can be interpreted in a monetary term. Suppose a gambling is set to given choices of taking 10,000 dollars for sure, or taking a 1% chance to win 1,000,000 and otherwise getting nothing. Normally, people would choose the first one, although on average the expected reward is the same. One may increase the chance to win to find at which value people would be indifferent with these choices, and the value is the utility of 10,000 dollars relative to unit utility at 1,000,000.

The other issue in ranking outcomes is that in most situations there are multiple, often conflicting, objectives to consider. For example, a higher dose can often increase not only drug efficacy but also the risk of AE. Therefore, dose selection should balance two conflicting objects: increasing efficiency and reducing the risk of AE. This type of task is known as multi-criteria decision analysis (MCDA), commonly used in health economics. A simple approach to dealing with multi-criteria is to find a measure that summarizes all criteria; the clinical utility index (CUI) is an example. For example, for cancer patients, an oncologist gave the following utility according to the efficacy and safety results Houede et al. [2010], as shown in Table 7.1. Here progressive disease means that the treatment cannot control tumor growth, while stable disease refers to the situation where the tumors are controlled at the current size. The best outcome is that the tumor responds to treatment and shrinks. The AE grade represents the severity of AEs, with 0 for no AE. But the grade is not cardinal; that is, a grade 2 AE may not be twice as severe as a grade 1. In the table, in addition to the values for the best and worst cases, the expert has to determine seven utility values. Clinical utility indices have been defined for a number of situations as the utility of clinical outcomes. Another example is the CUI in Ouellet et al. [2006] for insomnia treatments, takes 5 components: 1) Residual effect; 2) Wake after

Table 7.1
The utility of safety and efficacy outcomes of oncology patients of an oncologist Houede et al. [2010]. Numbers in the brackets are approximate utilities using additive weight approximation.

AE grade	Progressive disease	Stable disease	Tumor response
0	40 (46.7)	90 (73.3)	100 (100)
1	10 (23.3)	50 (50)	80 (76.7)
2	0 (0)	40 (26.7)	40 (5.33)

sleep onset; 3) Quality of sleep; 4) Latency to persistent sleep; 5) Sleep architecture, into account. All five terms have quantified criteria to measure if they are achieved. To summarize them into a single index, a weighted mean with relative weights 35, 25, 17, 13 and 10 was suggested. These CUIs are disease specific and cannot normally be used to compare outcomes across different indications.

The CUI of Ouellet et al. [2006] is an example of utilities constructed by weighting for multiple responses. Weighting is a common way to construct a summary reflecting the appropriate trade-off between them. Suppose that there are K aspects with sub-utility $U_1, ..., U_k, ..., U_K$, each representing one aspect of the overall outcome. A linear combination of them

$$U = \sum_{k=1}^{K} W_k U_k \tag{7.45}$$

provides a summary with relative importance of each aspect weighted by W_k. Then the DM may choose a decision to maximize U. The DM is often a panel of experts; hence, the weights may reflect views and judgments of multiple persons. The additive utility may not be accurate enough, but may be the only feasible way for a task with, e.g., $K = 5$. A K value as large as 5 is not hypothetical. Drug benefit-risk assessment is a typical example for decision-making considering several objectives.

To see how U_k and W_k are set based on utility values for multiple outcomes, consider the first example in which both the safety and efficacy endpoints have three categories. Therefore, the individual utility should take value 0 for the worst and 1 for the best, leaving the value for the middle category to be determined. After determining the individual U_k s, the only parameter to be determined is W_1, as $W_2 = 1 - W_1$. Therefore, there are in total three values to be determined. We use the additive utility (7.45) to approximate that given by Table 7.1. For this, we need to determine the utility of the middle category U_1 and U_2 and the relative weight. We can formally write the approximate utility as

$$U(\mathbf{U}, w) = wU_1 + (1 - w)U_2 \tag{7.46}$$

and try to find $\mathbf{U} = (U_1, U_2)$ and w to minimize

$$\sum_{i=1}^{n}(U_i - U(\mathbf{U}, w))^2 \tag{7.47}$$

where U_is are the individual utilities for all the categories in Table 7.1. The following codes find the best approximates, as shown in table 7.1.

```
yv=c(4,9,10,1,5,8,0,4,4)
fun=function(beta){
sdis=rep(c(0,beta[1],1),3)
sae=rep(c(1,beta[2],0),rep(3,3))
sum((yv-10*(beta[3]*sdis+(1-beta[3])*sae))^2)
}

opt=optim(par=c(13/17,6/15,0.5),fn=fun)

$par
[1] 0.7343702 0.3392987 0.5333230
```

Here, the marginal mean utilities 13/17 and 6/15 and the relative weight 0.5 are used as the initial values for U_1, U_2 and w. The optimal ones (given in "par") are not far away from them. However, the approximation for individual utility may be quite poor for some combinations (Table 7.1). This example also serves as a reminder of the difficulty in using a simple utility function to represent a utility that involves multiple aspects.

As another example, we consider the dose-selection problem in Neuenschwander et al. [2008] based on fitted logistic models with different priors. To put the problem in the BDA framework, they split the posterior probability of DLT into four intervals, with cutpoints (0.25,0.33,0.6). The interval (0.25,0.33) is considered as the zero-loss target. The other three intervals are considered as ranges of under-dosing or overdosing, each has a loss of different weights. For the four intervals, they proposed three loss sets: (1,0,1,1), (1,0,1,2) and (1,0,2,4). Since we have already obtained the posterior distribution with both weakly and strongly informative priors for this example, the Bayesian risk can be calculated from the posterior samples. The following code uses three different sets of weights for each model.

```
    Cut=c(0,0.2,0.35,0.6,1)
Risk=function(Prob,Cut,Wei){  #Prob is a vector of posterior sample
  nn=length(Prob)
  counts=hist(Prob, breaks=Cut, plot=F)$counts
  sum(counts*Wei)/nn
}

RMat=NULL
RMat=rbind(RMat,apply(PD,2,Risk,Cut=Cut,Wei=c(1,0,1,1)))
RMat=rbind(RMat,apply(PD,2,Risk,Cut=Cut,Wei=c(1,0,1,2)))
RMat=rbind(RMat,apply(PD,2,Risk,Cut=Cut,Wei=c(1,0,2,4)))
```

```
RMat=rbind(RMat,apply(PD0,2,Risk,Cut=Cut,Wei=c(1,0,1,1)))
RMat=rbind(RMat,apply(PD0,2,Risk,Cut=Cut,Wei=c(1,0,1,2)))
RMat=rbind(RMat,apply(PD0,2,Risk,Cut=Cut,Wei=c(1,0,2,4)))

plot(dname,RMat[1,],type="l",ylim=c(0,4),ylab="Risk",xlab="Dose",log="x")
lines(dname,RMat[2,],lty=2 )
lines(dname,RMat[3,],lty=3 )
lines(dname,RMat[4,],lty=4 )
lines(dname,RMat[5,],lty=5 )
lines(dname,RMat[6,],lty=6 )

legend(x=1,y=4,legend=c("Inform:weights=(1,0,1,1)",
   "Inform:weights=(1,0,1,2)","Inform:weights=(1,0,2,4)",
  "Weak:weights=(1,0,1,1)","Weak:weights=(1,0,1,2)","Weak:weights=(1,0,2,4)"))
```

Figure 7.5 shows the Bayesian risk of dose selection based on posterior samples with weakly and strongly informative priors for logistic models, with the three sets of weighted loss, which illustrate the importance of utility in dose selection when the response is subject to high uncertainty.

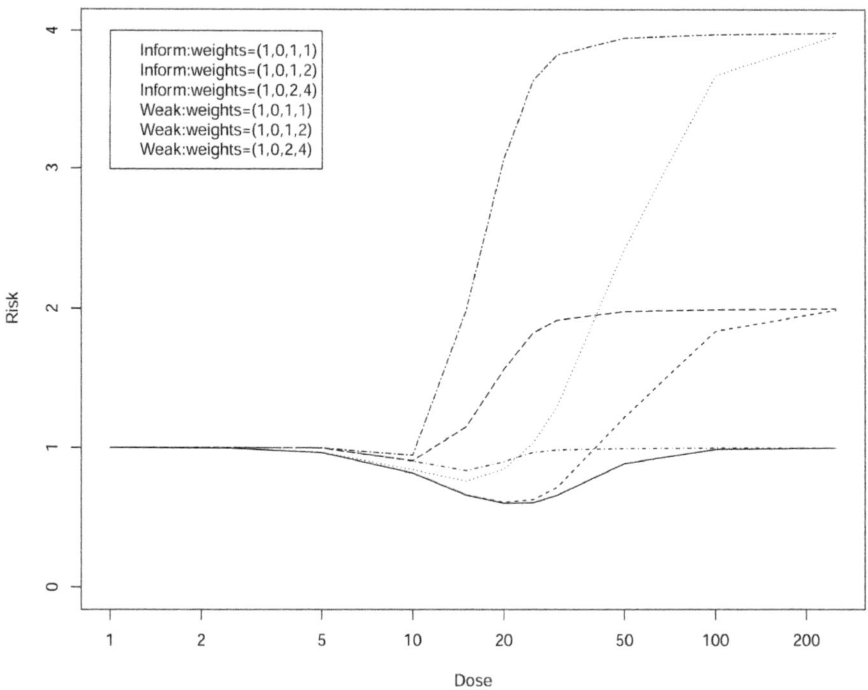

Figure 7.5
Bayesian risk of dose selection based on posterior samples with weakly and strongly informative priors for logistic models, with three sets of weighted loss.

7.6 Evidence synthesis and dose-response relationship in Bayesian meta-analysis

Multiple data sources, such as multiple clinical trials, observational studies, or a combination of them, may provide important information about DR relationship. The approach of synthesizing information from multiple sources is often called meta-analysis [Whitehead, 2002], which has been used for comparing treatments including dose levels. Although frequentist approaches can also be used, since meta data are typically of small sample size, the Bayesian approach has a clear advantage in this aspect.

DR data from multiple sources are often given by mean responses at each dose level. Hence, a common meta-analysis can be used to compare the response between doses. Alternatively, model-based meta-analysis uses regression (known as meta-regression) to fit mean responses for each dose and provides a marginal DR model for multiple sources. The key topic in meta-analysis is treatment heterogeneity, i.e., the variability in treatment effects of different studies or sources, and major technical advances in meta-analysis deal with this topic. Heterogeneity often occurs in the DER relationship, which is more difficult to deal with due to the complexity of the DER modeling. In meta-analysis, studies designed for different purposes may compare different treatments. Therefore, to compare specific treatments, we have to compare them indirectly if the treatments to be compared are not all from the same sources. The approach using direct and indirect treatment comparisons is called mixed treatment comparison, which has grown rapidly in recent years. Meta-analysis for the dose-response relationship has also been used increasingly [Langford et al., 2018; Crippa and Orsini, 2016].

7.6.1 Meta-analysis for non-parametric DR relationship

There are several excellent textbooks on meta-analysis, so we focus on its key aspects related to DR meta-modeling only. Suppose that we are interested in comparing the responses of a drug at multiple dose levels $\bar{D}$ with data from K sources. The DR relationship can be represented without a model by the difference in mean response between each pair of dose levels. Here we focus on a single pair of doses 1 and 2 and denote the mean difference between the doses in study k as Δ_{21k}. The meta data commonly includes its mean $\hat{\Delta}_{21k}$ with its SE $\hat{\mathbf{\Sigma}}_k$. We may assume that

$$\hat{\Delta}_{21k} = \Delta_{21} + U_k + \varepsilon_k \tag{7.48}$$

where Δ_{21} is the mean DR effect, $U_k \sim N(0, \mathbf{\Sigma}_u^2)$ represents heterogeneity, and $\varepsilon_k \sim N(0, \mathbf{\Sigma}_k^2)$ is the error in $\hat{\Delta}_{21k}$ carried over from the estimates with raw data. When $\mathbf{\Sigma}^2$ is the common residual variance for all K trials, $\mathbf{\Sigma}_k$ can be written as $\mathbf{\Sigma}/\sqrt{n_k}$, and n_k is the sample size of the kth study. Unlike the linear mixed models introduced in Chapter 3, here we assume that $\boldsymbol{\Sigma}_k^2$ is known, as it is often estimated in the analysis of individual sources. Therefore, we need only estimate Δ_{21} and $\boldsymbol{\Sigma}_u^2$. Fitting such a model is straightforward with common software, except for the need to specify the residual variance σ_k^2. This can be done in proc MIXED by inputting the variances from a dataset. It can also be fitted using proc NLMIXED, with a variable SEk=σ_k adding to a dataset include variables SEk and study, with the following code:

```
mud=Delta+ui;
random uk ~norma(0,sigmau) subject=study;
model dk ~normal(mud,var=SEk**2);
```

proc MCMC uses the same syntax, so this method can also be used in a Bayesian approach. Treatment heterogeneity U_k is the key component in the meta-analysis. The ideal situation is when $\sigma_u = 0$, i.e., treatment effects are the same in all trials. It has been common practice to test heterogeneity, or more specifically $H_0 : \sigma_u = 0$. However, since a meta-analysis hardly has sufficient power to detect heterogeneity, it is prudent to keep U_k in the model and to take its variability into account when interpreting and using the results of the meta-analysis.

The heterogeneity U_k in model (7.48) may depend on some observed covariates, particularly when they are quite different between studies. Meta-regression is an approach to model the relationship between the outcome and these factors, as well as the treatment. Meta regression adds covariates $\mathbf{X}_k$ into model (7.48):

$$\hat{\Delta}_{21k} = \Delta_{21} + \mathbf{X}_k^T \boldsymbol{\beta} + U_k + \varepsilon_k \tag{7.49}$$

where U_k is the residual heterogeneity after adjusting for $\mathbf{X}_k$, and we assume that $\boldsymbol{\beta}$ are constant for all dose pairs. This model can be fitted easily in the same way as previously described. Although we may still be mainly interested in Δ_{21}, $\boldsymbol{\beta}$ also contains very useful information, as $\mathbf{X}_k^T \boldsymbol{\beta}$ is the predictable part of heterogeneity. For example, if we are interested in the average treatment effect in a mixture population with covariates $\mathbf{X}_{01}, \mathbf{X}_{02}, ..., \mathbf{X}_{0K}$ with proportions $p_1, p_2, ..., p_K$, we can predict it with

$$\hat{\Delta}_{21m} = \hat{\Delta}_{21} + \sum_{k=1}^{K} p_k \mathbf{X}_{0k}^T \hat{\boldsymbol{\beta}}. \tag{7.50}$$

Its SE can also be easily calculated from the fitted model.

Sometimes summary data may be given as the mean response $\bar{Y}_{1k}$ and $\bar{Y}_{2k}$ treated with dose 1 and 2, respectively, rather than as their difference $\hat{\Delta}_{21k}$. One may work out the treatment differences and their SEs, or may fit the mean responses directly with model

$$\begin{aligned} \bar{Y}_{1k} &= (-\Delta_{21} + U_k)/2 + v_k + \varepsilon_{1k} \\ \bar{Y}_{2k} &= (\Delta_{21} - U_k)/2 + v_k + \varepsilon_{2k} \end{aligned} \tag{7.51}$$

where ε_{tk} is the SE of $\bar{Y}_{tk}, t = 1, 2$ and v_k is the baseline study effect that is canceled in (7.48). This model is called arm-based because it is based on meta-data by treatment arm. Note that here we allow for heterogeneity between ε_{tk}s, as the sample sizes of the two treatment arms are often different. The model fitting is also straightforward with any Bayesian software such as proc MCMC or Stan.

When meta-data from each study contain multiple doses, those without head-on comparison between, e.g., dose 1 and 2 may also be used for the estimation of Δ_{21}. For example, suppose that doses 1 and 2 are used in study 1, doses 1 and 3 in study 2, and doses 2 and 3 in study 3. Then Δ_{21} can also be estimated as $\hat{\Delta}_{233} - \hat{\Delta}_{132}$, bridging by the common dose 3 in both studies. Hence, it is often referred to as an indirect comparison and is often combined with a direct comparison $\hat{\Delta}_{211}$. Note that v_ks are canceled, so, the indirect comparison also eliminates confounding in v_k, if any. However, other random terms are doubled, compared with the direct comparison.

7.6.2 Bayesian meta regression for dose-response relationship

Although the non-parametric approaches are robust, we may still prefer to model the DR relationship from multiple data sources, which is straightforward with meta-regression. Suppose that the DR relationship in the jth arm of study k is described by

$$\bar{Y}_{jk} = \boldsymbol{\beta}_k D_{jk} + \varepsilon_{jk}, \tag{7.52}$$

with $\boldsymbol{\beta}_k = \boldsymbol{\beta} + U_k$, and the meta-analysis is to synthesis evidence about $\boldsymbol{\beta}$. We can adapt the model (7.48) for the estimate from individual trials as

$$\hat{\boldsymbol{\beta}}_k = \boldsymbol{\beta} + U_k + e_k. \tag{7.53}$$

The second stage for inference on $\boldsymbol{\beta}$ is exactly the same as in the previous subsection. If the outcome (e.g., occurrence of AEs) follows a GLM, then one can also use either a single-step or a two-step approach.

In the following, we use two examples to illustrate the approach. As the first example, we use the scenario in Zohar et al. [2011] where they reported a meta-analysis based on five phase I dose escalation trials for Sorafenib, an anti-cancer agent. The data are read into a SAS dataset and processed for analysis as:

```
data p1;
  input study d100 n100 d200 n200 d300 n300
              d400 n400 d600 n600 d800 n800;
cards;
1 0 3 0 3 . . 1 4 1 6 3 3
2  0 4 0 3 1 5 1 10 7 12 1 3
3 0 3 1 6 . .  0 8 3 7 . .
```

```
4 1 5 1 6 . .  0 15 4 14 2 7
5  0 3 1 12 . .  0 6 1 6 . .
;

data den (keep=study  n100   n200 n300 n400 n600  n800)
     num (keep=study  d100   d200 d300  d400 d600 d800);
  set p1;
run;
proc transpose data=den out=tden;
  by study;
run;
proc transpose data=num out=tnum;
  by study;
run;

data all;
  merge tden (rename=(col1=num)) tnum (rename=(col1=yi));
  dose=substr(_name_,2,3)+0;
  if num ne .;
run;
```

For the number of DLT Y_{jk} out of n_{jk} patients in trial k at the jth dose, we assume $Y_{jk} \sim Bin(n_{jk}, p_{jk})$. First, a GLMM that includes a random coefficient for dose

$$\text{logit}(p_{jk}) = \boldsymbol{\beta}_{0k} + (\boldsymbol{\beta} + U_k)D_{jk} \tag{7.54}$$

is fitted but the variation in U_k is close to zero. Consequently, a logistic model with individual baseline risk is fitted for each study to provide a better small sample property. We use a simple Bayesian approach with uniform prior for all parameters and run the following SAS proc GENMOD

```
proc genmod data=all;
  class study;
  model yi/num=dose study/d=b;
  bayes outpost=pred diag=all nbi=3000 nmc=5000 thinning=5;
run;
```

where the BAYES statement requires 1000 posterior samples generated from the MCMC procedure with 1:5 sampling ratio under the default uniform prior. From the posterior samples, we can calibrate the dose level corresponding to toxicity probability equal, e.g., 0.25. As the model allows different baseline risks for individual studies, suppose that we are interested in the average probability over these studies, we can take $\hat{\beta}_0 = \sum_{j=1}^{5} \hat{\beta}_{0k}/5$ and calculate the required dose as

$$d = (\log(0.25/0.75) - \hat{\beta}_0)/\hat{\boldsymbol{\beta}} \tag{7.55}$$

From the posterior sample of 1000, the median of d is 541(mg/m^2) (SD=65mg/m^2). The posterior samples can also be used to study the probability of overdose, e.g., the chance of the toxicity probability higher than

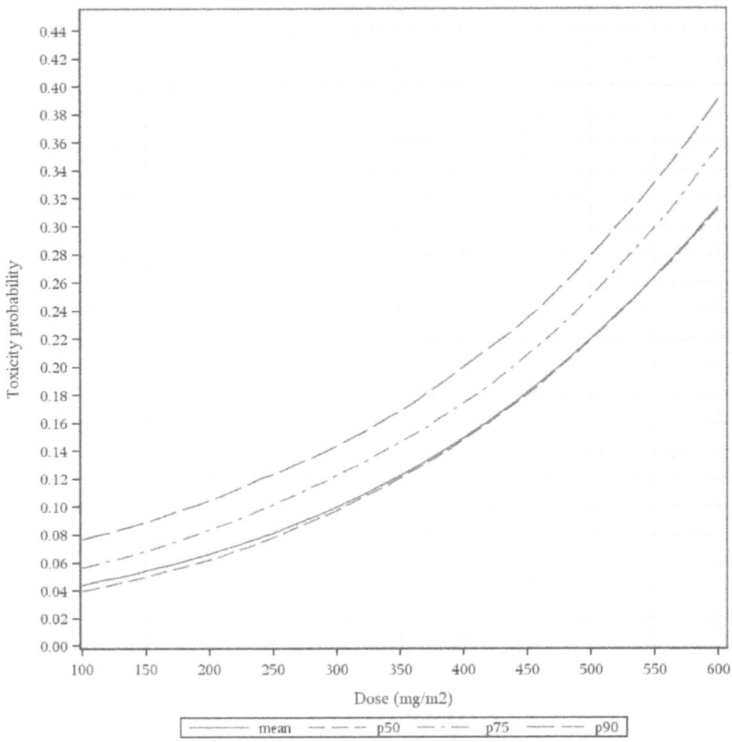

Figure 7.6
Mean, median (p50), 75% and 90% percentiles of toxicity probability at different dose level.

35 %. Figure 7.6 gives the mean, median, 75% and 90% percentiles of toxicity probability at several dose levels. It can be seen that the target dose is between 500-550 mg/m2 and, at that dose level, the chance of the toxicity probability higher than 35% is less than 10%, as the 90% line is lower than 35% in that dose range. In the analysis, we have not considered the issue that the selected dose is in the gap between 400 and 600mg/m2 doses, and at 400 mg / m2 dose the probability of toxicity was even lower than at 300 mg / m2 dose, although at which only a few patients were dosed. Therefore, the logistic model may not fit the data well locally.

As a more complex example, we consider the dataset in Langford et al. [2018] which consists of 14 multi-arm studies of alogliptin, an oral medication for lowering blood glucose in patients with type 2 diabetes mellitus. The response variable is HbA1c, a well-established biomarker for type 2 diabetes. They fitted a 3-parameter Emax model but did not take the study into account, except that in the contrast-based analysis, additive baseline factors are eliminated. The following code fits a mixed effect Emax model with study effect included. Since data are very sparse in some studies, we have to use a moderately informative prior.

```
library(rstan)
library(brms)
library(rstanarm)
library(gdata)
library(bayesplot)
library(lme4)
langford=read.csv(file="C:/Users/jixia/Projects/Warf/langford2.csv")
colnames(langford)=c("study","dose","nsub","resp","sd","Agel65"
                              ,"Male","numbase")
pmale=langford$Male/langford$numbase
pl65=as.numeric(langford$Agel65)/langford$numbase
pl65[is.na(pl65)]=mean(pl65,na.rm=T)

dataad=cbind(langford,pmale=pmale,pl65=pl65)
dataad=dataad[order(dataad$study),]

Istudy=as.vector(table(dataad$study))
nstudy=length(Istudy)
emax3=resp~b0+(bm-b0)*dose/(dose+exp(lb50))

gdata=dataad

n1 <- nls(emax3,
          data = dataad,
          start = list(b0=0, bm =-0.8, lb50 = 2))
coef0=summary(n1)$coef

jk=brm(bf(resp~b0+(bm-b0)*dose/(dose+exp(lb50)),
            b0+bm~1+(1|p|study),lb50~1|study,nl=T),
       prior=c(
         prior(normal(0, 3), nlpar = "b0"),
         prior(normal(-0.7, 3), nlpar = "bm"),
         prior(normal(1.1, 3), nlpar = "lb50")),data=dataad)

summary(jk)
> summary(jk)
 Family: gaussian
  Links: mu = identity; sigma = identity
Formula: resp ~ b0 + (bm - b0) * dose/(dose + exp(lb50))
         b0 ~ 1 + (1 | p | study)
         bm ~ 1 + (1 | p | study)
         lb50 ~ 1 | study
   Data: dataad (Number of observations: 45)
  Draws: 4 chains, each with iter = 2000; warmup = 1000; thin = 1;
         total post-warmup draws = 4000

Multilevel Hyperparameters:
~study (Number of levels: 14)
                 Estimate Est.Error l-95% CI u-95% CI Rhat Bulk_ESS Tail_ESS
sd(b0_Intercept)     0.22      0.07     0.12     0.39 1.00     1366     2255
sd(bm_Intercept)     0.17      0.05     0.09     0.28 1.00     1097     1516
sd(lb50_Intercept)   0.59      0.49     0.02     1.85 1.00      869     1120
cor(b0_Int,bm_Int)   0.16      0.34    -0.53     0.75 1.00     1269     1696
```

```
Regression Coefficients:
               Estimate Est.Error l-95% CI u-95% CI Rhat Bulk_ESS Tail_ESS
b0_Intercept      -0.06      0.08    -0.20     0.10 1.00     1061     1605
bm_Intercept      -0.86      0.06    -0.98    -0.74 1.00     1993     1900
lb50_Intercept     0.99      0.50    -0.20     1.70 1.00     1477      874

Further Distributional Parameters:
      Estimate Est.Error l-95% CI u-95% CI Rhat Bulk_ESS Tail_ESS
sigma     0.07      0.01     0.05     0.10 1.00     1131     1232

Draws were sampled using sampling(NUTS). For each parameter, Bulk_ESS
and Tail_ESS are effective sample size measures, and Rhat is the potential
 scale reduction factor on split chains (at convergence, Rhat = 1).
```

In the above models, we did not use the sample sizes and SD of the responses in the dataset. This information can be included in the model to give doses with more accurate response estimates and more weights. For this purpose, we calculated the SE of each dose based on its sample size and SD and name it as "sey". The following is a fitted model taking it into account.

```
 Family: gaussian
  Links: mu = identity; sigma = identity
Formula: resp | se(sey) ~ b0 + (bm - b0) * dose/(dose + exp(lb50))
         b0 ~ 1 + (1 | p | study)
         bm ~ 1 + (1 | p | study)
         lb50 ~ 1 | study
   Data: dataad (Number of observations: 45)
  Draws: 4 chains, each with iter = 2000; warmup = 1000; thin = 1;
         total post-warmup draws = 4000

Multilevel Hyperparameters:
~study (Number of levels: 14)
                              Estimate Est.Error l-95% CI u-95% CI Rhat Bulk_ESS Tail_ESS
sd(b0_Intercept)                  0.23      0.07     0.13     0.39 1.00     1728     2593
sd(bm_Intercept)                  0.16      0.05     0.06     0.27 1.01      674      255
sd(lb50_Intercept)                0.62      0.46     0.03     1.72 1.01      876     1381
cor(b0_Intercept,bm_Intercept)    0.23      0.34    -0.48     0.80 1.00     1043     1562

Regression Coefficients:
               Estimate Est.Error l-95% CI u-95% CI Rhat Bulk_ESS Tail_ESS
b0_Intercept      -0.05      0.08    -0.21     0.10 1.00     1187     1838
bm_Intercept      -0.86      0.06    -0.97    -0.75 1.00     1593     1821
lb50_Intercept     1.02      0.40     0.11     1.68 1.00     1445      561

Further Distributional Parameters:
      Estimate Est.Error l-95% CI u-95% CI Rhat Bulk_ESS Tail_ESS
sigma     0.00      0.00     0.00     0.00   NA       NA       NA
```

The results are very similar, except that due to the use of individual SE, the residual variance sigma is set to 0.

We can also predict the posterior means and quantile curves for each study. The following code generates the prediction and draws the mean and 0.25% and 97.5% quantile curves in Figure 7.7. Since these are quantiles based on the fitted model rather than the credible interval, they all decrease with dose.

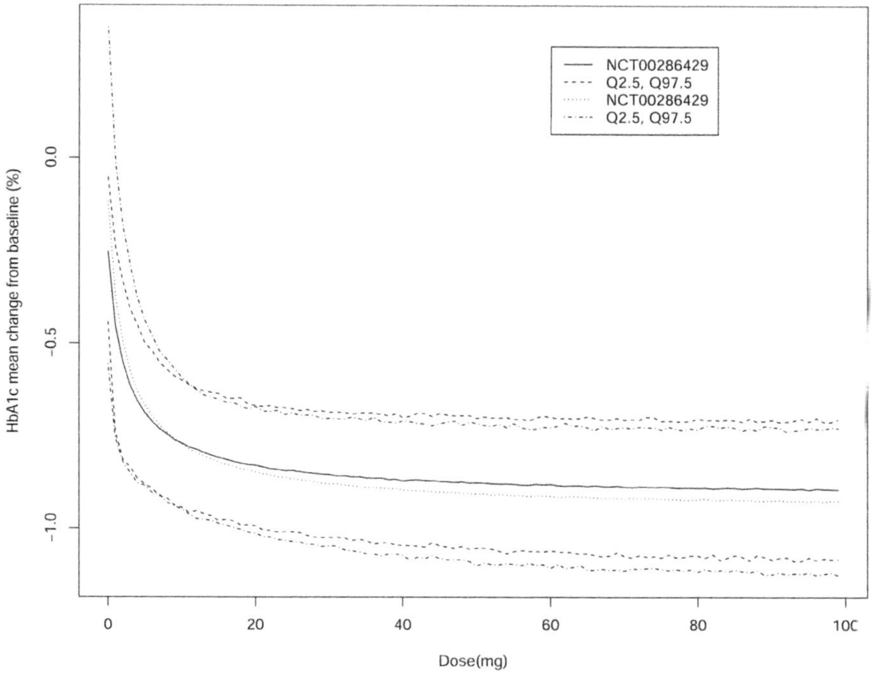

Figure 7.7
Predicted DR relationship for studies NCT00286429 and NCT00286429 in the dataset of Langford et al. [2018], with 0.025, 0.975 quantiles.

```
    alldose=(0:99)
newdata <- data.frame(
  dose = rep(alldose,2),
  study = c(rep("NCT00286429",100),rep("NCT01318122",100))
)
pred=predict(jk, newdata = newdata)
plot(alldose,pred[1:100,1],ylim=range(pred[,2:4]),type="l",
         xlab="Dose(mg)",ylab="HbA1c mean change from baseline (%)")
lines(alldose,pred[1:100,3],lty=2)
lines(alldose,pred[1:100,4],lty=2)

lines(alldose,pred[101:200,1],lty=3)
lines(alldose,pred[101:200,3],lty=4)
lines(alldose,pred[101:200,4],lty=4)
legend(x=60,y=0.3,legend=c("NCT00286429","Q2.5, Q97.5",
                  "NCT00286429","Q2.5, Q97.5"),lty=1:4)
```

7.7 Comments and bibliographic notes

This chapter attempts to introduce a number of topics on Bayesian approaches and decision analysis for DER modeling without much technical detail. There are several textbooks [Bernardo and Smith, 2009; Gelman et al., 1995; Robert et al., 2007] with different levels of technical difficulties. Parmigiani and Inoue [2009] provides extensive details in Bayesian decision analysis, including dynamic programming. Although there is no book specifically for (approximate) Bayesian analyses with model misspecification, many recent works such as [Lyddon et al., 2019; Pompe, 2021]cover this area.

The implementation of Bayesian approaches is highly dependent on the use of software. We have provided codes using multiple software, in particular, with Stan applications [Stan Development Team, 2023] added including those depending on it, such as R library arms, in this edition. These software often set default priors so we can run our dataset without specifying them. However, these priors and their impact on the analysis results should be carefully examined.

8

Causal dose-exposure-response analysis

Dose-exposure-response modeling plays an important role in many areas, particularly drug development, therapeutic drug monitoring, and post-marketing drug safety. Classical pharmacometric analyses typically use popPKPD modeling, for which NLMM are widely used to model DE and ER relationships. It is important to ensure that the relationships are causal in order to use these models to guide, e.g., therapeutic dose monitoring or optimal dose selection, since confounding factors may lead incorrect model fitting and prediction and consequently a wrong decision. Recent developments in causal inference provide means to mitigate the impact of confounders. This chapter shows how to consider causal DER relationships within and outside the pharmacometric framework and how to adapt it as needed. We argue that the use of causal analysis depends on the nature of DE, DR and ER models, the causal estimand and ultimately the purpose of the DER analyses.

8.1 Introduction

To set the scope of this chapter, we consider some typical aspects of causal DER modeling. We use causal DER relationships as a collection consisting of causal DE, ER and DR relationships, each may have its own use, and as an integrated entity that describes the overall causal relationship from dose to response. For example, in post-marketing study databases, the prescribed dose may depend on the patient's drug elimination function, hence the observed dose and exposure data may not reflect the causal DE relationship. The same may happen in DR data if dose is not randomized, e.g., the prescribed dose may depend on the risk of adverse events. The ER relationship may also be confounded even when dose levels are randomized, since often there are factors that affect both the exposure and the response. Causal inferences of each of the three relationships are similar; hence, we will often take one as an example, but point out the differences when discussing the others, since the causal inference principle and consideration can be adapted. One of our focus will be on using causal DE and ER modeling for a better estimation of the causal DR relationship, especially in dose finding trials with randomized dose levels.

DOI: 10.1201/9781003457008-8

A relevant topic that will not be covered in this chapter is response-dependent dose adjustment in both trials and clinical use of drugs. In this scenario, the adjustment introduces confounding biases between dose and response. One such example is the dose-titration paradox [Kristensen and Agersø, 2022]. This topic will be discussed in detail, including how to use modeling approaches for dose-adjustment in Chapter 9.

Causal inference is a key concept in statistics [Hernan and Robins, 2023] with rapid development and wide application in the last ten years since the first edition of this book. However, causal inference methods are developed mainly for binary or categorical treatment. The importance of causal dose-concentration-response relationship has also been noted in pharmacometrics works, e.g., Nedelman et al. [2007]; Sheiner [2002] and more recently Rogers et al. [2023]. Causal inference for the DR relationship has also been extensively considered in econometrics, although the dose (e.g., years of education received) has a very different meaning from that in our context. However, several approaches in this chapter are rooted in this area.

Often, the main confounders are known and may be observed. popPK and popPKPD modeling models DE and ER relationships by including them as covariates. Prediction of the relationship between DR and ER based on the popPK and popPKPD models can eliminate confounding biases when the models are correct and the model fitting is conducted correctly. In fact, this approach has a close link to direct adjustment and g-computation [Hernan and Robins, 2023], in the causal inference toolbox. The causal inference concept also plays an important role in the planning of popPK and popPKPD analyses.

To predict the response at a given dose level, the PK/PD modeling approach consists of two steps. First, we fit both the DE and ER models to the exposure and response data separately. For a given dose, we predict the exposure for individuals using the fitted DE model, then use the predicted exposure in the ER model to predict the response. The mean response can be estimated by averaging the predicted response. In addition to sensitivity to model misspecification, this approach is sensitive to potential confounding biases when fitting the ER model due to confounding factors that affect both the exposure and the response. An approach to diagnosing confounders in the PK/PD modeling was proposed by Nedelman et al. [2007], considered in Wadsworth et al. [2018, 2020] in pediatric trials, and reviewed in the ER antibody modeling [Kawakatsu et al., 2021].

To determine the optimal dose, comparisons of drug responses at different dose levels are fundamentally important [Food and Drug Administration, 2023]. For this purpose, a dose finding trial, in which subjects are randomized to a few fixed dose levels, is the most widely used trial design. An important topic in DER modeling is how to use it to improve the estimation of the causal DR relationship in a dose-finding trial and adjust for potentially unobserved confounders for the ER relationship. To mitigate the impact of confounding bias without knowing the confounders, a powerful approach is to use randomized dose as instrumental variable (IV), which leads to control function (CF) approaches, and has been used in the ER modeling with a few simple models Wang [2012a, 2014]. More recent development allows the use of more general models [Imbens and Newey, 2009; Zhang et al., 2024]. The CF function may also be used to improve non-parametric estimation of the dose-response relationship in an analysis of covariance (ANCOVA) adjustment in RCTs, with g-computation that includes CF in working models to improve the estimation of mean response in dose-finding trials.

Although a DR modeling approach can estimate the causal DR relationship directly, since only a few dose levels are tested in a dose-finding trial, the use of a model with even moderate complexity is infeasible. DER modeling is a more powerful and flexible alternative. Although people are rightly concerned about the potential confounding between exposure and response, we show that this approach may still be more efficient after adjustment for confounding.

This chapter starts from an introduction of causal inference for binary dose, since most causal inference theory and methods are developed in this setting. Then we extend our view to the ER and DR relationships with continuous dose/exposure and show how common approaches are adapted in the context of DER relationships.

8.2 Causal dose-exposure-response relationship

8.2.1 Causal inference and the counterfactual framework

The casual DER relationships represent the quantitative change in consequence due to a change in the cause. The consequence could be the response or the exposure, while the cause could be the dose or the exposure, depending on the individual context. A causal relationship differs from a correlation which simply means two quantities changing at the same time without knowing which causes the other. We start with a simple DR relationship with dose level 0 or 1, which is equivalent to a binary treatment. The causal DR relationship is best understood within the potential outcome framework [Rubin, 2005] in which we denote the response of the subject i under dose d as $Y_i(d)$, therefore, he has two potential responses $Y_i(1)$ and $Y_i(0)$, depending on the actual dose. The causal estimand for increasing the dose from 0 to 1 can be defined as

$$\Delta \equiv E(Y_i(1) - Y_i(0)) = \mu(1) - \mu(0) \tag{8.1}$$

with $\mu(d) = Y_i(d)$. However, when he can only be treated with one dose, the other response is a *counterfactual* which is never observed. The challenge is to estimate Δ. The sample mean response at dose d: $\bar{y}_d$ has a mean $E(\bar{y}_d) = E(Y_i(d)|D_i = d)$, but patients may have different characteristics that affect Y_i and also the chance of receiving dose 0 or 1, if the dose is not randomized;

therefore, $\bar{y}_1 - \bar{y}_0$ is a biased estimator of Δ. These characteristics are referred to as confounders and may or may not be observed. The most obvious way to overcome the problem is to randomize the dose so that $E(Y_i(d)|D_i = d) = E(Y_i(d)) = \mu(d)$, which is the approach of randomized dose-finding trials. However, the approach is difficult to apply to determine the ER relationship, as often we do not have direct control over exposure. Another approach is to make the counterfactual observable, e.g., to force the subject to receive both 0 and 1 doses. This can be done with a crossover trial in which a subject can receive multiple doses (e.g., to examine the proportionality of PK).

8.2.2 Directional acyclic graphs

When there are multiple variables, the causal relationships and confounding between them may be complex; hence a visual tool to represent the relationship is very useful. The development of directional acyclic graphs (DAG) (Figure 8.1) [Pearl, 2022] provides such a tool to investigate potential confounders and find approaches to deal with them. A DAG is a graph consisting of nodes, each representing a variable (e.g., a measure of exposure, a response, a factor or an intermediate measure), linked by directional edges (indicated by arrows), but do not form any directional circle, e.g., $A \rightarrow B \rightarrow C \rightarrow A$. For each arrow, the starting node is called a parent of the ending node, and the ending node is called a child of the starting node. From a node going along the direction by the arrow, we find its descendants, and going in the opposite

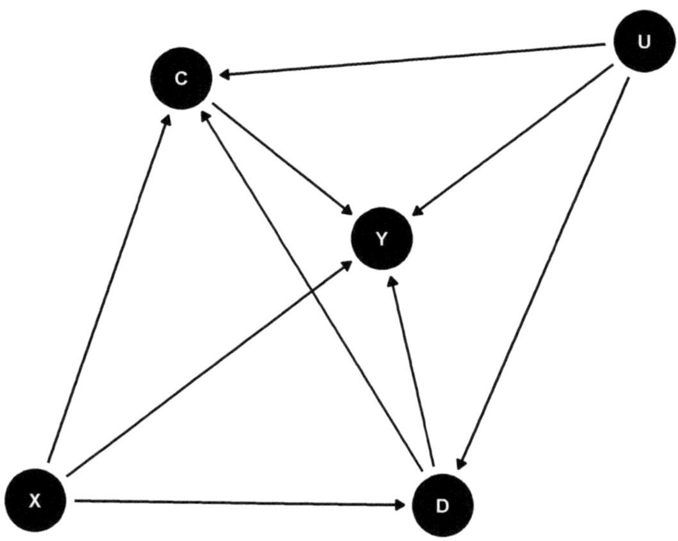

Figure 8.1
DAG for DER relationships with possible direct effect from D to Y, observed covariates X and unobserved covariates U.

direction, we find its ancestors. The DAG in Figure 8.1 shows the causal relationship between dose D, exposure C and response Y, and also variables X (observed) and U (unobserved) that may also have impacts on Y, C and D.

A DAG represents the dependence of the distributions of the variables on others, and an arrow indicates such a dependency. The distribution of a child conditional on its parents does not depend on anything else, based on the Markov assumption. Therefore, the joint distribution of all variables in a DAG can be factorized as a product of distributions of children conditional on their parents, whereas for those without any parent, their distributions are unconditional. Let $v_1, ..., v_K$ be all the nodes in a DAG, and $v_{pa(k)}$ be the parents of v_k, we can factorize the joint distribution of $v_1, ..., v_K$ as

$$p(v_1, ..., v_K) = \prod_k p(v_k | v_{pa(k)}) \tag{8.2}$$

The approach is known as Markov factorization, which is a DAG in the form of formulae.

An important concept related to dependency is the d-separation. In general, two sets of nodes A and B are d-separated by Z if 1) any path between a in A and b in B has a node in Z and 2) no z in Z is a collider (a path contains $a \to ... \to z \leftarrow ... \leftarrow b$) in any path between a and b. The reason for the latter is that two independent variables may become dependent if we condition on their common consequence, so 2) avoids creating a dependence by conditioning on Z. The importance of d-separation is that if A and B are d-separated by Z, then they are independent conditioning on Z.

The causal effects of a node v_j to v_k are presented by causal paths, which are paths with arrows pointing in the direction of v_k. For example, in Figure 8.1 D has a direct effect on Y ($D \to Y$) and an indirect effect ($D \to C \to Y$). To identify causal effects, we need to block confounding effects, as indicated by other paths between nodes regardless of their direction. The back-door criterion can identify the set of nodes blocking confounding paths [Pearl, 2022]. A set of nodes Z blocks confounding paths between a and b if: 1) no node in Z is a descendant of b and 2) Z blocks every path between a and b that has an arrow to b. Using the DAG in Figure 8.1 as an example, there is a causal path between C and Y and a confounding path of $C \leftarrow X \to Y$, hence the set of a single node X blocks it, according to the backdoor criterion. However, it does not block the path of $C \leftarrow U \to Y$.

The backdoor criterion suggests a way of adjustment for estimating causal effects: the back-door adjustment. Assuming that there is no U, and X takes a finite number of values, we can estimate

$$E(Y(c)) = \sum_{X=x} E(Y|C = c, X = x)P(X = x), \tag{8.3}$$

where the sum is taken over all possible x values. Since $E(Y|C = c, X = x)$ can be modeled using an ER model of C, X, this approach is essentially the same as the approach of averaging popPKPD model predictions at $C = c$ over X.

There is also a front-door version of the above criterion and adjustment. A set Z satisfying the front-door criteria if 1) it intercepts all directed paths from a to b, 2) there is no unblocked back-door path between a and Z, and 3) all back-door paths from Z to b are blocked by a. If such a Z exists, then the causal effect of a on b can be identified. Apply it on the DAG in Figure 8.1 with $a = D$ and $b = Y$ and assume that there is no arrow from X and U to C, then the following front-door formula estimates the causal effect of D on Y when D is not randomized:

$$\begin{aligned} E(Y(d)) &= \sum_{C=c} E(Y(c))p(C(d) = c) \\ &= \sum_{C=c} [\sum_{D=d'} E(Y(c)|D = d', C = c)P(D = d')]p(C = c|D = d) \quad (8.4) \end{aligned}$$

where we assume that C only takes a finite number of levels for simplicity. Otherwise, the sum can be replaced by an integral. We will see the application of this formula in the causal mediation analysis.

In a simple but important special case in which D has no direct effect given $C = c$, we have $\sum_{D=d'} E(Y(c)|D = d', C = c)P(D = d') = E(Y(c)|C = c)$, therefore $E(Y(d)) = \sum_{C=c} E(Y(c|C = c)p(C = c|D = d)$, which is a simple form of using popPK and popPKPD for the prediction of the DR relationship. This algorithm also supports popPK-popPKPD approaches with covariate adjustment when front-door criteria are satisfied by conditioning on covariates X.

8.2.3 Causal DER relationships with continuous dose and exposure

The causal DER relationship with a continuous cause has additional complexity. For example, the DR relationship for binary D can be defined as a single parameter Δ, while for continuous dose, $\mu(d)$ is a function. When D_i only takes a finite number of levels, we can define the causal DR relationship by

$$\Delta(d, d') = E(Y_i(d) - Y_i(d')) \quad (8.5)$$

where d and d' are a pair of D_i values. Then, the theory and methods for causal inference of binary treatment apply. However, it is often preferred to define it as a function of d. Under some assumptions, for example, a linear DR model $E(Y_i(d)) = \beta_d d$, it can be simplified as a single-number estimand

$$\Delta(d + 1, d) = E(Y_i(d + 1) - Y_i(d)) = \beta_d \quad (8.6)$$

the average mean response to an increase of d by 1 unit. But in general $\Delta(d, d')$ will depend on the dose levels.

We can also define a general DR relationship as a derivative of the mean response.

$$\Delta(d') = \lim_{\delta d \to 0} \frac{E(Y_i(d'+\delta d) - Y_i(d'))}{\delta d} = \frac{d\mu(d')}{dd'} \tag{8.7}$$

It represents the trend of $E(Y_i(d))$ for a small change δd in it and is a function of d. Taking the three-parameter Emax model $\mu(d) = b_0 + (b_m - b_0)/(b_n/d+1)$ as an example, $\Delta(d)$ is its derivative with response to d, i.e., $\Delta(d) = (b_m - b_0)b_n(b_n + d)^{-2}$ which reduces to zero when $d \to \infty$.

To see how $\Delta(d)$ is used, consider $\Delta_e(d)$ and $\Delta_s(d)$ defined for the efficacy and safety responses, respectively, and the goal is to determine the dose that maximizes the utility of the weighted efficacy and safety responses with weights w_e and $-w_s$, respectively. Then, the optimal dose makes $w_e\Delta_e(d) = w_s\Delta_s(d)$, assuming that both $\Delta_e(d)$ and $\Delta_s(d)$ increase monotonously with d. This approach is equivalent to maximizing an utility index $U(d) \equiv w_e\mu_e(d) - w_s\mu_s(d)$.

The above definitions apply to the causal ER relationship with d replaced by c. The causal ER relationship is an important topic in pharmacometrics, since exposure, or specifically drug concentration, generally cannot be randomized [Rogers et al., 2023]. Even in an RCT in which the dose is randomized, determining the causal ER relationship is still a challenging task. However, randomized doses might be useful for causal inference of the ER relationship [Zhang et al., 2024].

One may question the purpose of determining the causal ER relationship defined as $\mu(c)$, as it is often not feasible to force $C_i = c$. An obvious usage of the ER relationship is to confirm the DR relationship and drug action mechanisms. It can also be used to facilitate causal inference of the DR relationship, although often a conditional ER relationship is more useful. Nevertheless, in the following, we will mainly consider causal ER relationships.

8.2.4 Confounding and exposure decomposition

To determine the causal inference strategy for the ER relationship, an intuitive way is to decompose the variability in exposure C_i into three components,

1. that due to observed covariates,
2. that due to randomization (e.g., randomized dose),
3. the rest (which can be due to random variation or unobserved confounders).

They should be treated differently, as shown in this chapter.

The covariates in 1. may or may not be a confounder. Fitting the ER model may help to shed some light on this. In any case, adjusting for them is recommended if possible to reduce confounding bias and variability in the ER relationship. The second part does not need special treatment and is the power house for causal inference. The third part is the main concern in using observational studies, although some of it may not be confounded.

Some approaches can (partially) identify some of these parts. For example, a generalized propensity score (GPS) (or a popPK model) can identify the first part. The control function (CF) represents the third part. For the third part, a prudent approach is to adjust for it in the ER modeling. Prudence, however, may incur a high cost, as we will see in the CF approaches.

Some common DE models (e.g., drug concentration of a compartmental model specified by linear ODEs with coefficients independent of dose) have the following form on the log-scale:

$$\log(C_i(t)) = \gamma_d \log(D_i) + \log(h(X_i, \boldsymbol{\gamma}_x, t)) + V_i \tag{8.8}$$

with X_i observed. If D_i is randomized, $\gamma_d \log(D_i)$ is the part due to randomization, $\log(h(X_i, \boldsymbol{\gamma}_x, t))$ observed (assuming that the model can be fitted), and V_i the rest, which may include unobserved confounders. Intuitively, the first part can be used without additional adjustment, and the second needs adjustment in the ER model. The third one can be treated as part 1 if we assume that no unobserved confounders exist, but otherwise should be excluded. If D_i is not randomized, the first part may be divided into a predictable part by X_i, which can join part 2, and the rest can be combined with V_i. The rest of the chapter deals with identifying these parts and properly adjusting them.

The decomposition plays a key role in causal inference for both ER and DR relationships. It shows that with randomized D_i we can at least separate the randomized component in C_i, hence ER relationship can be identified without the assumption of no unobserved confounders (but with some technical conditions). It also shows that although there may be multiple confounding factors in the second part, their confounding effect is summarized in $h(X_i, \boldsymbol{\gamma}_x, t)$, which acts as a GPS. Therefore, it is sufficient to adjust for it in the ER model.

8.2.5 Linear structural models and causal mediation analysis

To make the above concept more concrete, we use some simple models, known as structural equation models (SEM), which represent the underlying mechanistic relationship between variables in the causal inference literature, in a way similar to the DAG in Figure 8.1. A simple linear one is

$$Y_i(C_i, D_i, X_i) = \beta_c C_i + \beta_d D_i + \boldsymbol{\beta}_x^T X_i + U_i \tag{8.9}$$

$$C_i(D_i, X_i) = \gamma_d D_i + \boldsymbol{\gamma}_x X_i + V_i \tag{8.10}$$

where we introduce zero-mean random terms U_i, V_i that are independent of the other variables. In this SEM, $Y_i(C_i, D_i, X_i)$ denotes the response of subject i who has C_i, D_i, X_i, hence $Y_i(C_i, D_i, X_i) = Y_i$: the observed response. Similarly, we have $C_i(D_i, X_i) = C_i$. In the model, D_i affects Y_i not only directly but also indirectly through C_i, and C_i acts as a mediator. The analysis of direct and indirect causal effects is known as mediation analysis [VanderWeele, 2015].

Using a SEM we can specify counterfactuals, although they cannot be all realized (observed). For example, one can replace C_i with any hypothetical exposure values, e.g., c or c' to obtain $Y_i(C_i = c, D_i, X_i)$ and $Y_i(C_i = c', D_i, X_i)$. With this model, the causal effects of C_i and D_i can be written as

$$\begin{aligned}\Delta_c(d, d+1) &= \beta_d \\ \Delta_d(c, c+1) &= \beta_c.\end{aligned} \tag{8.11}$$

where $\Delta_{c(d)}$ denotes holding $C_i = c(D_i = d)$ constant. Note that although we condition on c or d, with the linear model, the relationship does not depend on the one we condition on. For the total effect of D_i including direct and indirect ones, we need the DE model and assume that V_i is independent of U_i. Then the model (8.9) can be written as

$$Y_i = \beta_c(\gamma_d D_i + \boldsymbol{\gamma}_x X_i + V_i) + \beta_d D_i + \boldsymbol{\beta}_x^T X_i + U_i. \tag{8.12}$$

Hence, the total dose effect is

$$\Delta(d, d+1) = \beta_c \gamma_d + \beta_d. \tag{8.13}$$

When the ER model is nonlinear, the estimation of the direct, indirect and total effects become much more complex, and their estimation will be deferred to later sections. However, the above discussion suggests fitting an SEM with as many covariates as feasible and predicting the response of a given dose with the fitted model for the target population, then estimating the mean response of this dose by averaging, which is more or less the popPK and popPKPD approaches and is also known as the direct adjustment in causal inference [Hernan and Robins, 2023].

Although SEM allows direct and indirect effects, in the following, we assume that there is no direct effect, that is, the dose acts via exposure only, which is often assumed in popPK/PD modeling.

8.2.6 Nonlinear mixed-effect structure models

The data for DER modeling are often longitudinal with repeated measures of exposure and response, and sometimes dose, if it changes over time. Suppose that there are in total J_i repeated measures from subject $i, i = 1, ..., n$ subjects with response, exposure Y_{ij}, C_{ij} and dose D_{ij} at time t_{ij} and we assume $t_{i1} = 0$. We may also observe p baseline variables denoted by X_i that can affect exposure and response, or both. This notation is rather general and covers most types of data. Often Y_{ij} and C_{ij} are not measured all at the same time. In this case, we take J_i as the total number of measures of all types and set the one that was not measured at a given time as missing.

Typical NLMM for DER modeling can be written as

$$\begin{aligned} Y_{ij} =& g(C_{ij}, \boldsymbol{\beta}_i) + \epsilon_{ij} \\ C_{ij} =& h(D_{ij}, \gamma_i) + e_{ij}, \\ \boldsymbol{\beta}_i =& \boldsymbol{\beta}^T X_i + U_i \\ \gamma_i =& \gamma^T X_i + V_i \end{aligned} \tag{8.14}$$

where $g(.,.)$ and $h(.,.)$ are ER and DE models, ϵ_i and e_i are zero mean random independent variables. U_i and V_i are random subject effects that represent unobserved random variation in response and exposure and may be correlated. There may be elements in X_i that only affect $\boldsymbol{\beta}_i$ or γ_i. In these cases, we set the corresponding elements in $\boldsymbol{\beta}$ or γ zero. We find that the NLMM are SEMs, although the random effects are additional. One key variant of the first model is $Y_{ij} = g(h(D_{ij}, \gamma_i), \boldsymbol{\beta}_i) + \epsilon_{ij}$, which assumes that Y_{ij} depends on the latent exposure given by the DE model, rather than the observed one. We have discussed the two types of models in length in the section on ME models in Chapter 4 and will continue the discussion in this chapter.

In a phase II dose-finding trial, the doses are randomized at time zero, so we have $D_{ij} = D_{i1} \equiv D_i$, that is, a constant dose over time. The dose may change depending on the response, for example, with a dose reduction due to safety events. This topic will be discussed extensively in the next chapter.

Most popPK/PD modeling approaches are likelihood-based, requiring the distribution of all random components in the models. For example, a common assumption is $U_i \sim N(0, \boldsymbol{\Sigma}_u)$, $V_i \sim N(0, \boldsymbol{\Sigma}_v), e_{ij} \sim N(0, \sigma_e^2)$, and $\epsilon_{ij} \sim N(0, \sigma_\epsilon^2)$. With the full distributional assumption, the NLMM in (8.14) specifies the Markov decomposition for C and Y in Section 8.1. However, many approaches in this chapter do not need a full specification of the likelihood function.

SEMs can be used in two ways: when both DE and ER models can be specified and fitted correctly, the g-computation approach can be used to describe the causal DER relationship. When only partial SEM can be specified and fitted, they can be used for more efficient and robust estimation of the causal DER relationship using a semi-parametric approach. Therefore, fitting SEMs in the presence of confounding factors is an important topic in causal inferences. The details will be given in the next section.

Since our focus is on the causal DER relationship, we take some simple popPK and popPKPD models as examples of SEMs. One is the average concentration in steady state with repeated oral dosing of interval τ and the drug PK follows the two-compartmental model with first-order absorption, which is simply

$$C_{ss} = \frac{FD}{Cl\tau} \tag{8.15}$$

where F is bioavailability, clearance $Cl = K_e V_d$ with elimination coefficients K_e and volume of distribution V_d. Another is the steady-state trough concentration with repeated IV dosing (or oral dosing with rapid absorption) of interval τ:

$$C_{ss} = \frac{D\exp(-K_e\tau)}{V_d(1-\exp(-K_e\tau))}. \tag{8.16}$$

For the ER model, we use mostly logistic models because it represents the essential nonlinear part of the 4-parameter Emax model [An et al., 2019]. These models will be used later to illustrate some causal inference approaches.

8.3 Causal inference with adjustment for confounders

The key step of causal inference is the adjustment for confounders. This task needs different assumptions; among them, one may be more reasonable than another depending on the situation and adjustment methods. Some assumptions are on ER models particularly on the impact of covariates. Others are on the DE relationship and the impact of covariates. These assumptions may be more reasonable, since often the popPK relationship is well understood and can be verified when exposure data are rich. The third type of assumptions concerns randomized dose or exposure; the former is common in dose-finding trials, but the latter is rare, with few randomized concentration studies [Holford et al., 1993a]. Sometimes, combining two types of assumptions makes the adjustment more robust and the inference more efficient. For example, DR approaches that combine the first two types of assumptions are often more efficient when both hold and are still valid when only one is correct.

The causal inference methodology for binary or categorical treatment is well developed in all aspects, including its methods, algorithms and software, and experience of application. In some specific scenarios, e.g., comparing responses at a few fixed dose levels, the above approaches can be directly used. However, extending them to dealing with quantitative dose/exposure is much more difficult. Some approaches developed in econometrics are based on large sample sizes, which are rare in our context. The following explores approaches relying more on reasonable modeling assumptions.

8.3.1 Direct adjustment via structural models

We start from the linear model for the ER relationship

$$Y_i = \beta_c C_i + \boldsymbol{\beta}_x^T X_i + \epsilon_i, \tag{8.17}$$

where X_i includes all confounders so that ϵ_i is not correlated with C_i. In this case, the marginal causal ER relationship is represented by β_c, so fitting the above model is sufficient to estimate β_c, assuming that $\boldsymbol{\beta}_x^T X_i$ correctly represents the confounder effects.

When the model is nonlinear, e.g., a GLM:

$$E(Y_i|X_i) = g(\beta_c C_i + \boldsymbol{\beta}_x^T X_i) \tag{8.18}$$

β_c is the not sufficient to determine $\mu(c) = E(Y_i(c))$. However, after fitting the model, we can calculate it by

$$\hat{\mu}(c) = n^{-1} \sum_{i=1}^{n} g(\hat{\beta}_c c + \hat{\boldsymbol{\beta}}_x^T X_i) \tag{8.19}$$

where $\hat{\beta}_c, \hat{\boldsymbol{\beta}}_x$ are estimates of the coefficients by fitting the GLM.

Next, we consider the popPKPD model

$$Y_{ij} = g(C_{ij}, \boldsymbol{\beta}_i) + \epsilon_{ij} \tag{8.20}$$

$$\boldsymbol{\beta}_i = \boldsymbol{\beta}^T X_i + U_i \tag{8.21}$$

When $g(.,.)$ is a nonlinear function, the coefficients $\boldsymbol{\beta}$ alone are not sufficient to determine the marginal ER relationship. However, since we have

$$\mu_c(c) = E(Y_{ij}(c)) = E(g(c, \boldsymbol{\beta}_i)) \tag{8.22}$$

if estimates $\hat{\boldsymbol{\beta}}$ and $\hat{U}_i$ are available from popPKPD analysis, we can estimate

$$\hat{\mu}(c) = n^{-1} \sum_{i=1}^{n} g(c, \hat{\boldsymbol{\beta}}^T X_i + \hat{U}_i) \tag{8.23}$$

In some situations, an analytical solution for $E(g(c, \boldsymbol{\beta}_i))$ may exist, e.g., for Poisson regressions in which we have $E(g(c, \boldsymbol{\beta}_i)) = E(\exp(\beta_c c + \boldsymbol{\beta}^T X_i + U_i)) = \exp(\beta_c c + \text{var}(\boldsymbol{\beta}_i^T X_i + U_i)/2)$ with normally distributed X_i and U_i. However, the empirical mean estimator is more robust to misspecification of the distributional assumption in X_i and U_i, which is difficult to verify when n is not large.

If we assume that there is a parametric model for $\mu(c)$: $\mu(c) = m(c, \boldsymbol{\beta})$, an approach to estimate $\boldsymbol{\beta}$ is to generate $\hat{\mu}(c)$ for a set of c values using (8.19). Then we fit the model $m(c, \boldsymbol{\beta})$ to these $\hat{\mu}(c_k)$s to obtain $\hat{\boldsymbol{\beta}}$. Although in theory $m(c, \boldsymbol{\beta})$ should not be the same type of model as $g(C_{ij}, \boldsymbol{\beta}_i)$ due to non-collapsibility of nonlinear models in general, the approach is a useful way if we prefer a parametric form of the causal ER relationship. Note that the SE of $\hat{\boldsymbol{\beta}}$ given by normal regression software is incorrect, since it does not take into account all the variability in $\hat{\mu}(c_k)$s.

Suppose that there is no repeated measure for model (8.21), but $\mathbf{X}_i$ are observed. In this case, we can still fit model

$$Y_i = g^*(C_i, \boldsymbol{\beta}^T \mathbf{X}_i) + \epsilon_i \tag{8.24}$$

where $g^*(c, \boldsymbol{\beta}^T \mathbf{X}_i) = E(g^*(c, \boldsymbol{\beta}^T \mathbf{X}_i + U_i))$ and U_i is averaged over in the expectation. Although in general $g(.,.)$ is a different function from $g^*(.,.)$, we may take a pragmatic approach assuming that $g^*(.,.)$ is correct and this assumption can be verified by the data (with sufficient $\mathbf{X}_i$ data).

These approaches are closely linked to the g-computation in causal inference [Hernan and Robins, 2023]. Software such as stdReg fits common regression models such as logistic and Cox models, and provides the correct SE for $\hat{\beta}_c$.

Often, deciding which elements in $\mathbf{X}_i$ should be included in the ER model is still a difficult decision to make. When p is not small (e.g., when $\mathbf{X}_i$ contains a large number of genomics markers), including all of them in the ER model may be impossible (e.g., when Y_{ij} is an indicator of a rare event). In this case, DE modeling can help, since exposure data are often much richer than rare event data. If there are only a few with considerable impact in the DE model, one may include all of them in the ER model if possible. If not, the GPS approach below provides an alternative.

The same confounding issue also occurs when the DE model is fitted if the dose depends on factors that may affect the exposure. This may happen when the prescribed dose depends on some factors such as age or renal/liver functions. Therefore, the fitted DE model should also include sufficient factors in $\mathbf{X}_i$.

When the DE model is linear to $\mathbf{X}_i$ but the ER model has an additive nonlinear function of $\mathbf{X}_i$

$$\begin{aligned} C_i &= \mathbf{X}_i^T \boldsymbol{\gamma} + V_i \\ Y_i &= \beta_c C_i + g(\mathbf{X}_i) + \epsilon_i \end{aligned} \tag{8.25}$$

one may think that direct adjustment by a misspecified working model

$$Y_i = \beta_c C_i + \boldsymbol{\beta}_x^T \mathbf{X}_i + \epsilon_i \tag{8.26}$$

would be insufficient. In fact, for the estimation of β_c, it is sufficient. For easy illustration, we use the matrix form of the models and stack C_is as $\mathbf{C}$, $\mathbf{X}_i$ as $\mathbf{X} = (\mathbf{X}_1^T, ..., \mathbf{X}_n^T)^T$, a $n \times p$ matrix, V_is as $\mathbf{V}$, $g(\mathbf{X}_i)$ as $g(\mathbf{X})$ and Y_i as $\mathbf{Y}$. Then, by regression partition, we can write the estimate of β_c in (8.26) as

$$\hat{\beta}_c = (\mathbf{C}^T(I - \mathbf{P}_x)C)^{-1}(\mathbf{C}^T(I - \mathbf{P}_x)\mathbf{Y}) \tag{8.27}$$

where $\mathbf{P}_x = \mathbf{X}^T(\mathbf{X}^T\mathbf{X})^{-1}\mathbf{X}$ is the projection matrix to the space of $\mathbf{X}$ and $I - \mathbf{P}_x$ projects to its orthogonal space. With the weak law of large numbers, we know that $\mathbf{C}^T(I - \mathbf{P}_x)\mathbf{C}/n \to M_c$, a constant matrix. Therefore, the bias of $\hat{\beta}_c$ can be derived as

$$\begin{aligned} E((\mathbf{C}^T(I - \mathbf{P}_x)\mathbf{C})^{-1}(\mathbf{C}^T(I - \mathbf{P}_x)g(\mathbf{X}))) &\approx M_c^{-1}E(n^{-1}(\boldsymbol{\gamma}\mathbf{X}^T + \mathbf{V})(I - \mathbf{P}_x)g(\mathbf{X})) \\ &= M_c^{-1}n^{-1}E(\boldsymbol{\gamma}\mathbf{X}^T(I - \mathbf{P}_x)g(\mathbf{X})) = 0 \end{aligned} \tag{8.28}$$

where the last equation is due to $\mathbf{X}^T(I - \mathbf{P}_x) = 0$. A numerical example can be found below.

Finally, we consider situations where no adjustment for subject-level confounders is needed for causal ER modeling. This happens when there are sufficient repeated response measures for each subject to fit the popPKPD model (8.14) and the variability of C_{ij} is sufficient to estimate $\boldsymbol{\beta}_i$. The 2-stage approach is the simplest when the number of repeated measures J_i is sufficiently large, since $\boldsymbol{\beta}_i$ can be estimated individually by fitting data of each subject by nonlinear least squares (NLS) to obtain $\hat{\boldsymbol{\beta}}_i$. Following the asymptotic properties of NLS, we have $\hat{\boldsymbol{\beta}}_i \to \boldsymbol{\beta}_i$ when $J_i \to \infty$, and $\boldsymbol{\beta}$ can be estimated by regressing $\hat{\boldsymbol{\beta}}_i$ to covariates $\mathbf{X}_i$. Then, $\mu(c)$ can be estimated by the g-computation approach such as (8.23). Therefore, there is no need for adjustment for confounding at subject level. This is due to the fact that fitting the model to each subject is equivalent to conditioning on U_i and $\mathbf{X}_i$, so this approach blocks the backdoor path from C to Y in Figure 8.1. One may also think of this as an extreme case of stratification, that is, here we stratify by subjects. The precision of this approach depends on how accurately $\boldsymbol{\beta}_i$ can be estimated using within-subject data. However, often J_i is limited, hence calling for large sample properties within subject is risky. Also, when the variability in C_{ij} is low for some subjects, outliers can affect the estimation of $\boldsymbol{\gamma}$ and consequently $\mu(c)$,

Another approach commonly used in popPK/PD modeling is the MLE that maximizes the marginal likelihood of Y_{ij} and C_{ij}, assuming distributions for random terms. Although MLE is much more complex than the 2-stage approach and also needs distributional assumptions, by the NLMM theory, when $J_i \to \infty$, the MLE estimates converge to the same limit as the 2-stage approach, even when the distributional assumptions are misspecified. Therefore, when $J_i \to \infty$, adjustment for confounding factors at the subject level is not required for MLE as well. However, we prefer to adjust for potential confounding rather than relying on the large sample properties that are often in question.

8.3.2 Generalized propensity scores

Propensity scores (PS) have been widely used in causal inference [Rosenbaum and Rubin, 1983]. The basic PS is for binary treatment and is defined as the probability of being treated, as a function of $\mathbf{X}_i$. It can be used as a measure of the confounding effect in treatment allocation and can be used for matching and weighting so that after adjustment by PS, each subject would have the same chance of being treated.

When exposure has only a few levels, say $c^1, c^2, ..., c^K$, to estimate causal ER relationship, the PS can be extended to GPS, following the same idea. For example, a GPS can be defined as

$$e(c^k|\mathbf{X}_i) \equiv P(C_i = c^k|\mathbf{X}_i). \tag{8.29}$$

An assumption (known as the positivity assumption) is that for any $\mathbf{X}_i$, $P(C_i = c^k|\underline{\mathbf{X}}_i)$ is not degenerate. This type of GPS (PS for multilevel exposure) has been widely used, including the original work proposed it

[Imbens, 2000; Wang et al., 2001; Zhang et al., 2016]. However, these approaches cannot be applied to continuous exposure, such as concentration or PK parameters.

GPS for continuous exposure is much more complex even without repeated measures. Starting from a simple situation with constant dose D and only one pair of C_i and Y_i from subject i. In this case, a GPS can be defined as the conditional density function of exposure, given $\mathbf{X}_i$ [Imai and Van Dyk, 2004; Hirano and Imbens, 2004; Zhao et al., 2020]: $e(c|\mathbf{X}_i) \equiv f_{c|x}(c|\mathbf{X}_i)$. Hirano and Imbens [2004] assumed a normal distribution for $e(c|\mathbf{X}_i)$ with mean $\gamma^T\mathbf{X}_i$. Imai and Van Dyk [2004] consider a more general situation in which $e(c|\mathbf{X}_i)$ can be uniquely parameterized, that is, by a parametric function that can uniquely determine $e(c|\mathbf{X}_i)$. For example, if C_i follows a standard normal distribution with mean $\gamma^T\mathbf{X}_i$, then $e(c|\mathbf{X}_i)$ is uniquely determined by $\gamma^T\mathbf{X}_i$.

Some key assumptions are needed to use GPS for confounding adjustments. We assume the following, although there are several alternatives:

1. (Consistency) $Y_i(C_i) = Y_i(c)$ when $C_i = c$ for any c in its range.
2. (Ignobility)

$$P(C_i|Y_i(c), \mathbf{X}_i) = P(C_i|\mathbf{X}_i) \tag{8.30}$$

$$\text{or}: \quad P(Y_i(c)|C_i, \mathbf{X}_i) = P(Y_i(c)|\mathbf{X}_i) \tag{8.31}$$

3. There is a unique parametric function $\theta(\mathbf{X}_i, \gamma)$ that fully specifies $P(C_i|\mathbf{X}_i)$.

Among them, the second, with two options, is the most important as it means that the concentration C_i does not depend on the potential outcome $Y_i(c)$ given $\mathbf{X}_i$. The two options are not equivalent, and which one is needed depends on the method of using GPS. The third one is not necessary for all GPS based adjustments, but very useful in our context. With these assumptions, we have [Hirano and Imbens, 2004]

$$p(Y_i(c)|\mathbf{X}_i, e(c|\mathbf{X}_i)) = p(Y_i(c)|e(c|\mathbf{X}_i)), \tag{8.32}$$

that is, it is sufficient to condition on $e(\mathbf{X}_i)$ to control confounding effects in C_i.

The PS approach has the advantage of adjusting potentially many covariates using a single score; an obvious issue is that it does not guarantee the balance of these factors themselves. An approach to its improvement is the covariate balancing PS, which adds covariate balancing conditions when fitting the PS model. Similar problems occur in GPS adjustment, and the same remedy has also been proposed [Fong et al., 2018]. A less obvious approach is to balance for a sample of $\hat{\gamma}$ using bootstrap when fitting the PS model [Brown et al., 2021], based on the idea that subjects with exactly the same $\mathbf{X}_i$ always have the same bootstrapped GPS.

Although GPS is often estimated by an empirical model, in popPK/PD modeling, the popPK model is a mechanistic GPS model. For example, for intravenous bolus administration, a popPK model for steady-state trough after multiple doses:

$$C_i = \frac{D_i^{\gamma_d} \exp(-K_{ei}\tau)}{V_{di}(1 - \exp(-K_{ei}\tau))}\epsilon_i, \tag{8.33}$$

where ϵ_i is a positive random term, τ is the dosing interval, γ_d allows non-proportional PK. V_{di}, K_{ei} are the volume of distribution and elimination rate as a function of $\mathbf{X}_i$

$$\begin{aligned} \log(V_{di}) =& \gamma_v^T \mathbf{X}_i \\ \log(K_{ei}) =& \gamma_e^T \mathbf{X}_i. \end{aligned} \tag{8.34}$$

The popPK model has a multiplicative random error since $C_i > 0$ by its nature. The model can be written on the log-scale:

$$\log(C_i) = \gamma_d \log(D_i) + \log(\frac{\exp(-K_{ei}\tau)}{V_{di}(1 - \exp(-K_{ei}\tau))}) + V_i, \tag{8.35}$$

where $V_i = \log(\epsilon_i)$ is a zero mean random error. In terms of the decomposition in Section 8.2.4, the second term is the observed part $h(\mathbf{X}_i, \gamma)$ and is a complex nonlinear function of $\mathbf{X}_i$, but it represents their confounding effects on C_i.

A nonlinear mixed model normally also includes random effects, but they are omitted here since there are no repeated measurements to identify them. Even in this simple situation, we have two linear predictors, rather than one in the GLM model. To simplify, we take

$$e(\mathbf{X}_i) = \frac{\exp(-K_{ei}\tau)}{V_{di}(1 - \exp(-K_{ei}\tau))}, \tag{8.36}$$

in which the dependence on $\mathbf{X}_i$ is via V_{di}, K_{ei}. It may not fully specify $P(C_i|\mathbf{X}_i)$ since it also depends on ϵ_i, but it captures all effects of $\mathbf{X}_i$.

8.3.3 Adjustment by Generalized propensity scores

There are multiple approaches to using GPS for adjustment, some may be more appropriate than others for a specific purpose. Most are rooted in the key result (8.32). For example, let

$$g(c, e) = E(Y_i(C_i)|C_i = c, e(c|\mathbf{X}_i) = e) \tag{8.37}$$

then

$$E(Y_i(c)) = E(g(c, e(c|\mathbf{X}_i))). \tag{8.38}$$

One way to use the result is to adjust $e_i \equiv e(C_i|\mathbf{X}_i)$ in an ER model, e.g., $g(C_i, e_i) = \beta_c C_i + \beta_e e_i$. A more complex function of e_i can also be used, e.g., as in Hirano and Imbens [2004] that included e_i^2 and $e_i^2 C_i$ in the model.

In general, we can specify an ER model conditional on both C_i and e_i (and other covariates if appropriate):

$$E(Y_i|C_i, e_i) = g(C_i, e_i, \boldsymbol{\beta}) \tag{8.39}$$

with unknown parameters $\boldsymbol{\beta}$. Hirano and Imbens [2004] used the density function as e_i in the model. Zhao et al. [2020] show that a more stable approach is to use the parametric form $\boldsymbol{\gamma}^T\mathbf{X}_i$ to replace e_i.

Since $g(c, e)$ is conditional on e, to obtain the marginal ER model, g-computation can be used as below (8.43). After obtaining the parameter estimate $\hat{\boldsymbol{\beta}}$, $\mu(c)$ can be estimated by

$$\hat{\mu}(c) = n^{-1}\sum_{i=1}^{n} g(c, e_i, \hat{\boldsymbol{\beta}}) \tag{8.40}$$

which uses the principle of (8.32) with $E(Y_i|C_i, e_i)$ as integrand.

If the final goal of DER modeling is to predict the outcome for a given dose: $\mu(d)$, the g-computation can also be used. For this purpose, we also need the DE model to predict C_i for a given dose. Denote the predicted C_i under dose d by $\hat{C}_i(d)$, $\mu(d)$ can be estimated by

$$\hat{\mu}(d) = n^{-1}\sum_{i=1}^{n} g(\hat{C}_i(d), e_i, \hat{\boldsymbol{\beta}}) \tag{8.41}$$

The above approach is based on the correct specification of the model $g(C_i, e_i, \boldsymbol{\beta})$. Alternatively, stratification and matching by GPS are simple semi-parametric approaches. Taking the former as an example, we divide the GPS value range into K intervals $(L_k, U_k), k = 1, ..., K$ and assign all subjects to these K strata, then we can fit a stratified ER model. The rational of stratification is that approximately within a stratum, the probability of having exposure $C_i = c$ rather than $C_i = c'$ does not depend on $\mathbf{X}_i$. For example, if the ER model is a logistic model, the stratified analysis fits a model

$$E(Y_i|C_i, S_{ik}) = \text{expit}(\beta_0 + \sum_{k=1}^{K} \beta_k S_{ik} + \beta_c C_i) \tag{8.42}$$

where β_k is the coefficient for the indicator $S_{ik} \equiv I(L_k \leq e_i < U_k)$. Then β_c is a causal exposure effect conditional on S_{ik}. $E(Y_i|C_i, S_{ik})$ can be considered as an approximation to $E(Y_i|C_i, e_i)$.

The interpretation of β_c is tricky as it is the causal effect of subjects within strata, not a marginal causal effect. However, g-computation can be used to estimate $\mu_(c) = E(Y(c))$ by

$$\hat{\mu}(c) = n^{-1}\sum_{i=1}^{n} \text{expit}(\hat{\beta}_0 + \sum_{k=1}^{K} \hat{\beta}_k S_{ik} + \hat{\beta}_c c) \tag{8.43}$$

in which the response to exposure c is averaged throughout the population. Then it can be used to estimate the rate difference or ratio of $\mu(c)$ and $\mu(c')$, and even their marginal OR by

$$\hat{OR}(c, c') = \frac{\hat{\mu}(c)(1 - \hat{\mu}(c'))}{\hat{\mu}(c')(1 - \hat{\mu}(c))}. \tag{8.44}$$

However, since the logistic model is not collapsible, even if the conditional log-OR is constant, the marginal OR depends on c and c'. The GPS matching follows a similar idea as stratification, that is, to compare $\mu(c)$ and $\mu(c')$ we find a pair of subjects with $c_i = c$ and $c_{i'} = c'$ with the same or similar GPS values. But it is rarely used due to the difficulty in matching GPS.

Inverse probability weighting (IPW) can also be used for GPS adjustment by weighting each subject with the inverse of GPS. To see how it works, we first consider how to estimate $E(Y_i(c^k))$ when C_i only takes K possible levels. It can be estimated by an IPW estimator [Imbens, 2000]

$$\hat{\mu}(c^k) = n^{-1} \sum_{i=1}^{n} I(C_i = c^k) Y_i / P(c^k | \mathbf{X}_i), \tag{8.45}$$

since $E(\hat{\mu}(c^k)) = E(I(C_i = c^k)Y_i(c^k)/P(C_i = c^k|\mathbf{X}_i)) = E(Y_i(c^k))$. Although for continuous C_i, $P(C_i = c) = 0$, with a proper GPS model $e_i > 0$, the same intuition applies without dealing with technical difficulties. For example, to adjust by GPS in a logistic model with

$$E(Y_i|C_i) = \text{expit}(\beta_0 + \beta_c C_i), \tag{8.46}$$

we can estimate β_0 and β_c by solving the inverse GPS weighted EE

$$\sum_{i=1}^{n} w_i (1, C_i)^T (Y_i - \text{expit}(\beta_0 + \beta_c C_i)) = 0 \tag{8.47}$$

where $w_i = 1/e_i$ is the inverse GPS weight. The weights can have extreme values, since some e_i may be close to zero. Therefore, in practice, we use a stable weight $w_i = f(C_i)/e_i$, where $f(c)$ is the marginal density function of C_i, which can be estimated by averaging GPS over $\mathbf{X}_i$. See the R-code later for how the stable weight is implemented. The key difference between the IPW and the conditional approach that includes e_i as a covariate is that the IPW estimator directly estimates the marginal ER relationship, while the other estimates the conditional ER relationship.

Estimated β_0 and β_c are consistent under some technical conditions; see, e.g., Zhang et al. [2016]. Note that although for stratification, using the density version e_i or its parametric form $\gamma^T \mathbf{X}_i$ does not make much difference, for IPW, only using the density is valid. This fact also indicates the sensitivity of the IPW approach to the DE model misspecification. Although one can use a non-parametric approach to estimate e_i, the estimated e_i and the corresponding weight may become even more unstable.

Next, we add dose D_i to the model and examine how the above approaches should be changed to accommodate it, assuming that D_i has no direct effect. When D_i is not randomized and its assignment can depend on $\mathbf{X}_i$, the DE model can also be subject to confounding bias. However, if a popPK model is performed correctly with $\mathbf{X}_i$ including all confounders, direct adjustment is sufficient to eliminate the confounding effect. Therefore, we can assume that, e.g., the IV steady-state model

$$C_i = \frac{D_i \exp(-K_{ei}\tau)}{V_{di}(1 - \exp(-K_{ei}\tau))}\epsilon_i, \tag{8.48}$$

is correctly fitted and the estimated parameters are consistent. For simplicity, we assume again that C_i takes only K possible level $c^1, ..., c^K$, and also D_i only takes K levels $d^1, ..., d^K$ with the propensity of taking d^k as

$$p_k(\mathbf{X}_i) \equiv P(D_i = d^k|\mathbf{X}_i) = h(\mathbf{X}_i, \gamma) \tag{8.49}$$

where we assume a model $h(.,.)$ and parameters γ. For simplicity we denote the GPS with dose d by $e^d(c^k|\mathbf{X}_i)$, we can derive

$$e^d(c^k|\mathbf{X}_i) = E(e(c^k|D_i, \mathbf{X}_i)P(D_i|\mathbf{X}_i)) = \sum_{j=1}^{K} e(c^k|D_i = d^j, \mathbf{X}_i)p_j(\mathbf{X}_i) \tag{8.50}$$

where $e(c^k|D_i, \mathbf{X}_i)$ is the GPS (8.36) with $D_i, \mathbf{X}_i$ as covariates, and $e^d(c^k|\mathbf{X}_i)$ can be used as the GPS.

When D_i is randomized, there is no need to adjust for $\mathbf{X}_i$ for dose allocation. However, we still need to take $p_k \equiv P(D_i = d^k)$ into account in the adjustment. Specifically, to estimate $E(Y_i(c^k))$ we should weight Y_i of subject i who had $D_i = d^j$ in the sample mean by $(P(c^k|\mathbf{X}_i, d^j)p_j(\mathbf{X}_i))^{-1}$. For continuous C_i, $P(c^k|\mathbf{X}_i, d_j)$ can be replaced by the density of C_i conditional on $\mathbf{X}_i, d^j$.

To verify this approach, we can write the weighted mean of Y_i with $C_i = c^k$ as

$$\begin{aligned}
&E(n^{-1}\sum_{i=1}^{n} \frac{I(C_i = c^k, D_i = d^j)Y_i}{P(c^k|\mathbf{X}_i, d_j)p_j(\mathbf{X}_i)}) \\
=&E(E(\frac{I(C_i = c^k, D_i = d^j)Y_i(c^k)}{P(c^k, d^j|\mathbf{X}_i)}|\mathbf{X}_i)) \\
=&E(Y_i(c^k)).
\end{aligned} \tag{8.51}$$

in which the second equation is due to the absence of direct effect from D_i to Y_i.

Finally, we consider models with repeated measurement and will introduce random effects into the models step by step. Suppose that we have repeated trough measures in steady state, but only one outcome measure. Then C_{ij} is still given by (8.48), but random coefficients can be introduced as

$$\begin{aligned}\log(V_{di}) =& \gamma_v^T \mathbf{X}_i + V_{vi} \\ \log(K_{ei}) =& \gamma_e^T \mathbf{X}_i + V_{ei}\end{aligned} \tag{8.52}$$

where we assume that $V_{vi} \sim N(0, \sigma_v^2)$ and $V_{ei} \sim N(0, \sigma_e^2)$, as typically assumed for a popPK model. The GPS can be obtained by averaging over the random coefficients

$$e(c|\mathbf{X}_i) = E(f(c|V_{di}, K_{ei})|\mathbf{X}_i) \tag{8.53}$$

in which a numerical calculation may be needed to evaluate the right-hand side. It seems that since the random components are independent of $\mathbf{X}_i$, we may still use $e(c|\mathbf{X}_i)$ based on (8.34).

If there are repeated outcome measures Y_{ij}, we can also introduce random coefficients as in the original ER models (8.24). Here, we focus on a logistic model without $\mathbf{X}_i$:

$$E(Y_{ij}|C_{ij}, U_i) = \text{expit}(\beta_{0i} + \beta_{ci} C_{ij}) \tag{8.54}$$

where $\boldsymbol{\beta}_i = (\beta_{0i}, \beta_{ci}) = \boldsymbol{\beta} + U_i$. Again, we assume that the confounded components in U_i can be represented by the random term in the DE model, so fitting a model $E(Y_{ij}|C_{ij}, e_i) = \text{expit}(\beta_{0i} + \beta_{ci} C_{ij} + \beta_e e_i)$ is sufficient to adjust for confounding effects. Again, we note that the logistic model is not collapsible; hence, when the model for $E(Y_{ij}|C_{ij}, e_i)$ is logistic, the model for $E(Y_{ij}|C_{ij}, U_i)$ is not. This problem generally occurs in nonlinear conditional ER models and the corresponding marginal ER relationship may not have a parametric form.

Adjustment with general NLMMs (8.21) and (3.17) needs further discussion. As discussed above, when there are many repeated measures with sufficient variation in C_{ij}, $\hat{\boldsymbol{\beta}}_i$ can be estimated consistently with no impact of subject-level confounders. However, even without repeated measures, models (8.21) and (3.17) are more general than the logistic models above, since potential confounders can occur in multiple places in model (8.21), rather than in the linear predictor only in the logistic model. To extend our approach to these models, we consider a model with a structure similar to NLMMs, but without repeated measures and random effects. That is, we assume that

$$\begin{aligned}Y_i &= g(C_i, \boldsymbol{\beta}_i) + \varepsilon_i \\ \boldsymbol{\beta}_i &= \boldsymbol{\beta} + \boldsymbol{\beta}_x^T \mathbf{X}_i + U_i\end{aligned} \tag{8.55}$$

where $\mathbf{X}_i$ are potential confounders that may or may not be observed. Our goal is to model the marginal ER relationship without explicitly adjusting for $\mathbf{X}_i$ in this model. Due to non-collapsibility of general nonlinear models, the marginal ER model may not have an analytical form; hence, approximation or the use of empirical models is necessary.

We first consider a first-order approximation around $\boldsymbol{\beta}$ as (3.23).

$$Y_i \approx g(C_i, \boldsymbol{\beta}) + \dot{g}_\beta(C_i, \boldsymbol{\beta})(\boldsymbol{\beta} + U_i) + \varepsilon_i \tag{8.56}$$

This is a good approximation only when U_i is small, but the adjustment based on it requires fewer assumptions. For the adjustment with GPS e_i following Imai and Van Dyk [2004], we assume that

$$E(Y_i|C_i, e_i) \approx g(C_i, \boldsymbol{\beta}) + E(U_i|e_i) = g(C_i, \boldsymbol{\beta}) + \beta_e e_i + U_i^* \tag{8.57}$$

where we have assumed that $U_i = \beta_e e_i + U_i^*$ and $C_i \perp U_i^*$. This approximation allows us to fit a model $g(C_i, \boldsymbol{\beta})$ and adjust for e_i.

A possible improvement can be based on the assumption of

$$E(Y_i|C_i, e_i) = g(C_i, e_i, \boldsymbol{\beta}, \boldsymbol{\beta}_e) \tag{8.58}$$

which can be considered a more accurate approximation than (8.56) if e_i represents a part of the prognostic effects of $\mathbf{X}_i$. A model based on this approximation is $\boldsymbol{\beta}_i = \boldsymbol{\beta} + \boldsymbol{\beta}_e e_i + U_i^*$. For example, with $\boldsymbol{\beta}_i = (Emax_i, EC_{50i})$, the model includes two coefficients in $\boldsymbol{\beta}_e$ to adjust for e_i in each of the two components.

$$E(Y_i|C_i, e_i) \approx g(C_i, \boldsymbol{\beta}, \boldsymbol{\beta}_e) + \beta_e e_i + U_i^*, \tag{8.59}$$

With this approximation, we can fit a model

$$Y_i = g(C_i, \hat{e}_i, \boldsymbol{\beta}, \boldsymbol{\beta}_e) + \varepsilon_i. \tag{8.60}$$

It is not a marginal causal ER model and the parameter estimates conditioning on $\hat{e}_i$ do not have a causal interpretation. However, the marginal DR relationship can be estimated as

$$\hat{\mu}(Y_i(c)) = \sum_{i=1}^{n} g(C_i, \hat{e}_i, \hat{\boldsymbol{\beta}}, \hat{\boldsymbol{\beta}}_e) \tag{8.61}$$

which is a g-computation approach.

When there are a few repeated measures, the task of adjustment becomes more complex. One approach is to use the approximation of Lindstrom and Bates [1990] (3.24) and add $\hat{e}_i$ as an additional adjustment. However, this approximation is known to be unstable due to the need to fit a nonlinear model to a few data points for each subject. Its performance needs careful evaluation.

8.3.4 Covariate balancing

IPW eliminates confounding effects by balancing the distribution of $\mathbf{X}_i$ in the weighted population. Alternatively, we can also directly balance the covariates as proposed by entropy balance [Vegetabile et al., 2021] and CBGPS

[Fong et al., 2018], both balancing the cross product $\mathbf{X}_i^* C_i^*$, where $X_i^*(C_i^*)$ is centered $\mathbf{X}_i(C_i)$, that is, we find w_i such that

$$\sum w_i \mathbf{X}_i^* C_i^* = 0. \tag{8.62}$$

To see how it works, suppose that the data generation model is

$$Y_i^* = \beta_c C_i^* + \boldsymbol{\beta}_x \mathbf{X}_i^* + \epsilon_i. \tag{8.63}$$

Our goal is to estimate β_c without directly adjusting $\mathbf{X}_i^*$, that is, to fit a linear model $Y_i^* = \beta_c C_i^* + \epsilon_i$. Fitting the model without adjustment does not result in a consistent estimator of β_c, since $\mathbf{X}_i^*$ is a confounder. However, a weighted LS estimator with weights w_i satisfying (8.62) is a consistent. The weighted LS method solves the EE

$$S(\beta_c) = \sum_{i=1}^n w_i C_i^* (Y_i^* - \beta_c C_i^*) = 0. \tag{8.64}$$

Since $E(S(\beta_c)) = E(\sum_{i=1}^n w_i C_i^* (\boldsymbol{\beta}_x^T \mathbf{X}_i^* + \epsilon_i) = E(w_i C_i^* \epsilon_i) = 0$, where the second equation is due to (8.62), we have $\hat{\beta}_c \to \beta_c$ when $n \to \infty$. Note that this property relies on the linear ER model.

Although any w_i that balances $\mathbf{X}_i^* C_i^*$ can be used, GPS-based weights have an additional advantage. As we have seen above, even when the ER model is not linear in $\mathbf{X}_i$, the IPW with GPS can still adjust for confounding. For simplicity, we consider $w_i = 1/e_i$ rather than the stable weight and assume a simple DE model $C_i^* = \boldsymbol{\gamma}_x^T \mathbf{X}_i^* + V_i$ where $V_i \sim N(0, \sigma_v^2)$ is independent of $\mathbf{X}_i$. To calculate the weight $w_i = 1/e_i$, we can estimate $\boldsymbol{\gamma}_x$ by solving the equation

$$S(\boldsymbol{\gamma}_x) = n^{-1} \sum_{i=1}^n \exp((C_i^* - \boldsymbol{\gamma}_x^T \mathbf{X}_i^*)^2 / 2\sigma_v^2) \mathbf{X}_i^* C_i^* = 0. \tag{8.65}$$

When the DE model is correctly specified, its solution $\hat{\boldsymbol{\gamma}}_x \to \boldsymbol{\gamma}_x$, since for an arbitrary $\boldsymbol{\gamma}'_x$ $(C_i^* - \boldsymbol{\gamma}_x'^T \mathbf{X}_i^*)^2$ is a function of $\mathbf{X}_i^*$, hence $E(S(\boldsymbol{\gamma}'_x)) \neq 0$, unless $\boldsymbol{\gamma}'_x = \boldsymbol{\gamma}_x$. Therefore, with this approach, we obtain a GPS that is the density of C_i^* and its weights balance $\mathbf{X}_i^* C_i^*$.

Looking at (8.64), we find that if the confounding term $\boldsymbol{\beta}_x C_i^*$ in the model (8.63) is replaced by an arbitrary function $f(C_i^*)$, then to eliminate its impact, we need a balancing condition.

$$\sum w_i f(\mathbf{X}_i^*) C_i^* = 0. \tag{8.66}$$

Although this seems not feasible without knowing $f(\mathbf{X}_i^*)$, there may be other data sources that allow us to fit a flexible model for $f(\mathbf{X}_i^*)$ without the dose part. Then the fitted model can be used for balancing. This approach is well known in survey sampling as model-assisted calibration [Breidt and Opsomer, 2017]. In addition, if the data generation model has a term $C_i^* \mathbf{X}_i^*$, we also have to balance the term $C_i^{*2} \mathbf{X}_i^*$. Therefore, covariate balancing may not be sufficient to adjust if an arbitrary nonlinear model is assumed.

8.3.5 Doubly robust approaches

The GPS estimator for ER modeling can be made doubly robust, that is, it is consistent when either the GPS model, or a ER model is correct. We start from the case where only finite levels $C_i \in (c^1, ..., c^K)$ are possible. An IPW-based DR estimator has the following form:

$$\hat{\mu}(c^k) = \sum_{i=1}^{n} \frac{I(C_i = c^k)Y_i}{e_i(c^k)} - \frac{I(C_i = c^k) - e_i(c^k)}{e_i(c^k)} m(\mathbf{X}_i, c^k, \hat{\boldsymbol{\beta}}) \tag{8.67}$$

$$= \sum_{i=1}^{n} \frac{I(C_i = c^k)(Y_i - m(\mathbf{X}_i, c^k, \hat{\boldsymbol{\beta}}))}{e_i(c^k)} + m(\mathbf{X}_i, c^k, \hat{\boldsymbol{\beta}}) \tag{8.68}$$

where $m(\mathbf{X}_i, c, \boldsymbol{\beta})$ is an ER model and $\hat{\boldsymbol{\beta}}$ are estimated by fitting the model to the data. It can be seen that $E(\hat{\mu}(c^k)) = \mu(c^k)$ when either $m(\mathbf{X}_i, c, \boldsymbol{\beta})$ or the $e_i(c^k)$ model is correct, hence $\hat{\mu}(c^k) \to \mu(c^k)$, under some additional technical conditions. To confirm $E(\hat{\mu}(c^k)) = \mu(c^k)$, first consider the situation of the correct GPS model, hence $E(I(C_i = c^k)) = e_i(c^k)$. Therefore, the expectation of the second term in (8.67) tends to zero. Second, if the ER model $m(\mathbf{X}_i, c^k, \boldsymbol{\beta})$ is correct, then $E(Y_i(c^k)) = \mu(c^k)$ and the expectation of the first term in (8.68) tends to zero and $\hat{\mu}(c^k) \to \mu(c^k)$.

When C_i is continuous, the above estimator cannot be applied directly, since there are no data to provide a model-independent estimate for $\mu(c)$. However, a non-parametric approach can be applied to provide such an estimator. Let $K((C_i - c)/\rho)$ be a kernel function with parameter ρ and a doubly robust estimator for $\mu(c)$ is

$$\hat{\mu}(c) = (n\rho)^{-1} \sum_{i=1}^{n} \frac{K((C_i - c)/\rho)(Y_i - m(\mathbf{X}_i, c, \hat{\boldsymbol{\beta}})}{e_i(c)} + \sum_{i=1}^{n} m(\mathbf{X}_i, c, \hat{\boldsymbol{\beta}}) \tag{8.69}$$

where ρ can be determined by, e.g., cross-validation.

A more specific approach for continuous exposure is based on probabilistic GPS

$$e(c|\mathbf{X}_i) = P(c - \delta \leq C_i < c + \delta|\mathbf{X}_i) \tag{8.70}$$

with a pre-specified δ in [Graham et al., 2015], but they used a different construction for the DR relationship with continuous dose. They proposed a doubly robust approach to estimate $\mu(c)$ combining stratification and IPW with probabilistic GPS and showed that their estimator is approximately consistent if the ER model or the probabilistic GPS model is correct.

CBGPS is another approach to construct a doubly robust estimator. Due to its flexibility to balance X_i^*s even when the GPS model is incorrect, the EE (8.64) is unbiased regardless of whether the GPS is correct or not. When GPS is correct, even when the true model is $Y_i^* = \beta_d C_i^* + g(\mathbf{X}_i^*) + \epsilon_i$, EE (8.64) is also unbiased, since w_i balances the distribution of $\mathbf{X}_i$ by the definition of GPS. See the numerical example below. However, the difference between the two scenarios is that in the first, the balance is guaranteed for the specific dataset, while in the second, the balance is in probability, so the imbalances in the individual components in $\mathbf{X}_i$ may still be considerable.

8.3.6 A numerical example

This example is to illustrate the direct adjustment and GPS approaches with a large simulated dataset so that we can examine the (large sample) bias and robustness to model misspecification. We consider both a linear ER model so that the coefficient for the exposure represents the ER relationship, and a logistic model which captures the essential nonlinear part of the Emax model. For the GPS model, we assume that the exposure (expos) in the code below has a normal distribution, and the GPS and ER models all have two covariates in $\mathbf{X}_i$, in a linear combination $\mathbf{X}_i^T\boldsymbol{\beta}$. To generate scenarios of misspecified models, we also generate the data with $\exp(\mathbf{X}_i^T\boldsymbol{\beta})$ in the GPS or ER models. The methods we compare here are the direct adjustment with $\mathbf{X}_i$, IPW, stratification, and direct adjustment with GPS and IPW with CBGPS, compared with those without adjustment. The causal estimand is the coefficient for the exposure, which represents both subject-specific and marginal effects.

The code for the simulation and the result when both models are correct is given below. The unadjusted estimate (1.18) is obviously biased, compared to true value 1. All adjusted methods have negligible bias.

```
> library(CBPS)
> set.seed(123456)
> n <- 10000
> np=2 # Two covariates
> X <- mvrnorm(n, mu = rep(0,np), Sigma = diag(np))
> beta <- c(0,1,1) # Coefficients including intercept
> expos <- cbind(1,X)%*%beta + rnorm(n, sd = 3) #Exposure
> # Wrong GPS model
> #expos <- exp(0.5*cbind(1,X)%*%beta) + rnorm(n, sd = 3)
> sigt=sd(expos)
> mt=mean(expos)
> fitde=lm(expos~X)   #Fit GPS model
> prede=predict(fitde) #GPS
> sig=sd(fitde$residuals)
> expos.effect <- 1 #  #True exposure effect in ER model
> y <- expos.effect*expos +X%*%effect.beta+ rnorm(n, sd = 3)
> #Wrong ER model
> #y <- expos.effect*expos +exp(0.7*X%*%effect.beta)+ rnorm(n, sd = 3)
>
> lm(y~expos)  #No adjustment
(Intercept)        expos
    0.03181      1.17818

> wei=dnorm(expos,mt,sigt)/dnorm(expos,prede,sig)  #GPS robust weights
> lm(y~expos,weights = wei)  #IPW with GPS
```

```
(Intercept)        expos
   0.007846     0.976867

> strata=discretize(prede,breaks=5) # Strata (5) by GPS
> lm(y~expos+strata)  # Stratified analysis
         (Intercept)  expos  strata[-1.26,-0.383)  strata[-0.383,0.35) ..
              -2.001  1.011                 1.271                 2.109
>
> lm(y~expos+X)    #Direct adjustment by X

(Intercept)        expos           X1           X2
    0.01633      0.98577      1.01123      1.05335

> lm(y~expos+prede)  #Direct adjustment by GPS

(Intercept)        expos        prede
    0.04747      0.98577      1.01610

> fit2 <- CBPS(expos ~ X)   #CBGPS
> lm(y~expos,weights=fit2$weights)  # IPW by CBGPS

(Intercept)        expos
   0.008623     0.979349
```

The second block presents the results when the ER model is incorrect. The unadjusted estimate is 0.76, while all the adjusted ones are almost unbiased, except that of the stratified, which has moderate bias that might be due insufficient stratification. The direct adjusted estimate is unbiased, although the ER model is misspecified in the $\mathbf{X}_i$ part, as we have shown by the regression partition (8.28).

```
> #Wrong ER model
> y <- expos.effect*expos +exp(0.7*X%*%effect.beta)+ rnorm(n, sd = 3)
> lm(y~expos)  #No adjustment

Coefficients:
(Intercept)        expos
      2.067        0.759

> wei=dnorm(expos,mt,sigt)/dnorm(expos,prede,sig)  #GPS robust weights
> lm(y~expos,weights = wei)  #IPW with GPS

(Intercept)        expos
      2.066        1.008

> strata=discretize(prede,breaks=5) # Strata (5) by GPS
> lm(y~expos+strata)  # Stratified analysis

  (Intercept)     expos  strata[-1.26,-0.378) strata[-0.378,0.378) ...
     5.3233     0.9515               -3.1240                -3.9307
```

```
> lm(y~expos+X)    #Direct adjustment by X

(Intercept)        expos           X1           X2
     2.0694       1.0043      -0.2039      -2.4432

> lm(y~expos+prede)  #Direct adjustment by GPS

(Intercept)        expos        prede
      2.067        1.004       -1.235

> fit2 <- CBPS(expos ~ X)    #CBGPS
> lm(y~expos,weights=fit2$weights)  # IPW by CBGPS

(Intercept)        expos
      2.063        1.007
```

The next block shows results when the GPS model is misspecified, since the data are generated with a linear and a quadratic term of $\gamma^T \mathbf{X}_i$, but the ER model is correct. The unadjusted estimate is 0.85, and the IPW with GPS is biased upwards (1.23). The estimator stratified by GPS has a small bias and perhaps benefits from its robustness. Direct adjustment by GPS also results in unbiased estimate. This is mainly due to that the GPS model is linear and we use $\mathbf{X}_i^T \hat{\gamma}$ as a covariate The CBGPS remains unbiased due to its nature of covariate balancing.

```
# ....
> linx=cbind(1,X)%*%beta
> expos <- linx+linx^2/2 + rnorm(n, sd = 3) #GPS model misspecified
#...
> lm(y~expos)  #No adjustment

(Intercept)        expos
     0.1659       0.8513

> wei=dnorm(expos,mt,sigt)/dnorm(expos,prede,sig)  #GPS robust weights
> lm(y~expos,weights = wei)  #IPW with GPS

(Intercept)        expos
      0.333        1.231

> strata=discretize(prede,breaks=5) # Strata (5) by GPS
> lm(y~expos+strata)  # Stratified analysis

Coefficients:
(Intercept)  expos  strata[-0.189,0.634)    strata[0.634,1.36) ..
  1.9555     0.9783                -1.2768                -1.9854

> lm(y~expos+X)    #Direct adjustment by X
```

```
(Intercept)        expos          X1          X2
    0.02222      0.99841    -0.15553    -1.71036

> lm(y~expos+prede)  #Direct adjustment by GPS

(Intercept)        expos       prede
     0.9735       0.9984     -0.9530

> fit2 <- CBPS(expos ~ X)    #CBGPS
> lm(y~expos,weights=fit2$weights)  # IPW by CBGPS

(Intercept)        expos
      0.225        1.009
```

The next part of this example uses a logistic regression for a response in the range of (0,1). These responses include binary and proportional responses. It also represents the essential nonlinear part of the Emax model, in which two additional parameters are linear to the response. In the logistic model, we assume that confounders affect the intercept, which is equivalent to EC50 in the Emax model. One major problem to evaluate nonlinear models with confounders is their non-collapsibility, that is, even if we can adjust for confounders, their randomness makes the marginal model different from a logistic model. Here we take a pragmatic approach to use a logistic model approximation to the marginal model when $\mathbf{X}_i$ are not confounders but have the same variability.

The following block presents results when both GPS and ER models are correct. The gold standard β_c is 0.70.

```
> set.seed(123456)
> n <- 20000
> np=2 # Two covariates
> X <- mvrnorm(n, mu = rep(0,np), Sigma = diag(np))
> X0 <- mvrnorm(n, mu = rep(0,np), Sigma = diag(np))
> beta <- c(0,1,1) # Coefficients including intercept
> expos <- cbind(1,X)%*%beta + rnorm(n, sd = 3) #Exposure
> # Wrong GPS model
> #expos <- exp(0.5*cbind(1,X)%*%beta) + rnorm(n, sd = 3)
> #linx=cbind(1,X)%*%beta
> #expos <- linx+linx^2/2 + rnorm(n, sd = 3)
> sigt=sd(expos)
> mt=mean(expos)
> fitde=lm(expos~X)   #Fit GPS model
> prede=predict(fitde) #GPS
> sig=sd(fitde$residuals)
> expos.effect <- 1 #  #True exposure effect in ER model
> p <- expos.effect*expos +X0%*%effect.beta
> y=1/(1+exp(-p))
> # Gold standard
```

```
> glm(y ~ expos, family = "quasibinomial")$coef[2]
    expos
0.700133
> p <- expos.effect*expos +X%*%effect.beta
> y=1/(1+exp(-p))
> wei=dnorm(expos,mt,sigt)/dnorm(expos,prede,sig)
> glm(y ~ expos, weights=wei, family = "quasibinomial")
(Intercept)        expos
   -0.01543      0.69929
# Direct adjustment with g-computation
> betada=glm(y ~ expos+X, family = "quasibinomial")$coef
> Sdata=cbind(rep(1,n),expos,X0)
> lp=Sdata%*%betada
> glm(1/(1+exp(-lp)) ~ expos, family = "quasibinomial")$coef
(Intercept)       expos
0.003341887 0.700133045
> fit2 <- CBPS(expos ~ X)  #GCBPS
> glm(y ~ expos, weights = fit2$weights, family = "quasibinomial")
(Intercept)        expos
   -0.01553      0.69992
```

The next block shows the results when the GPS model is incorrectly specified. The data generation model includes not only $\gamma^T \mathbf{X}_i$, (linx in the code) but also a quadratic term of it. The gold standard is still 0.70. The IPW estimate 0.743 is slightly biased, while the CBGPS estimate 0.706 is almost the same as the gold standard. The direct adjustment estimate is unbiased.

```
> # Wrong GPS model
> linx=cbind(1,X)%*%beta
> expos <- linx+linx^2/2 + rnorm(n, sd = 3)
> wei=dnorm(expos,mt,sigt)/dnorm(expos,prede,sig)
> glm(y ~ expos, weights=wei, family = "quasibinomial") #GPS

(Intercept)        expos
     0.0720       0.7432
> betada=glm(y ~ expos+X, family = "quasibinomial")$coef
> Sdata=cbind(rep(1,n),expos,X0)
> lp=Sdata%*%betada
> glm(1/(1+exp(-lp)) ~ expos, family = "quasibinomial")$coef #Direct adj.
(Intercept)       expos
0.003154264 0.699536121

> fit2 <- CBPS(expos ~ X)
> glm(y ~ expos, weights = fit2$weights, family = "quasibinomial") #CBGPS
(Intercept)        expos
    0.07565      0.70588
```

The last scenario is when the ER model is misspecified because the ER data generation model includes $\exp(0.5\mathbf{X}_i^T\boldsymbol{\beta}_x)$, rather than $\mathbf{X}_i^T\boldsymbol{\beta}_x$. Since the ER model has changed, we need to recalculate the gold standard, which is now 0.852. Both the IPW and the CBGPS estimates are 0.836, very similar to the gold standard, while the direct adjustment estimate is 0.792, with a considerable bias.

```
> p <- expos.effect*expos +exp(0.5*X0%*%effect.beta)
> y=1/(1+exp(-p))
> gold=glm(y ~ expos, family = "quasibinomial")$coef[2]
> gold
   expos
0.851721
...
> #Wrong ER model
> p <- expos.effect*expos +exp(0.5*X0%*%effect.beta)
> y=1/(1+exp(-p))
> gold=glm(y ~ expos, family = "quasibinomial")$coef[2]
> p <- expos.effect*expos +exp(0.5*X%*%effect.beta)
> y=1/(1+exp(-p))
> wei=dnorm(expos,mt,sigt)/dnorm(expos,prede,sig)
> glm(y ~ expos, weights=wei, family = "quasibinomial") #GPS
(Intercept)        expos
     1.1335       0.8357
> betada=glm(y ~ expos+X, family = "quasibinomial")$coef
> Sdata=cbind(rep(1,n),expos,X0)
> lp=Sdata%*%betada
> glm(1/(1+exp(-lp)) ~ expos, family = "quasibinomial")$coef #Direct adj
(Intercept)       expos
  1.1135282   0.7918054
> fit2 <- CBPS(expos ~ X)
> glm(y ~ expos, weights = fit2$weights,  family = "quasibinomial") #CBGPS
(Intercept)        expos
    1.133530       0.835541
```

8.4 Randomized dose-finding trials and instrumental variables

Randomized dose-finding trials, in which subjects are randomized to a few fixed doses, are frequently used to select the optimal dose in drug development. In this section, we consider the following special questions concerning DER modeling in such trials.

1. Can randomized dose help identify causal ER relationships?
2. How much benefit (if any) can we obtain from DER modeling, compared to using the DR model directly?
3. Is there a safe (robust to model misspecification) way to use DER modeling for better estimation of the DR relationship?

The use of randomized doses for causal ER modeling is more complex than comparing mean responses between dose levels. A key approach is based on instrumental variable (IV). We start from Question 1, as it is the key to the other questions.

8.4.1 Dose randomization and instrumental variable

We introduce IV in a non-technical manner and will add technical details when they are needed. An IV is a variable that affects exposure C_i, but has no direct impact on response Y_i and is independent of confounders [Cameron and Trivedi, 2005]. To see why randomized dose D_i satisfies the request as an IV, taking models (8.9) and (8.10) as an example, D_i has impacts on C_i as long as $\gamma_d \neq 0$ in the DE model (8.10), and D_i has no direct effect as specified in the ER model (8.9). The second condition is satisfied since D_i is independent of $\mathbf{X}_i$ and V_i by randomization.

Suppose that we are interested in the marginal ER relationship when the true models are (8.9) and (8.10), but all confounders $\mathbf{X}_i$ and U_i are not observed. For a centered linear ER model $Y_i = \beta C_i + U_i$ (hence it has no intercept), the EE $S(\beta) = \sum_{i=1}^n C_i(Y_i - \beta C_i)/n$ is not unbiased, i.e., with $E(S(\beta)) \neq 0$, since C_i and $\mathbf{X}_i, V_i$ are correlated. An IV approach here is to replace C_i with D_i in a suitable place in the EE for the ER model. An IV estimate for β is the solution to the following EE (with one C_i in $S(\beta)$ replaced with D_i):

$$S_{IV}(\beta) = \sum_{i=1}^{n} D_i(Y_i - \beta C_i)/n = 0. \tag{8.71}$$

Condition $E(S_{IV}(\beta)) = 0$ is satisfied because of $E(S_{IV}(\beta)) = E(D_i(\boldsymbol{\beta}_x \mathbf{X}_i + U_i)) = 0$, so the solution to $S_{IV}(\beta) = 0$:

$$\hat{\beta}_{IV} = \frac{\sum_{i=1}^n D_i Y_i}{\sum_{i=1}^n C_i D_i} \tag{8.72}$$

is a consistent estimator of β if it is the unique solution to $E(S_{IV}(\beta)) = 0$. This condition means that not all parametric models can be identified by dose as IV.

The IV has advantages over those introduced in the previous sections, as it does not need the assumption of no unobserved confounder. However, although the IV estimate is consistent, its precision may be poor. Its variance

$$\text{var}(\hat{\beta}_{IV}) = \frac{\sum_{i=1}^n D_i^2}{(\sum_{i=1}^n D_i C_i)^2} \text{var}(Y_i|C_i) \tag{8.73}$$

is typically higher than the variance of the LS estimate. Therefore, using a weak IV with low correlation to C_i may have a high variance. Furthermore, with small sample sizes, $\hat{\beta}_{IV}$ may also have a higher finite sample bias than the LS estimator without adjustment. If the true model is (8.9), $\text{var}(Y_i|C_i)$ is the sum of variances of $\boldsymbol{\beta}_x \mathbf{X}_i$ and U_i, therefore, without adjusting $\mathbf{X}_i$ not only leads to confounding bias, but also to higher variability if the IV approach is used. Hence, if $\mathbf{X}_i$ is observed, it should be included in the model in (8.71).

The IV estimator $\hat{\beta}_{IV}$ can also be obtained using the two-stage LS (2SLS) approach [Cameron and Trivedi, 2005]. For linear DE and ER models, the 2SLS method first fits the ER model $C_i = \gamma D_i + V_i$ to obtain $\hat{\gamma}$ and the predicted exposure $\hat{C}_i = \hat{\gamma} D_i$. The next stage fits a model $Y_i = \beta \hat{C}_i + U_i$, and the obtained LS estimate is exactly $\hat{\boldsymbol{\beta}}_{IV}$. To see this, taking $\hat{C}_i = \hat{\gamma} D_i$ and $\hat{\gamma} = (\sum_{i=1}^n D_i^2)^{-1} \sum_{i=1}^n D_i C_i$ into the stage 2 LS estimator

$$\hat{\boldsymbol{\beta}}_{2sls} = (\sum_{i=1}^{n} \hat{C}_i^2)^{-1} \sum_{i=1}^{n} \hat{C}_i Y_i \tag{8.74}$$

then we find the right-hand side in (8.72). The 2SLS approach can be implemented in standard statistical packages; however, the SE given in the second stage is incorrect. For linear models, the variance of the 2SLS estimate is the same as the estimator by solving the EE (8.72). Some software for using IV approaches provides the correct SE for statistical inference. An alternative is to use bootstrap, which is often more accurate in practical problems.

For nonlinear regression models with additive confounding factors, the EE for IV estimates has the following form

$$S_{IV}(\boldsymbol{\beta}) = \sum_{i=1}^{n} \mathbf{Z}_i (Y_i - g(C_i, \boldsymbol{\beta})) = \sum_{i=1}^{n} \mathbf{Z}_i \delta_i = 0 \tag{8.75}$$

where $\mathbf{Z}_i$ is a set of IVs, including dose, and $\delta_i \equiv Y_i - g(C_i, \boldsymbol{\beta})$. Note that a non-confounded covariate can be an IV itself, hence $\mathbf{Z}_i$ can include these covariates. For nonlinear models using dose itself, as the IV is not optimal, but we can derive the optimal IV from the dose. As introduced in Chapter 4, for a nonlinear model $Y_i = g(C_i, \boldsymbol{\beta}) + \varepsilon_i$ the optimal estimator for $\boldsymbol{\beta}$ is the solution to EE:

$$S_{IV}(\boldsymbol{\beta}) = \sum_{i=1}^{n} E(\frac{\partial g(C_i, \boldsymbol{\beta})}{\partial \boldsymbol{\beta}} | \mathbf{Z}_i)(Y_i - g(C_i, \boldsymbol{\beta})) = 0 \tag{8.76}$$

where $E(\partial g(C_i, \boldsymbol{\beta})/\partial \boldsymbol{\beta} | \mathbf{Z}_i)$ is the optimal IV. As it contains parameters to be estimated, a two-stage approach can be used. In the first stage, we can fit the y-part model, e.g., ignoring the confounding factor, or using d_i as the IV to obtain a preliminary estimate for $\boldsymbol{\beta}$. In the second stage, the estimated $\boldsymbol{\beta}$ is used to calculate $E(\partial g(C_i, \boldsymbol{\beta})/\partial \boldsymbol{\beta} | \mathbf{Z}_i)$, then we use the optimal EE to obtain a refined estimate for $\boldsymbol{\beta}$. Some software such as SAS proc MODEL implement this approach and offers several options.

We have shown that the IV approach can eliminate confounding bias for ER models with additive confounding terms. For models with multiplicative confounding factors, such as Poisson type models (e.g., negative binomial models), due to a confounding factor in the linear predictor, $S_{IV}(\boldsymbol{\beta})$, (8.76) does not have zero mean. The following EE was proposed by Terza et al. [2008]

$$S(\boldsymbol{\beta}) = \sum_{i=1}^{n} \mathbf{Z}_i (1 - Y_i^{-1} \exp(\beta_0 + \beta_c C_i)) = 0, \tag{8.77}$$

and it can be shown that $E(S(\boldsymbol{\beta})) = 0$. However, the main drawback of using this EE is that the general GLS software cannot be used to estimate $\boldsymbol{\beta}$. In fact, it has been shown that even a standard IV EE of Poisson regression

$$S(\boldsymbol{\beta}) = \sum_{i=1}^{n} \mathbf{Z}_i(Y_i - \exp(\beta_0 + \beta_c C_i)) = 0, \tag{8.78}$$

is used, confounders only make the estimated intercept β_0 biased. The estimated relative risk β_c is still consistent [Wang, 2012a]. The IV approach has also been shown to eliminate the confounding in the heterogeneity of the treatment effect for simple models such as the linear model and multiplicative models such as a Poisson or negative binomial model with a log-link function[Wang, 2012a].

Recall that the decomposition of the variability in C_i divides it into three parts. The IV approach uses the part due to D_i. To improve the efficiency of the IV approach, we can adjust $\mathbf{X}_i$ if observed in the ER model so that its variability is also eliminated in the ER mode conditional on $\mathbf{X}_i$. If the marginal ER relationship is the final goal, we may also use g-computation to average the distribution of $\mathbf{X}_i$ in the conditional ER model.

8.4.2 Control function methods

We consider very general DE and ER models

$$\begin{aligned} Y_i &= g(C_i, U_i) \\ C_i &= h(D_i, V_i). \end{aligned} \tag{8.79}$$

and assume that V_i and U_i are correlated, hence C_i is confounded by U_i in the ER model. The idea of the control function (CF) method is to construct V_i by the DE model such that C_i and U_i are independent conditional on V_i. That is,

$$C_i \perp U_i | V_i. \tag{8.80}$$

Then, we can eliminate the confounding effect of U_i by adjusting for V_i. The CF approach is also a two-stage method very similar to the two-stage IV method, but uses IVs in a different way. To adjust for V_i, we need to obtain its estimate $\hat{V}_i$. When the DE model has additive V_i

$$C_i = h(D_i, \gamma) + V_i \tag{8.81}$$

we can take advantage of V_i being separable from the model part and take the residual of the fitted DE model as $\hat{V}_i$.

When U_i is available, we can include U_i as a covariate to adjust for the confounding bias. But U_i may not be completely confounded. It is the component correlated with V_i that causes bias and must be adjusted for. The CF method uses the IV model to predict this component and then includes its prediction to adjust the ER model. To this end, we assume that U_i can be written as

$$U_i = aV_i + \varepsilon_i \tag{8.82}$$

where ε_i is a random term independent of V_i. Therefore, U_i has two components; aV_i is the source of confounding and the error term ε_i is independent of C_i. The relationship (8.82) is valid when U_i and V_i are jointly normally distributed. However, it may also be empirically correct without the distributional assumption. Although we cannot fit model (8.82), because U_i is not observed. However, there is no need to know parameters in this model. To adjust for the confounded part in U_i, we simply include a predicted V_i in the ER model.

The following is the CF algorithm as a two-stage approach:

- fit the DE model to obtain $\hat{V}_i$s as the residuals of the fitted model.
- fit the ER model including C_i and $\hat{V}_i$.

The difference between the IV and CF methods is that in the ER model, the former replaces the exposure with a predicted (hence not confounded) one and the latter adds a predicted confounding effect to adjust for it. As the nature of this approach suggests, it is also known as two-stage residual inclusion [Cameron and Trivedi, 2005]. Interestingly, if both the ER and DE models are linear, the CF approach is equivalent to the IV approach. However, for multiplicative models, the CF estimate may have a significantly lower SE than the IV estimate [Wang, 2012a, 2014].

Until now, we have taken the residual of the DE model as the CF. In fact, CF can be constructed using general models (8.79), where the confounding error V_i is not separable from the other part [Imbens and Newey, 2009; Zhang et al., 2024]. Formally, we can implement a CF approach based on the general DE and ER models (8.79) with the following assumptions.

1. D_i is independent of U_i, V_i.
2. V_i is continuously distributed with a strictly increasing distribution function.
3. The DE model is strictly increasing in V_i for every $D_i = d$.

In this case, we can take $V_i \sim F_{v|d}^{-1}(v)$, where $F_{v|d}(v)$ is the conditional distribution of V_i given $D_i = d$. It can be shown that C_i and U_i are independent conditional on V_i [Imbens and Newey, 2009]. Estimates $\hat{V}_i$ can be constructed from their empirical distribution. This $\hat{V}_i$ weakly converges to V_i: $\hat{V}_i \sim_d V_i$, which is a key to the asymptotic properties of the CF-adjusted estimation [Imai and Van Dyk, 2004; Zhang et al., 2024]. In fact, it is also equivalent to the residual CF, since there is a one-one mapping between them.

As above, to adjust for V_i, we assumed an ER model that includes $\hat{V}_i$ as a covariate. For example, a logistic model fits $E(Y_i|C_i, \hat{V}_i) = \text{expit}(\beta_c C_i + \beta_v \hat{V}_i)$. As a general model, we denote $m(C_i, V_i) = E(Y_i|C_i, V_i)$. This is a subject-specific model conditional on $\hat{V}_i$. If the marginal ER model for $\mu(c) \equiv E(Y_i|C_i = c)$ is our target, we can derive it from $m(c, V_i)$ by averaging over V_i. That is, $\mu(c) = E(m(c, V_i))$. The marginal model often has no closed form, with exception of linear, Poisson and probit models. However, with $\hat{V}_i$, we can calculate it numerically. For example, with the logistic model we can estimate $\mu(c)$ by

$$\hat{\mu}(c) = n^{-1} \sum_{i=1}^{n} \text{expit}(\hat{\beta}_c c + \hat{\beta}_v \hat{V}_i). \tag{8.83}$$

Since V_i does not have a specific mechanistic meaning, a mechanistic ER model conditional on V_i is not easy to find and justify. We may use a flexible model, e.g., spline functions of C_i and V_i [Zhang et al., 2024].

An interesting question is whether, with randomized doses of a few fixed levels, we can identify the causal ER relationship without model assumption or not? The general answer is negative [Imbens and Newey, 2009; Zhang et al., 2024]. In principle, partial identification by constructing bounds that limit $\mu(c)$ in a region is possible; see Zhang et al. [2024] for a specific construction for ER modeling. However, with only a few dose levels, the bounds are often not sufficiently narrow for practical use, given the variability in C_i.

The CF approach may also be used to adjust for confounders in models (8.55). Interestingly, a similar approximation to (8.56) applies to the CF approach. Let V_i be the CF, we may assume

$$E(Y_i|C_i, V_i) = g(C_i, V_i, \boldsymbol{\beta}, \boldsymbol{\beta}_v) \tag{8.84}$$

which is an extension of the approach in Zhang et al. [2024]. Although GPS and CF all represent potential confounding effects, the two approximations are generally different, since the GPS represents observed confounders, while the CF unobserved confounders. To implement this model, we also need assumptions under which (8.80) is sufficient to adjust for multiple $\boldsymbol{\beta}_i$ with the same construction, if $\boldsymbol{\beta}_i = \boldsymbol{\beta} + \mathbf{U}_i$ and $\mathbf{U}_i = \boldsymbol{\beta}_v V_i + \mathbf{U}_{0i}$, with an unconfounded part $\mathbf{U}_{0i}$. This allows adjusting for V_i in different components in the popPK/PD models. In an Emax mode, e.g., if both EC50 and Emax depend on age, and age is also a predictor of exposure. Then CF contains age effects on exposure. An adjustment for it is to fit the NLMM including $\hat{V}_i$ in

$$\boldsymbol{\beta}_i = \boldsymbol{\beta} + \boldsymbol{\beta}_v \hat{V}_i \tag{8.85}$$

where $\boldsymbol{\beta}_v$ is a vector that represents the impact of V_i on all elements of $\mathbf{U}_i$, and $\boldsymbol{\beta}_v \hat{V}_i$ may be replaced by more complex functions of $\hat{V}_i$.

We present a numerical example to show how to use the CF approach to estimate $\mu(c)$. We take the steady-state trough level model (8.35) as the DE model and assume that both V_d and K_e depend on age and weight: two hypothetical covariates. They also have an impact on a binary response Y_i, age and weights are confounders, and their joint effect is $\boldsymbol{\beta}_x^T \mathbf{X}_i$ on the logit scale. If they are observed, we can adjust for them in a logistic model, and hence this approach becomes the approach based on popPKPD modeling. Now suppose that the data from a randomized dose-finding trial with three dose levels, but age and weights are (hypothetically) not recorded. However, a DE model for the trough level can be fitted, then the residuals $\hat{V}_i$ contain the effect of the two confounders and can be used as a CF. Then, the task is equivalent to predicting $\boldsymbol{\beta}_x^T \mathbf{X}_i$ with $\hat{V}_i$. Since the ER model may be a complex nonlinear function of $\mathbf{X}_i$, we use natural spline functions of $\hat{V}_i$ for the prediction.

The following is a simulation code to evaluate large sample biases of the proposed approach. The data are generated with three dose levels and two confounders named age and weights are generated, with parameter setting in the code below. The empirical ER model uses cubic spline functions for CF and $\mu(c)$ is calculated for a wide range of c values using g-computation with the R package stdReg, compared to direct adjustment assuming age and weight are observed as the gold standard. The summary of the difference shows that the biases are negligible.

```
> nsub=10000
> tau=1
> library(splines)
> library(stdReg)
> Di=sample(1:3,size=nsub,replace = T)
> age=18+runif(nsub)*(65-18)
> weight=rnorm(nsub,70,15)
> Vd=exp(-1+age/60+weight/100)
> Ke=exp(-age/90-weight/100)
> cf=(tau*Ke-Vd)-log(1-exp(-tau*Ke))
> lci=cf+log(Di)+rnorm(nsub)
> cf=lm(lci~log(Di))$residuals
> plot(cf,age,ylim=c(20,120))
> lines(cf,weight,type="p",pch="+")
>
> yi=1/(1+exp(-lci-age/90-weight/100))
> cfdata=data.frame(yi,cf,lci)
> fit=glm(yi~lci+ns(cf,3), family = "quasibinomial",data=cfdata) #CF
> Stdfit=stdGlm(fit,data=cfdata,X="lci", x=seq(from=-2,to=4,by=0.2))
>
> gdata=data.frame(yi,lci,age,weight) #Adj by age+weight
> fitg=glm(yi~lci+age+weight, family = "quasibinomial",data=gdata)
> Stdfitg=stdGlm(fitg,data=gdata,X="lci", x=seq(from=-2,to=4,by=0.2))
>
> summary(Stdfit$est-Stdfitg$est) # Diff between CF and gold standard
      Min.    1st Qu.     Median       Mean    3rd Qu.       Max.
-2.124e-03 -5.182e-04 -6.095e-05 -4.196e-04 -8.631e-06  1.014e-04
```

8.4.3 DER modeling for estimation of DR relationship

A classical pharmacometric approach to determine the DR relationship is to combine popPK and popPKPD modeling approaches to predict the response for a given dose. An interesting question is whether DER modeling is more efficient than DR modeling, which is not affected by confounding when the dose is randomized. There seems an obvious yes answer to this question, since we use more information (exposure data) for DER modeling. Indeed, without confounding factors, the answer is correct, although the efficiency gain is bounded. However, the following question is whether the answer is still yes if adjustment for confounders is needed. When all confounders are observed, the answer is still generally positive, since direct adjustment not only removes confounding bias, but also increases the accuracy of prediction. However, it is less obvious whether the same answer holds if confounders are not observed and a general IV or a CF approach is used for adjustment.

We consider this question in the context of dose-finding trials, in which DR modeling, when feasible, is valid due to the absence of confounding in the DR relationship. In particular, the mean response of each dose represents the causal DR relationship, although they may be highly variable. Suppose that the CF approach is used to adjust for potential confounding in the ER model, is there still an efficiency gain by using DER modeling? The answer depends on the specific setting of the model. A part of this subsection is extracted from Wang et al. [2025b].

8.4.4 Linear models

We first consider simple linear DE and ER models

$$\begin{aligned} Y_i =& \beta_c C_i + U_i \\ C_i =& \gamma_d D_i + V_i \end{aligned} \tag{8.86}$$

with centered data so that there is no intercept in the models. U_i and V_i are independent zero-mean random variables with variances $\text{var}(U_i) = \sigma_u^2$ and $\text{var}(V_i) = \sigma_v^2$. This setting leads to a marginal DR model

$$Y_i = \beta_c \gamma_d D_i + \beta_c V_i + U_i \equiv \alpha_d D_i + U_i^* \tag{8.87}$$

where $U_i^* = \beta_c V_i + U_i$ and a_d can be estimated either by fitting the DR model (8.87) by LS to Y_i and D_i only, or by $\hat{\gamma}_d \hat{\beta}_c$, where $\hat{\gamma}_d$ and $\hat{\beta}_c$ estimated by fitting the DE and ER models separately. They are valid estimates since we have assumed independent V_i and U_i at the moment. One interesting question is: is the DER modeling more efficient than the DR modeling, if so, by how much? For the product of two random variables, its asymptotic variances of $\hat{\gamma}_d \hat{\beta}_c$ can be written as

$$\begin{aligned} \text{var}(\hat{\gamma}_d \hat{\beta}_c) =& (E(\hat{\beta}_c))^2 \text{var}(\hat{\gamma}_d) + (E(\hat{\gamma}))^2 \text{var}(\hat{\beta}_c) \\ \approx& (\beta_c^2 \sigma_v^2 / \sigma_d^2 + \gamma_d^2 \sigma_u^2 / \sigma_c^2)/n \end{aligned} \tag{8.88}$$

where $\sigma_d^2 = \text{var}(D_i)$ and $\sigma_c^2 = \text{var}(C_i) = \gamma_d^2 \sigma_d^2 + \sigma_v^2$. The variance of $\hat{\alpha}_d$ is $\text{var}(\hat{\alpha}_d) = n^{-1}(\beta_c^2 \sigma_v^2 + \sigma_u^2)/\sigma_d^2$. Then the ratio of the variance of the two estimators is

$$\frac{\text{var}(\hat{\gamma}_d\hat{\beta}_c)}{\text{var}(\hat{\alpha}_d)} \approx \frac{\beta_c^2\sigma_v^2/\sigma_d^2 + \gamma_d^2\sigma_u^2/\sigma_c^2}{(\beta_c^2\sigma_v^2 + \sigma_u^2)/\sigma_d^2}$$
$$= 1 - \frac{\sigma_v^2\sigma_u^2}{(\beta_c^2\sigma_v^2 + \sigma_u^2)(\gamma_d^2\sigma_d^2 + \sigma_v^2)} \tag{8.89}$$

As the second term of the second equation is positive, the DER estimator is always more efficient than the DR model one. In addition, the second term tends to zero when $\sigma_v^2 \to 0$ or $\sigma_v^2 \to \infty$. The maximum gain occurs in between the extremes.

The above result is based on independent U_i and V_i, i.e., there is no confounding in the ER model. Next, we examine the relative efficiency of the DER estimator using the CF approach when V_i and U_i are correlated. Let $\hat{\beta}_c^{cf}$ be the estimate of the fitting model $Y_i = \beta_c C_i + \beta_v \hat{V}_i + \epsilon_i$, where we ignore the difference between $\hat{V}_i$ and V_i [Imbens and Newey, 2009; Zhang et al., 2024]. We compare the variance ratio of the DER estimator $\hat{\beta}_c^{cf}\hat{\gamma}_d$ to that of $\hat{\alpha}_d$, the parameter estimated in the linear DR model using only data D_i and Y_i. For the variance of $\hat{\beta}_c^{cf}$, we take a shortcut using the equivalence between the CF and the 2SLS estimators [Cameron and Trivedi, 2005]. Hence, the asymptotic variance of the CF estimator is the same as that of the 2SLS estimator

$$\text{var}(\hat{\beta}_c^{cf}) \approx n^{-1}\sigma_v^2\text{cov}(D_i, \mathbf{X}_i)^{-1}\text{var}(D_i)\text{cov}(D_i, \mathbf{X}_i)^{-1}. \tag{8.90}$$

Also, with the DE model in (8.86), we have $\text{cov}(D_i, C_i) = \gamma_d\text{var}(D_i) = \gamma_c\sigma_d^2$, hence $\text{var}(\hat{\beta}_c^{cf}) = n^{-1}\gamma_d^{-2}\sigma_v^2/\sigma_d^2$. Taking it to (8.88) to obtain $\text{var}(\hat{\gamma}_d\hat{\beta}_c^{cf})$ and replacing the numerator in (8.89), we find

$$\frac{\text{var}(\hat{\gamma}\hat{\beta}_c^{cf})}{\text{var}(\hat{\alpha}_d)} \approx \frac{\beta_c^2\sigma_v^2/\sigma_d^2 + \sigma_v^2/\sigma_d^2}{(\beta_c^2\sigma_v^2 + \sigma_v^2)/\sigma_d^2} = 1 \tag{8.91}$$

That is, with linear models (8.86), there is no gain (and no loss) in using DER if the IV adjustment is needed to adjust for potential confounders. Note that although we only show equal asymptotic variance, the two estimators in the linear model situation are, in fact, numerically identical.

8.4.5 ER models with a sigmoid curve

A general nonlinear ER model may not lead to a marginal model of the same kind, so the comparison between the DR and DER approaches may not have a gold reference. However, the probit model allows for a parameter conversion between the two approaches, assuming that all the random terms, confounded or not, are normally distributed. Suppose that $Z_i = \beta_0 + \beta_c C_i + U_i$, in which $U_i \sim N(0, 1)$, is a latent variable and $Y_i = I(Z_i > 0)$ is a binary response. We also assume that $C_i = \gamma_d D_i + V_i$ and $V_i \sim N(0, \sigma_v^2)$. Since given D_i, all other random variables are normally distributed, the marginal DR model for Y_i is a probit DR model

$$E(Y_i|D_i) = \Phi(\alpha_0 + \alpha_d D_i). \tag{8.92}$$

where (α_0, α_d) can be estimated directly by fitting the model to Y_i, D_i data.

Another way to estimate them is the DER model approach that combines the DE and ER parameters in a similar way as for the linear ER model in the above section. The first step is to use $\hat{V}_i$ to adjust for the confounder U_i. We can write

$$Z_i = \beta_0 + \beta_c C_i + U_i = \beta_0 + \beta_c C_i + \beta_v \hat{V}_i + \xi_i \tag{8.93}$$

where $\xi_i = U_i - \beta_v \hat{V}_i$ is the residual error term after adjusting for the CF with $\text{var}(\xi_i) = 1 - \beta_v^2 \sigma_v^2$. In particular, $\rho = \text{Corr}(U_i, V_i)$ $\beta_v = \text{cov}(U_i, V_i)/\sigma_v^2 = \rho/\sigma_v$ (since $\text{var}(U_i) = 1$) is the coefficient of $\hat{V}_i$ in the regression of U_i on $\hat{V}_i$ and can be written as $\beta_v = \text{cov}(U_i, V_i)/\sigma_v^2 = \rho/\sigma_v$. Therefore, we have $\rho^2 = \beta_v^2 \sigma_v^2$ and $\text{var}(\xi_i) = 1 - \rho^2$. The parameters in (8.93) cannot be estimated directly, since Z_i is a latent variable. However, given C_i and $\hat{V}_i$, Z_i is normally distributed, hence it is valid to fit a probit ER model

$$E(Y_i|C_i, \hat{V}_i) = \Phi(\beta_0^* + \beta_c^* C_i + \beta_v^* \hat{V}_i) \tag{8.94}$$

where the right-hand side is equivalent to $P((\beta_0 + \beta_c C_i + \beta_v \hat{V}_i + \xi_i)/\sqrt{1-\rho^2} \geq 0) = \Phi((\beta_0 + \beta_c C_i + \beta_v \hat{V}_i)/\sqrt{1-\rho^2})$. Therefore, the relationship between $\boldsymbol{\beta} \equiv (\beta_0, \beta_c, \beta_v)$ and $\boldsymbol{\beta}^* \equiv (\beta_0^*, \beta_c^*, \beta_v^*)$ is $(1-\rho^2)^{1/2}\boldsymbol{\beta}^* = \boldsymbol{\beta}$.

Although V_i is not observed, ρ can be estimated using the following relationship

$$\beta_v^* = \beta_v(1-\rho^2)^{-1/2} = \frac{\rho}{\sigma_v(1-\rho^2)^{1/2}} \tag{8.95}$$

which leads to

$$\rho^2 = \frac{C\sigma_v^2}{1 + \beta_v^* \sigma_v^2} \tag{8.96}$$

in which β_v^* can be estimated by the CF probit model (8.94) and σ_v^2 is the residual variance in the DE model.

To find the marginal DR model based on the fitted DE and ER probit models, we replace C_i in the ER model with that in the DE model and take the average over all random terms

$$\begin{aligned} E(Y_i|D_i) =& P(\beta_0 + \beta_c(\gamma_0 + \gamma_d D_i + \hat{V}_i) + \beta_v \hat{V}_i + e_i \geq 0) \\ =& P(\beta_0 + \beta_c\gamma_0 + \beta_c\gamma_d D_i + (\beta_c + \beta_v)\hat{V}_i + e_i \geq 0) \\ =& \Phi(\frac{\beta_0 + \beta_c\gamma_0 + \beta_c\gamma_d D_i}{\sqrt{1-\rho^2 + (\beta_c+\beta_v)^2\sigma_v^2}}). \end{aligned} \tag{8.97}$$

which has an equivalent form of the probit DR model (8.92). Comparing the two probit DR models, we find the relationship between the two sets of parameters:

$$(\alpha_0, \alpha_d) = (\beta_0 + \beta_c\gamma_0, \beta_c\gamma_d)(1 - \rho^2 + (\beta_c + \beta_v)\sigma_v^2)^{-1/2} \tag{8.98}$$

where γ_0 and γ_d can be estimated in the DE model and $\boldsymbol{\beta}$ can be estimated by $\boldsymbol{\beta} = (1-\rho^2)^{1/2}\boldsymbol{\beta}^*$.

Inference based on IV approaches can be based on asymptotic normality of the estimators, which is well developed [Cameron and Trivedi, 2005]. In practice, one can also use bootstrap, which is often more robust than the asymptotic property-based ones, and may also be easier for implementation.

Although in principle DER and DR estimators can be compared based on the asymptotic properties of the estimated parameters in both models and the relationship between them as in (8.98), we prefer to use simulation for comparisons of the properties of small samples.

8.4.6 A simulation study

To examine the benefit of using the combined DER estimator, compared to using a DR model directly, we conduct a simulation study to compare the two approaches and focus on probit models so that a fair comparison can be made between them. Results using a logistic model for the empirical mean approach to response estimation are also presented.

For simulation, we generate Y_i using a probit model with different levels of confounding effect and sample sizes. We set $\beta_0 = -3, \beta_c = 1, \gamma_0 = 0, \gamma_d = 1$, $\sigma_u = 1, \sigma_v = 1$, with ρ varying from 0 to 0.9 and the sample size from 40 to 120. This model setting gives $(\alpha_0, \alpha_d) = (-2.12, 0.71)$ when $\rho = 0$. We also assume that the dose levels are (1,2,3,4,5) units. This dose range gives a symmetric pattern $E(Y_i|d) = (0.08, 0.24, 0.50, 0.76, 0.92)$ when $\rho = 0$. For each setting, 10000 simulation runs are performed. To examine efficiency, we compare the bias and variance of $\hat{\mu}_d$ of the DER approach with the CF adjustment and without it ($\rho = 0$ only) with those of the DR approach. Extensive simulation results for multiple scenarios can be found in Wang et al. (2024).

The results with varying sample size and ρ are summarized in Table 8.1. Both the DR and DER parameters have moderate biases, especially when $n = 40$, which are likely due to nonlinearity, since the parameter estimation of the DR model is not affected by confounding. Interestingly, in general, the bias of the DER estimator is lower than the DR one. The variance ratios are all less than one, which shows the benefit of DER approaches in general, although in some situations the efficiency gain is small. The benefit is higher when sample sizes are small, which is expected, since the extra information in DER modeling may be more important with small sample sizes. When $\rho = 0$ there is no confounding error such that the DER estimator without CF adjustment is also valid. Therefore, comparing the first two rows of each block shows the impact of CF adjustment when it is not necessary. For all sample sizes, the loss of efficiency due to the CF adjustment is substantial.

Table 8.1
Summary of biases and variances of DER estimator (with and without CF adjustment ($\rho = 0$ only)) to the DR estimator using Probit regressions by ρ the proportion of confounded variation in exposure in terms of variances, with sample sizes 40, 80 and 120: Scenario 1.

			Bias (DR)		Bias (DER)		Var(DR)		V(DER)/V(DR)	
n	ρ	Adj.	α_0	α_d	α_0	α_d	α_0	α_d	α_0	α_d
40	0.0	No	-0.305	0.101	-0.114	0.037	1.805	0.188	0.146	0.119
40	0.0	Yes	-0.305	0.101	-0.227	0.075	1.805	0.188	0.659	0.631
40	0.3	Yes	-0.288	0.094	-0.212	0.069	1.437	0.150	0.569	0.559
40	0.6	Yes	-0.214	0.069	-0.154	0.049	0.884	0.087	0.591	0.580
40	0.9	Yes	-0.159	0.051	-0.094	0.029	0.557	0.056	0.604	0.589
80	0.0	No	-0.091	0.031	-0.040	0.013	0.248	0.024	0.474	0.415
80	0.0	Yes	-0.091	0.031	-0.070	0.023	0.248	0.024	0.916	0.914
80	0.3	Yes	-0.107	0.034	-0.087	0.027	0.233	0.022	0.907	0.911
80	0.6	Yes	-0.089	0.027	-0.067	0.020	0.196	0.019	0.887	0.890
80	0.9	Yes	-0.078	0.024	-0.051	0.015	0.175	0.016	0.798	0.803
120	0.0	No	-0.053	0.017	-0.022	0.007	0.146	0.014	0.497	0.433
120	0.0	Yes	-0.053	0.017	-0.039	0.013	0.146	0.014	0.928	0.932
120	0.3	Yes	-0.065	0.020	-0.052	0.016	0.140	0.013	0.922	0.928
120	0.6	Yes	-0.053	0.016	-0.039	0.011	0.123	0.012	0.897	0.904
120	0.9	Yes	-0.048	0.014	-0.032	0.009	0.108	0.010	0.786	0.795

8.4.7 Dose-response estimation with Sigmoid ER models

We have shown that the DER approach can generally provide more accurate estimation of the DR model parameters when probit models are assumed. However, the model-based DER approach using the probit model is sensitive to model misspecification. An alternative is to use empirical means that average over $\hat{V}_i$. After fitting the probit ER model, $\mu(d)$ can be estimated by

$$\hat{\mu}_{pb}(d) = n^{-1}\sum_{i=1}^{n} \Phi(\hat{\beta}_0^* + \hat{\beta}_c^* \hat{C}_i(d) + \hat{\beta}_v^* \hat{V}_i) \tag{8.99}$$

where $\hat{C}_i(d) = \hat{\gamma}_0 + \hat{\gamma}_d d + \hat{V}_i$. This estimator does not depend on the normality of V_i, but still assumes a probit ER model. The drawback is obvious: the DR model is not parametric and $\hat{\mu}_{pb}(d)$ is a semi-parametric estimator.

In fact, this approach can be applied to other types of ER models, e.g., the logistic regression ER model

$$E(Y|C_i, V_i) = \text{expit}(\beta_0 + \beta_c C_i + \beta_v V_i). \tag{8.100}$$

Although the marginal odds ratio may not exist, the logistic model-based estimator for the mean response at a given dose d

$$\hat{\mu}_{lg}(d) = n^{-1}\sum_{i=1}^{n} \text{expit}(\hat{\beta}_0^* + \hat{\beta}_c^* \hat{C}_i(d) + \hat{\beta}_v^* \hat{V}_i) \tag{8.101}$$

is a valid semi-parametric estimator for $\mu(d)$.

The following is a simple simulation for comparisons of small-sample properties of the above approaches. Without the setting of the double probit model, we do not have the gold standard to compare. Therefore, we have to compare them with the mean response by dose levels. The simulation setting is mostly the same as those for the previous simulation except the following changes: 1) the dose levels are 1, 2 and 3 which is more feasible than the 5-level setting; 2) sample sizes reduce to 30 and 60. First, we consider a logistic ER model and compare the DER modeling approach with the mean response by dose with and without CF adjustment. The variance ratio of the DER modeling estimator to that of the mean response is presented in Figure 8.2. DER modeling approaches are more efficient than sample means at all dose levels. The CF-adjusted DER modeling have the highest relative efficiency at the middle dose, whereas the unadjusted one, as expected, is more efficient than the CF adjusted ones. The impact of ρ is generally very small, although the variance ratio tends to reduce with ρ generally.

In the above situation, since there are three doses, we can still fit a logistic DR model, although there is little room for model diagnosis. In the next example, we generate data from a 4-parameter Emax ER model with a confounder on EC50 and still with three doses. In this case, fitting the Emax DR model is no longer feasible. However, a 4-parameter Emax ER model can be used in the DER modeling, and the estimator (8.101) can be adapted for the Emax model. The distribution of the biases of the estimated response using DER modeling and the mean response by dose is given in Figure 8.3. The model-based approach is generally more efficient with less outliers, compared with the sample means at each dose, although the difference is generally small.

8.4.8 CF as a covariate in ANCOVA for dose-response modeling

In some situations, CF can also be used as a covariate to improve the estimation of the DR relationship even when simple approaches are valid due to randomized dose. We consider two situations: the first assumes that there is no DR model, while the other is based on a semi-parametric model with a linear part for the dose. For the first situation, we combine the IV approach and the ANCOVA estimators by including the CF as a covariate in the ANCOVA model for a more accurate DR relationship than the unadjusted one. Much of this subsection is extracted from Wang et al. [2025c] where more details and simulation results are presented.

To construct our estimator, we need the following assumption:

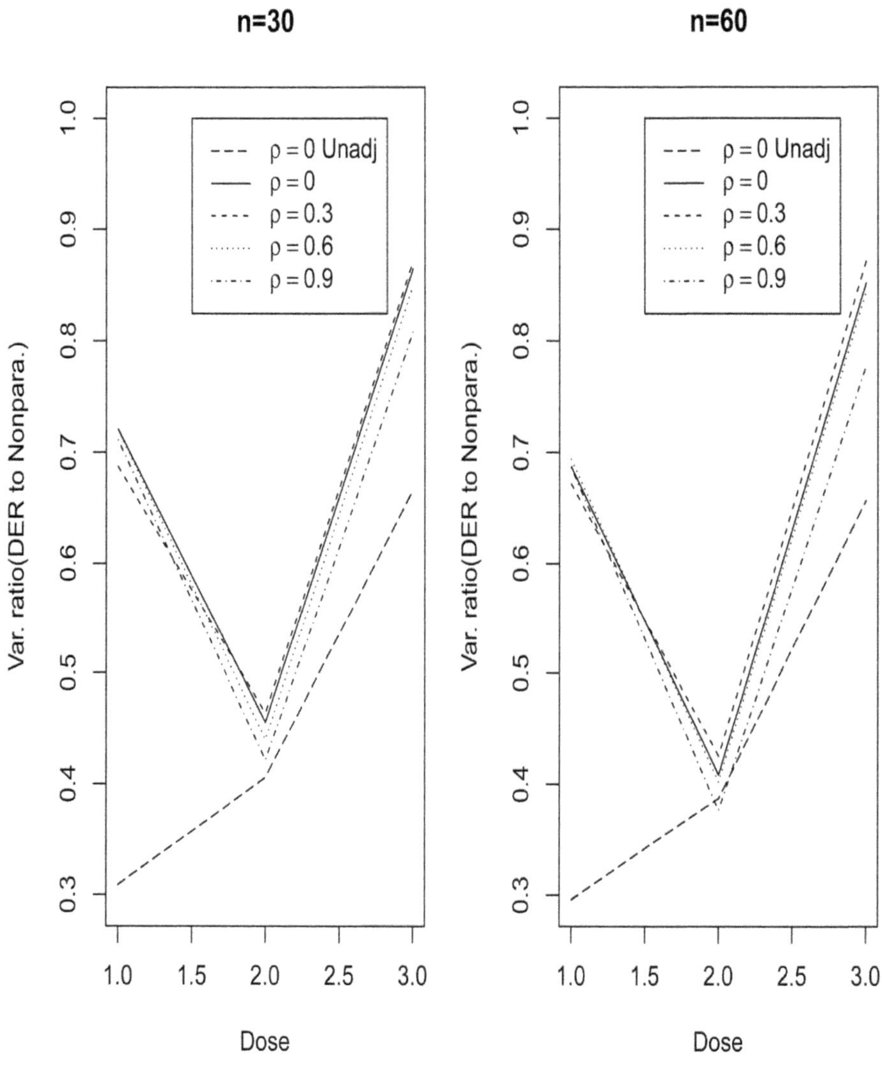

Figure 8.2
Variance ratio of DER estimators with and without CF adjustment to that of mean response by dose, with linear DE and logistic ER models, with three dose levels.

Assumption 3 There exists a CF V such that

$$V \perp D|X \tag{8.102}$$

for any given X.

Randomized D alone is not sufficient for this assumption, since although in principle the conditional distribution of C_i: $F_{C|D,X}(.)$ can be constructed as

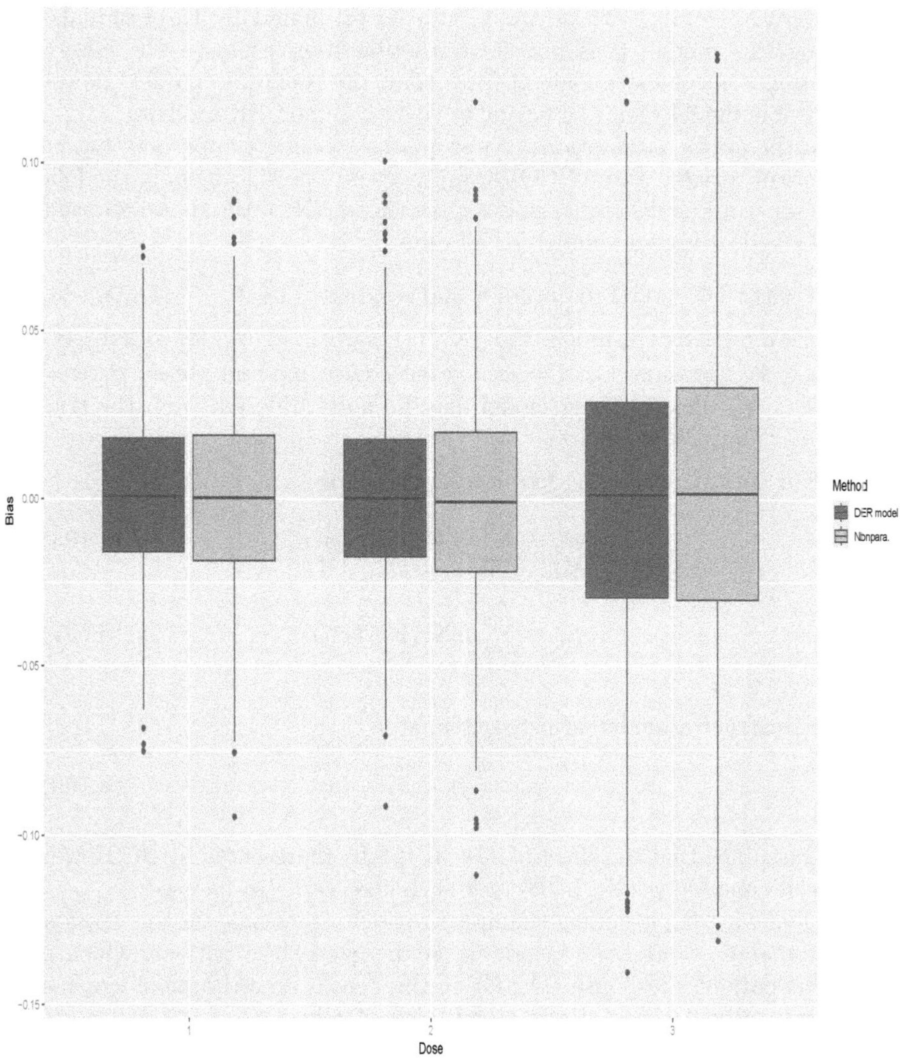

Figure 8.3
Distribution of bias of DER estimator using 4-parameter Emax model with CF adjustment to that of mean response by dose, with linear DE and logistic ER models, with three dose levels.

a CF, it may still depend on D. A sufficient condition is a separable structure for the DE model. For example, this assumption holds with DE model

$$C_i = (\gamma_0 + \boldsymbol{\gamma}_x \mathbf{X}_i)D_i + V_i \tag{8.103}$$

With this model, the residual $C_i - (\gamma_0 + \boldsymbol{\gamma}_x \mathbf{X}_i)D_i = V_i$, and $V_i \perp D_i$. In fact, the assumption holds with all separable models in the form of

$C_i = h(D_i, \mathbf{X}_i) + V_i$, with which V_i can be estimated by the residuals after fitting this model. It is not clear whether there exists a CF satisfying Assumption 3 for a more general form than the separable model. However, the separable model seems sufficient to cover common PK models.

With the above assumptions, we propose a two-stage approach that combines control variable and ANCOVA approaches. The algorithm in the following uses separate models for each dose, known as ANCOVA II. An alternative is ANCOVA I, using one model for all doses.

1. Fit the DE model to obtain $\hat{\gamma}$ and residuals $\hat{V}_i = C_i - h(D_i, \mathbf{X}_i, \hat{\gamma})$.
2. Fit a working DR model $E(Y_i|\mathbf{X}_i, \hat{V}_i) = g(\mathbf{X}_i, \hat{V}_i, \boldsymbol{\beta}_k)$ for n_k subjects $i \in S_k$: the subset of $i = 1, ..., n$ with $D_i = d_k$, and obtain $\hat{\boldsymbol{\beta}}_k, k = 1, ..., K$. This working model may be quite different from the true marginal DR model.
3. For each d_k of the K dose levels, calculate

$$\hat{\mu}_k = \sum_{i \in S_k} g(\mathbf{X}_i, \hat{V}_i, \hat{\boldsymbol{\beta}}_k)/n_k; \tag{8.104}$$

$$\hat{\mu}_k^a = \sum_{i=1}^{n} g(\mathbf{X}_i, \hat{V}_i, \hat{\boldsymbol{\beta}}_k)/n, \tag{8.105}$$

4. Construct a model adjusted estimator

$$\hat{\mu}_k^m = \bar{y}_k + \hat{\mu}_k^a - \hat{\mu}_k. \tag{8.106}$$

We have assumed that the effect of dose d_k is fully represented by $\boldsymbol{\beta}_k$. However, dose-specific models $g_k(\mathbf{X}_i, \hat{V}_i, \boldsymbol{\beta}_k)$ for each dose can also be used.

The following hypothetical example provides a rationale for this approach. Suppose that $C_i = \beta_d D_i + V_i$ and V_i is the age of the patient, which also affects the patient's response. The CF in this case is an estimate of age, hence the CF adjustment is essentially an adjustment for age.

Assumption 3 is the key to the robustness of $\hat{\mu}_k^m$ to misspecified model $g(\mathbf{X}_i, V_i, \boldsymbol{\beta}_k)$, as we need $E(g(\mathbf{X}_i, V_i, \boldsymbol{\beta}_k)|D_i = d_k) = E(g(\mathbf{X}_i, V_i, \boldsymbol{\beta}_k))$ such that $\hat{\mu}_k^a - \hat{\mu}_k \to 0$ with $n_k \to \infty$ even when the model is misspecified. This assumption can be examined in practice, at least in principle.

To see why $\hat{\mu}_d^m$ is generally more accurate than $\bar{y}_d$, consider the simple situation where $C_i = \gamma D_i + V_i$ with an unknown prognostic factor V_i as a random error. Then we can fit this model to obtain the residuals $\hat{V}_i = C_i - \hat{\gamma} D_i \approx V_i$. With a working model $g^*(V_i, \boldsymbol{\beta}_k) = \boldsymbol{\beta}_k + V_i$, that is, a model for dose level d_k with V_i as a covariate, the above algorithm is asymptotically equivalent to the ANCOVA II adjustment for V_i [Lin, 2013], which is known to be at least as efficient as $\bar{y}_k$.

In the special situation of only two dose levels and the DE model contains only group means, the sum of residual of the DE model is zero, then we have

$\sum_{i:D_i=1} \hat{V}_i + \sum_{i:D_i=0} \hat{V}_i = 0$. Consequently, when $n_0 = n_1$, $\hat{V}_i$ is already balanced, and therefore adjusting for $\hat{V}_i$ makes no difference in this situation.

Next, we consider using $\hat{V}_i$ to adjust for covariates in linear DR models so that, under some conditions, the adjustment may improve efficiency but is robust to a certain model misspecification. We use the following ANCOVA I working model

$$Y_i = \beta_0 + \beta_d D_i + \beta_v \hat{V}_i + \epsilon_i \tag{8.107}$$

Our goal is to estimate $E(Y(d))$ as a linear function of d, adjusting for $\hat{V}_i$. Fitting this model to obtain the parameter estimates $\hat{\beta}_d$ and $\hat{\beta}_v$ is straightforward. It is well known from standard linear model theory that when the model is correct, adjusting for V_i is beneficial. But the adjustment might harm when the model is misspecified [Lin, 2013]. The simulation below shows that $\hat{\beta}_d$ is robust to model misspecification to some extent.

The working model can also be extended by replacing $\beta_d D_i$ in (8.107) with a nonlinear function $g_d(D_i, \beta_d)$, and $\hat{\beta}_d$ still has some robust properties. It is also possible to use a nonlinear model such as a generalized linear model including D_i and V_i as covariates. Then, the marginal DR model can be estimated by g-computation. However, the estimated DR model is no longer robust to model misspecification.

8.4.9 Simulation evidence

We conducted a simulation to compare the proposed estimator with the unadjusted one. The following models and parameters are used.

- Fixed dose levels $d_k = 1, 2, 3$ with 1:1:1 random allocation to either 60 or 100 subjects.
- The data are generated by the following models

$$C_i = D_i + V_i, \quad V_i \sim N(0, 1) \tag{8.108}$$
$$Y_i = C_i + b_1 \exp(C_i + b_2 V_i) + 0.5V_i + U_i, \quad U_i \sim N(0, 1) \tag{8.109}$$

  With this setting, μ_3 is roughly 95%. The models are misspecified when b_1 and b_2 are non-zero.

- The true mean response at each d_k is estimated by a simulation sample of 100000 subjects.
- For each scenario, relative biases and variances are calculated using 5000 simulation runs.

For analysis, we use three approaches: 1) A linear ANCOVA I DR model with $\hat{V}_i$ and D_i as covariates, 2) A linear ANCOVA II DR model with $\hat{V}_i$ and D_i as covariates for each dose level.

Table 8.2
Relative bias and variance of unadjusted and adjusted estimators responses based on ANCOVA I, II models at doses 1, 2 and 3, with varying n, b_1 and b_2 and 5000 simulation runs each scenario: normally distributed outcome.

			Bias× 10 (unadjusted)			Bias× 10 (adjusted)			Var ratio (adj/unadj)		
n	b_1	b_2	μ_1	μ_2	μ_3	μ_1	μ_2	μ_3	μ_1	μ_2	μ_3
ANCOVA I											
60	0.3	0.2	-0.02	-0.02	-0.02	-0.00	-0.01	-0.03	1.42	0.68	0.76
60	0.1	0.2	-0.02	-0.01	-0.02	-0.01	-0.01	-0.02	0.60	0.58	0.73
60	0.3	0.0	-0.02	-0.01	-0.01	-0.01	-0.01	-0.02	0.99	0.58	0.73
60	0.0	0.0	-0.02	-0.01	-0.00	-0.01	-0.01	-0.00	0.39	0.54	0.76
100	0.3	0.2	-0.01	-0.01	-0.01	-0.01	-0.01	-0.02	1.53	0.68	0.81
100	0.1	0.2	-0.01	-0.01	-0.01	-0.01	-0.00	-0.01	0.61	0.57	0.78
100	0.3	0.0	-0.01	-0.01	-0.01	-0.01	-0.00	-0.01	0.97	0.57	0.77
100	0.0	0.0	-0.01	-0.00	-0.00	-0.01	-0.00	-0.00	0.39	0.53	0.79
ANCOVA II											
60	0.3	0.2	-0.02	-0.02	-0.02	-0.05	-0.05	-0.05	0.33	0.54	0.73
60	0.1	0.2	-0.02	-0.01	-0.02	-0.03	-0.04	-0.04	0.30	0.48	0.71
60	0.3	0.0	-0.02	-0.01	-0.01	-0.04	-0.04	-0.04	0.27	0.47	0.71
60	0.0	0.0	-0.02	-0.01	-0.00	-0.01	-0.01	-0.00	0.38	0.53	0.75
100	0.3	0.2	-0.01	-0.01	-0.01	-0.03	-0.03	-0.03	0.38	0.55	0.79
100	0.1	0.2	-0.01	-0.01	-0.01	-0.02	-0.02	-0.02	0.31	0.48	0.77
100	0.3	0.0	-0.01	-0.01	-0.01	-0.02	-0.02	-0.02	0.29	0.47	0.76
100	0.0	0.0	-0.01	-0.00	-0.00	-0.01	-0.00	-0.00	0.37	0.50	0.77

The relative biases and variance ratios (adjusted to unadjusted) of the ANCOVA I and II estimators compared to those of the unadjusted estimator $\hat{\mu}^m$ at the three doses are presented in Table 8.2. With the ANCOVA I estimator (upper panel), although the working ER model is misspecified in all but one scenario, the adjusted estimator had comparable bias to those of unadjusted, while its variances were generally lower. However, when there is severe model misspecification (rows 1 and 5), the variance of the adjusted one at dose level 1 may be higher than that of the unadjusted one. The results of the ANCOVA II estimator are given in the lower panel. Its bias is slightly larger than the ANCOVA I estimate, but it has consistently lower variance ratios, except when there is no model misspecification, in which situation the two perform very similarly.

8.5 Bayesian causal inference for DER relationship

To end this chapter, we give the above a Bayesian twist and explore ways to use Bayesian approaches for causal inference of DER relationships. The pioneer work in Bayesian causal inference is Rubin [1978], who introduced the framework and concept which are still widely used now. However, much controversy arises from the conflict of the classical Bayesian approach which assumes correct prior and model specification and pragmatic approaches for adjusting confounding with, e.g., Bayesian propensity score. Li et al. [2023] giving a brief review in binary treatment settings. The same applies, perhaps in a more complex way, to continuous treatment such as dose or exposure. We will take the causal ER relationship as an example, but most approaches can be easily adapted to the DR relationship when the dose is not randomized. As Bayesian causal inference is a big topic, we will concentrate on the GPS, IC and CF approaches and discuss their Bayesian counterparts.

Since classical Bayesian approaches are based on likelihood, we start from the likelihood function based on data $(Y_i, C_i, D_i, \mathbf{X}_i)$ and assume that D_i is randomized and $\mathbf{X}_i$ is fixed. We can decompose the likelihood as

$$L(\boldsymbol{\beta}, \gamma) = \prod_{i=1}^{n} f(Y_i|\mathbf{X}_i, C_i, \boldsymbol{\beta}) f(C_i|\mathbf{X}_i, D_i, \gamma) p(D_i) \tag{8.110}$$

Note that here we have used a key assumption: ignorability, that is, C_i does not depend on the potential outcome $Y_i(c)$ conditional on $\mathbf{X}_i$ [Rubin, 1978], which means the ER model has no unobserved confounders. Assuming $\pi_0(\boldsymbol{\beta}, \gamma) = \pi_0(\boldsymbol{\beta})\pi_0(\gamma)$, we can write the posterior density as

$$p(\boldsymbol{\beta}, \gamma|H^n) \propto \prod_{i=1}^{n} f(Y_i|\mathbf{X}_i, C_i, \boldsymbol{\beta})\pi_0(\boldsymbol{\beta}) f(C_i|\mathbf{X}_i, D_i, \gamma)\pi_0(\gamma) \tag{8.111}$$

where we use H^n to denote all data. Therefore, for the causal relationship between C_i and Y_i, if a model based on $f(Y_i|\mathbf{X}_i, C_i, \boldsymbol{\beta})$ can be fitted, we do not need the DE part $P(C_i|\mathbf{X}_i, D_i, \gamma)\pi_0(\gamma)$. However, we will focus on situations in which the $f(Y_i|\mathbf{X}_i, C_i, \boldsymbol{\beta})$ model cannot be fitted.

First, we consider the GPS adjustment with which we can write the conditional density of Y_i as $f(Y_i|e(\mathbf{X}_i, \gamma), C_i, \boldsymbol{\beta})$ with GPS $e(\mathbf{X}_i, \gamma)$ and replace it in (8.111). This may not be a valid full Bayesian approach, but can be considered as an approximate Bayesian approach based on quasi-likelihood in Section 7.3.2. Now we are in a similar situation to that with joint or sequential modeling, since due to the presence of $e(\mathbf{X}_i, \gamma)$ in $f(Y_i|e(\mathbf{X}_i, \gamma), C_i, \boldsymbol{\beta})$, the posterior of γ in (8.112) also depends on the ER model

$$p(\boldsymbol{\beta}, \gamma|H^n) \propto \prod_{i=1}^{n} f(Y_i|e(\mathbf{X}_i, \gamma), C_i, \boldsymbol{\beta})\pi_0(\boldsymbol{\beta}) f(C_i|\mathbf{X}_i, D_i, \gamma)\pi_0(\gamma) \tag{8.112}$$

Note that $f(C_i|\mathbf{X}_i, D_i, \gamma)$ is the GPS model. Although this might be a benefit if all model specifications are correct, we may prefer a more prudent way to "cut the feedback" from the ER model to the DE model in joint modeling. This results in the sequential modeling approach in that we fit the DE model separately, but with a Bayesian approach, then fit the ER model conditional on a posterior sample of $e(\mathbf{X}_i, \gamma)$.

Posterior samples from (8.112) can be drawn with MCMC approaches. An easier alternative is Bayesian bootstrap (BB), which generates BB a posterior sample for $\boldsymbol{\beta}$ with the following steps:

1. Generate BB weights $w_i^b, i = 1, ..., n; b = 1, ..., B$ and repeat the following B times using weight set w_i^b each time
2. Fit GPS model using weights w_i^b to obtain $\hat{\gamma}^b$ based on $f(C_i|\mathbf{X}_i, D_i, \gamma)$. Then estimate $e(\mathbf{X}_i, \hat{\gamma}^b)$.
3. Fit ER model with GPS adjustment and weights w_i^b to obtain $\hat{\boldsymbol{\beta}}^b$, based on $f(Y_i|e(\mathbf{X}_i, \hat{\gamma}^b), C_i, \boldsymbol{\beta})$ by including $e(\mathbf{X}_i, \hat{\gamma}^b)$ as a covariate.
4. If the marginal ER relationship is the estimand of interest and the mean response model is $E(Y_i|C_i, \hat{e}_i(\mathbf{X}_i)) = m(C_i, e_i, \boldsymbol{\beta})$, a BB posterior sample of the marginal ER model can be generated by

$$\hat{m}^b(c) = n^{-1} \sum_{i=1}^{n} -1m(c, e(\mathbf{X}_i, \hat{\gamma}^b), \hat{\boldsymbol{\beta}}^b). \tag{8.113}$$

The same algorithm can be easily adapted for IPW adjustment by replacing step 3 with GPS-based weighting in step 3.

The validation of this approach follows the approximate Bayesian methods 10.5, for which we have shown under minimum distributional assumption that the posterior distribution of $\boldsymbol{\beta}$ is consistent. Recall that under a general loss function, a BB sample $\hat{\boldsymbol{\beta}}^b$ has the following asymptotic property

$$\sqrt{n}(\hat{\boldsymbol{\beta}}^b - \hat{\boldsymbol{\beta}}) \sim_d \sqrt{n}(\boldsymbol{\beta} - \hat{\boldsymbol{\beta}}), \tag{8.114}$$

that is, it weakly converges to the posterior distribution centered around the minimum loss function estimates $\hat{\boldsymbol{\beta}}$. Applying the same argument here, the same properties hold when the conditions in Section 8.3.2 are satisfied.

The same approach can be used for the CF adjustment. This is not a classical Bayesian approach, but leads to a general posterior distribution with asymptotic properties given in Section 7.3.2, and the BB approach can generate a posterior sample of it. Since it is based on the adjustment for the CF by including it as a covariate, it is similar to the approach that includes GPS as a covariate. To use the above algorithm, we generate $\hat{v}_i^b = C_i - h(D_i, \mathbf{X}_i, \hat{\gamma}^b)$ in Step 2, and in Step 3, $\hat{v}_i^b$, rather than $e(\mathbf{X}_i, \hat{\gamma}^b)$, is included in the conditional ER model to obtain the posterior sample $\hat{\boldsymbol{\beta}}^b$. Then, a posterior sample BB for the marginal ER relationship represented by $E(Y_i(c))$ can be estimated by

$$\hat{m}^b(c) = n^{-1} \sum_{i=1}^{n} m(c, \hat{v}_i^b, \hat{\boldsymbol{\beta}}^b). \tag{8.115}$$

GPS and CF approaches can be used to predict the marginal DR relationship based on the conditional ER model. Taking the CF approach as an example, a posterior sample of $E(Y_i(d))$ can be generated by

$$\hat{m}^b(d) = n^{-1}\sum_{i=1}^{n} \hat{m}^b(\hat{C}_i^b(d), \hat{v}_i^b, \hat{\boldsymbol{\beta}}^b), b = 1, ..., B \tag{8.116}$$

where $\hat{C}_i^b(d) = h(d, \mathbf{X}_i, \hat{\gamma}^b) + \hat{v}_i^b$,

We have omitted $\mathbf{X}_i$ in the ER models in the discussion above for simplicity. In practice, key prognostic factors should be directly adjusted in the ER model; the algorithms still apply by adding them to the ER model, and, for the estimation of the marginal DR or ER model, we average $m(c, \mathbf{X}_i, \hat{v}_i^b, \hat{\boldsymbol{\beta}}^b)$.

Some other frequentist causal adjustment approaches can also be adapted as an (approximate) Bayesian approach [Stephens et al., 2023]. For example, the IV regression approach can be considered as a GMM approach, for which Bayesian approaches have been developed [Yin et al., 2019]. Associated with the IPW approach is the doubly robust estimator for $E(Y_i(c))$ or $E(Y_i(d))$, for which an easy Bayesian approach to obtain a posterior sample is the BB [Graham et al., 2016]. The covariate balancing approach is slightly different. If the balancing is based on empirical likelihood, the likelihood-based Bayesian approach can be easily applied. For the general covariate-balancing approach, it has been shown, although in a different context, that the BB approach also provides a valid posterior sample for binary treatments [Wang and Tiwari, 2025a]. We have only briefly stated some simple adjustment for Bayesian DER approaches. These approaches can be classified as semiparametric Bayesian inference with more technically involved approaches and theory [Ray and van der Vaart, 2020]. Without going to the technical details, we have just shown that most of the causal inference approaches can be made Bayesian by BB or some other Bayesian computation approaches.

8.6 Causal DER relationship and time-to-event models

Causal DER relationships for TTE are more difficult to model and estimate than other types of response. In the Cox model, although dose as a covariate can be fitted, its coefficient is not a causal parameter even for data from a randomized dose trial. The reason is, as we discussed, that during the trial the subjects at risk change continuously and those with different doses, e.g., are no longer comparable. Therefore, for causal DER relationship for TTEs, we need alternative causal estimands. The following are commonly used two.

1. Survival probability causal effect (SPCE): $\Delta^{d,d'}(t) \equiv S^d(t) - S^{d'}(t)$, where d, d' are two constant dose levels.

2. Restricted average causal effect (RACE): $\Delta_R^{d,d'}(\tau) \equiv \int_0^\tau S^d(t)dt - \int_0^\tau S^{d'}(t)dt$

We can also define the above as ratios rather than differences between $S(t)$ of each dose. In fact, the above definitions are valid when d and d' are dosing rules, e.g., starting with 1mg dose and reducing to 0.5mg after occurrence of the first AE. The corresponding estimate is known as that of the "treatment policy".

Although the Cox model does not have the causal interpretation we like, it can be a powerful tool to derive, e.g., $\Delta^{d,d+1}(t)$. Suppose that a (correct) Cox model

$$h_0(t)\exp(\beta_d d_i + \boldsymbol{\beta}_x \mathbf{X}_i) \tag{8.117}$$

is fitted and $\hat\beta_d, \hat{\boldsymbol{\beta}}_x$, together with the baseline survival function $\hat S_0(t)$, are estimated. Then we can estimate

$$\hat S^d(t) = n^{-1}\sum_{i=1}^n \hat S_0(t)^{\exp(\hat\beta_d d + \hat{\boldsymbol{\beta}}_x \mathbf{X}_i)} \tag{8.118}$$

for a given d. This is an application of the g-computation approach, which has been implemented in the R package stdReg, which gives not only the estimate but also its SE and CI.

Approaches for subject-level confounding adjustment described in this chapter can be used for both SPCE and RACE. For example, the g-computation approach above can be used for direct adjustment for confounders in $\mathbf{X}_i$. The model can also include estimated GPS or CF in the model. GPS-based weighting and stratification can also be applied directly on the Kaplan-Meier estimator [Kalbfleisch and Prentice, 2002]. Alternatively, we may use a model for some causal estimands such as RACE and apply the above adjustment to it.

Although these causal estimands can be defined, they all have similar issues in both application and methodology. One is that none of them is a single number measure, as is HR in Cox models, because they all depend on t or τ. We may define them as limits when $t(\tau) \to \infty$, but these equations are often not estimable. Second, the DR relationship for one unit dose increase $\Delta^{d,d+1}(t)$ depends on d, as the same issue when we define causal OR for binary responses. Therefore, DER analysis becomes much more complex than fitting a Cox model with dose as a covariate.

8.7 Comments and bibliographic notes

Causal inference is a fast-developing field with such a large volume of literature that this chapter can only cover a small fraction of it. Some excellent textbooks include Hernan and Robins [2023]; Pearl [2022], but focus on causal inference of binary and categorical treatments. Researches and applications of causal dose-response modeling have been seen in social sciences, particularly econometrics. Although their methodology can be adapted, most of them focus on scenarios of large sample sizes that are often infeasible in our context. This chapter presents several simulation results. However, the readers should do their own simulations based on their scenarios to assess the performance of each method. The R codes for the simulation results presented in Table 8.1, Figures 8.2 and 8.3 are available in the online Appendix and can be downloaded from the book website.

We have seen a close link between direct adjustment approaches and the classical popPK and popPKPD approaches. One purpose of this chapter is to show how to evaluate the classical approaches in view of causal inference and to search for improvement. Since most of the approaches depend on assumptions that are not verifiable with the data, an important approach is to apply multiple approaches to assess the sensitivity of the models to their assumptions.

9

Learning dose-exposure-response relationships: dose allocation and optimization

This chapter concerns dual goals: learning the DER relationship and dose allocation, particularly response-dependent allocation, using the DER relationship. Previous chapters have covered them individually. The challenge we face is to perform them in parallel. That is, we learn the DER relationship in parallel to using it for dose allocation, which is also crucial to learning the DER relationship. In this context, dose allocation often depends on previous responses of the same patient, or previous patients, hence it is often referred to as dose-adjustment. Most of the chapter focuses on the DR relationship, but we also show that DE and ER modeling also helps for dose allocation. Dose finding is a process of learning the DER relationship. This concept can be traced back to the seminal paper of Sheiner [1997] long before the current use of modern machine learning (ML) methods and dynamic programming and control theory [Bertsekas, 2012] in pharmacometrics. The learning of DER relationship has its specific aspect, often driven by feasibility, which is the main topic of this chapter.

9.1 Dose-response relationship and dose allocation

We start with dose allocation for different purposes using the DR relationship. Let D be the dose and $Y(d) \equiv Y(D = d)$ be the potential response to dose $D = d$. Here we consider doses that may be confounded, hence generally $E(Y(d)) \neq E(Y|D = d)$. Often the DR relationship of interest is the mean DR function

$$E(Y(d)) = g(d) \tag{9.1}$$

where $g(d)$ is an unknown function. Depending on the practical context, the optimal dose d^* may be the solution of

$$g(d) = y^0 \tag{9.2}$$

where y^0 is a target level of response (e.g., 25% toxicity in a Phase I dose escalation trial). Alternatively, it may be defined as the maximum dose whose

DOI: 10.1201/9781003457008-9

toxicity is not higher than the target level p^*:

$$d^* = \max(d : g(d) \leq p^*). \tag{9.3}$$

Sometimes, a treatment is to keep the response between the lower limit L and the upper limit U, e.g., $L = 2$ and $U = 3$ of the international normalized ratio (INR) for warfarin dosing for certain patients. Therefore, d^* may be defined as

$$d^* = \text{argmax}_d P(L < Y(d) < U). \tag{9.4}$$

In this case, the mean DR relationship may not be sufficient, as the probability depends on the distribution of $Y(d)$. Then, the dose-response relationship in terms of the quantile effect may be more relevant.

The DR relationship can be derived from the DE and ER models, if they are available, as we have shown in previous chapters. The same approaches can be used to determine the dose to achieve a certain exposure level using the DE model:

$$d^* = \text{argmax}_d P(L < C(d) < U). \tag{9.5}$$

Likewise, the ER model may help determine the target exposure to achieve the target response level. Although the exposure level is difficult to accurately control, in practice, dose titration to a certain exposure window is sometimes used for drugs with highly variable exposure.

Recently, clinical utility indices that represent a summary of efficacy and toxicity have been used as a single measure of the clinical benefit of a drug at a given dose. If $E(Y(d)) = g(d)$ is the expected clinical index at dose d, the optimal dose that maximizes the expected clinical utility can be defined as

$$d^* = \text{argmax}_d g(d). \tag{9.6}$$

However, often only prefixed doses $\bar{D} = (d^1, ..., d^K)$ can be used, the optimal dose defined based on $g(d)$ may not be among them. A practical definition of the optimal dose is the best dose among $\bar{D}$. Formally, taking the utility-based definition as an example, we define

$$d^* = \text{argmax}_{d \in \bar{D}} g(d). \tag{9.7}$$

For model-based dose allocation, there are generally three modeling options in order to determine the dose.

1. Modeling DR relationship: this includes modeling DER relationships based on mechanistic or empirical models aiming at the estimation of DR relationship. This is a classical approach in both the biostatics and pharmacometric fields.
2. Modeling dose-objective relationship: This approach bypasses the response and directly models how the objective (e.g., $P(L < Y(d) < U)$) changes with dose. The objective may be more difficult to model than the DR relationship, but it directly relates to our objective.

3. One step further from the second is to directly model the optimal dosing rule. This can be a direct modeling if the optimal doses are known, or can be indirectly, e.g., for a linear dosing rule with unknown parameters, we can find the parameters that lead to the optimal dosing, as we will see later.

9.2 Dose allocation and learning DR relationship in parallel

9.2.1 Adaptive trial designs for dose allocation

Adaptive trial designs are sequential approaches that allocate the next patient based on existing results. The goal of these studies is often double: to maximize the clinical benefit of patients in the trial, and also to find the best dose at the end of the trial. This sequential approach can be considered as a process of leaning the DR relationship and often leads to more patients treated at more adequate dose levels with a greater clinical benefit for these patients. Examples of such a design include the simple 3 + 3 dose-escalation design which does not need a model and model-based approaches such as the CRM and Bayesian logistic model approaches for phase I dose-escalation trials [Daimon et al., 2019] to find the maximum tolerant dose defined as in (9.3). For example, denoting $\hat{p}(d)$ as the predicted probability of dose-limiting toxicity (DLT) at dose d based on a fitted DR model, we can assign dose $d^k \in \bar{D}$ with its $\hat{p}(d^k)$ closest to, but not higher than, the target DLT level p^*.

Adaptive model-based dose allocation approaches generally fit the model in parallel with dose allocation, and the model is updated sequentially. Suppose that $\hat{\boldsymbol{\beta}}^n$ is the parameter estimate based on the data H^n from the first n subjects, a simple myopic rule is to allocate to the $n+1$th subject the dose that best meets the given criteria. For example, if the goal is to maximize the mean utility $E(U_i(d)|\hat{\boldsymbol{\beta}}^n) = g(d, \hat{\boldsymbol{\beta}}^n)$ then a myopic optimal dose for the next patient is

$$D_{n+1} = \text{argmax}_{d \in \bar{D}} g(d, \hat{\boldsymbol{\beta}}^n) \tag{9.8}$$

This approach is similar to the play-the-winner role to allocate discrete treatments (including doses). If the goal is to find the dose with the closest DLT level to the target level p^*, then the next myopic dose can be chosen as

$$D_{n+1} = \text{argmin}_{d \in \bar{D}} (g(d, \hat{\boldsymbol{\beta}}^n) - p^*)^2 \tag{9.9}$$

The myopic rule seems a reasonable sequential allocation rule; however, it may be trapped at a suboptimal dose level, even if the model $g(d, \boldsymbol{\beta})$ is correct. The reason is the lack of exploration of other doses, which is important not only for finding the optimal dose but also for estimating model parameters.

In contrast, a model-free method for finding the dose d^* with which $g(d^*) = p^*$, assuming that $g(d)$ is not decreasing, is Robins-Minor's stochastic search

$$D_{n+1} = D_n + \alpha_n (p^* - Y_n) \tag{9.10}$$

where $\alpha_n \geq 0$ is a real number sequence. This algorithm does not depend on any model. Under some technical conditions, $D_n \to d^*$. The choice of α_n is tricky, but it should converge to 0 at a certain rate, as described in the next section.

9.2.2 Exploration versus exploitation

Recall that our goal is to select the optimal dose and also to maximize the benefit of the patients in the trial. The first requires exploration to obtain information; for that, information on suboptimal doses is also needed. The second needs to exploit the information already obtained in order to allocate the current optimal dose to the remaining patients. The conflict between exploration and exploitation also occurs for other reasons, such as modeling. The problem of the Bayesian logistic model approach is an example of exploration dominated by exploitation [Iasonos et al., 2016]. This is also a key topic in ML, particularly reinforcement [Sutton et al., 1998], which will be applied in this chapter in multiple sections.

An easy approach that balances both is to do them sequentially, with the first stage focusing on exploration, while the second on exploitation. Let Y_{ij} and D_{ij} be the response (e.g., the clinical benefit) and the dose of patient $i, i = 1, ..., n_j$ in stage $j, j = 1, 2$. In the first stage, we can assign subjects to all doses in $\bar{D}$ (e.g., by randomization). At the end of stage 1, we fit a DR model

$$E(Y_{i1}|D_{i1}) = g(D_{i1}, \boldsymbol{\beta}_1) \tag{9.11}$$

and obtain $\hat{\boldsymbol{\beta}}_1$, then the dose of the second stage can be optimized according to the purpose of the trial. For example, if we want to maximize the clinical benefit of the trial population, the stage 2 dose may be $d^* = \text{argmax}_{d \in \bar{D}} g(d, \hat{\boldsymbol{\beta}}_1)$. If the purpose is to finally determine the optimal dose for future trials, a model-based approach is to use c-optimal dose levels that minimize $det(c_d^T \text{var}(\hat{\boldsymbol{\beta}}) c_d)$, with c_d consisting of contrasts between a subset of candidate dose levels, determined based on $g(d, \hat{\boldsymbol{\beta}}_1)$, which provides information for dose selection using MCPmod [Bretz et al., 2005]. Often, the goal is a compromise between the two purposes. In this case, an allocation rule with a good balance of exploration and exploitation can be used, as shown in the next section.

When no model is assumed, this two-stage approach leads to the common practice of a dose finding trial with an extension phase in which only one or two selected doses are used. In this case, although fitting a DR model is not possible to the second-stage data, a DER model approach may still be useful.

The two-stage approach can be a simple and good option if the relative sample size of each stage, i.e., the proportions for exploration and expectation, are determined correctly. This is obviously not an easy task, since the amount of information needed for exploration depends on the complexity of the DR relationship, which is unknown at the design stage.

9.2.3 Bandits and Thompson sampling

The balance between exploration and exploitation can be illustrated by the bandits problem. Here, bandits refer to mathematical models that mimic bandit gambling machines, which may give different amounts of reward when they are played. The question is how to decide which one to play, given the information from previous plays. We start with such a model in our context without assuming any DR model, hence the dose levels are treated as individual treatments. Our goal is to find the optimal sequential dose allocation rule that maximizes the overall benefit of all patients in the trial. In fact, for binary and normal responses, [Gittins, 1979] have given analytical solutions. Its application in clinical trial designs has been found in recent publications such as Villar et al. [2015], although the use of such designs in a real trial seems rare. Gittins algorithm is rather complex, but the allocation rule can be tabulated, and software can be used to generate the dose allocation rule. Gittins rule is deterministic, i.e., the dose for the next patient completely depends on the dose and response of existing patients.

A simple solution to deal with the balance of exploitation and exploration is Thompson sampling (TS), widely used in machine learning [Russo et al., 2018]. Suppose that a higher response is better, TS samples from the posterior distribution of the mean response of all doses, then take the dose with highest posterior sample. The posterior distribution is updated each time new data are added. Intuitively, when information is lacking, the posterior sample has high variability, so that the algorithm explores different dose levels. With increasing information, the posterior sample converges to the optimal dose, hence exploration reduces, and the algorithm converges to the optimal dose (if it exists and is unique). Since the TS rule is random, it is more feasible in clinical trials than deterministic dosing rules.

The key step of TS is to generate posterior samples of the mean response. A classical approach is to use MCMC with fully specified likelihood functions and priors. However, this approach is not efficient for TS, since MCMC needs a large number of iterations to achieve the steady state of all variables before taking the posterior sample. Although the posterior sample can be very large, TS only uses one (or a small number if multiple patients are randomized together). For this purpose, the BB approach is much more efficient. As described in Section 7.3.3, it does not need a full specification of likelihood and priors. Furthermore, prior information can be included as pseudo-prior data, and the whole BB algorithm does not need special software.

As an example, we consider a design to use 3 doses 1, 2 and 3 with utility $Y_i(d) \sim N(\mu_d, 1)$, (μ_1, μ_2, μ_3)=(2, 1.5, 1). We treat 100 patients sequentially, with the dose of the next patient depending on the response of previous patients following the TS rule. To do this, we need a posterior sample of each

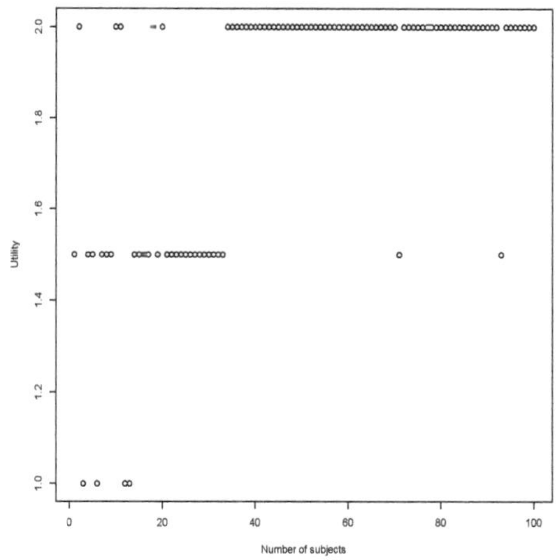

Figure 9.1
Trajectory of utility over number of subjects used to learn the optimal dose.

dose based on, say, m patients who are uniformly assigned to all doses. Recall that a BB sample is simply

$$\hat{\mu}_k = \sum_{D_i=k} w_i Y_i / \sum_{D_i=k} w_i \tag{9.12}$$

where $w_i \sim \exp(1)$. Then the dose for the $m+1$ patient is

$$D_{m+1} = \text{argmax}_k \hat{\mu}_k, k = 1, ..., 3. \tag{9.13}$$

The codes show how this algorithm works.

```
mu=c(2,1.5,1)
idose=rep(ddose,3)  # unifrom dose allocation to 9 patients
ndose=length(idose)
yi=rnorm(ndose,mean=mu[idose])
Mout=data.frame(yi=yi,di=ddose) # Data of 9 patients to run TS
xopt=NULL
uti=NULL
nb=100
for (k in 1:nb){
  len=dim(Mout)[1]
  bwei=rexp(len)
  hatmu=as.numeric(lm(yi~as.factor(di)-1, weights = bwei, data=Mout)$coef)
  nxdose=which(hatmu==max(hatmu))                #The next dose
  xopt=c(xopt,nxdose)
  uti=c(uti,mu[nxdose])   # True response rate of the next dose
  Mout=rbind(Mout,c(rnorm(1,mean=mu[nxdose]),nxdose)) # Append the data
}
plot(1:nb,uti)
```

The plot in Figure 9.1 shows the utility trajectory for the number of patients enrolled in a simulation, in which the optimal dose is identified for most patients after 40 of them are treated. However, the trajectory may be rather different in another simulation run. If we run the code many times, we may find that the TS method may also be trapped at a suboptimal dose. The reason is the same as for the failure of the play-the-winner rule, just it happens much less frequently. There is a small chance that the initial batch of patients shows very biased estimates that make the probability of the allocation of the true optimal dose almost impossible, even with random sampling variation. One remedy for this problem is to increase the size of the initial set of patients. Another is the so-called ϵ-greedy allocation in that the next patient has a ϵ (small) probability of being assigned to other doses rather than the one selected by the TS rule. Both remedies reduce the frequency of using the optimal dose in the trial in most scenarios; hence, we pay the cost of preparing for the worst.

In the above example, the posterior distribution of μ_ds has a closed form (See Chapter 7), from which we can directly take a posterior sample without MCMC or BB. The code serves as an illustration of the use of BB in more general situations. An easy way to use closed form without BB is to assume that μ_d has a t-distribution with df, mean and variance given by the first m patients. Then a sample from the t-distribution can replace the line "hatmu=..." in the code.

TS has some notable large sample properties, as shown by multiple approaches in ML [Russo et al., 2018]. Among them, a key one in the context of ML is that its learning rate achieves the upper bound [Lai and Robbins, 1985], that is, in general, no other algorithm can learn uniformly faster than TS. However, this advantage may not be applicable to dose-ranging trials. With a small n, information may never be enough to determine which dose is the best, while to maximize the benefit of the n patients, the allocation rule should move to exploitation long before all n patients are treated. To improve its small sample properties, accelerated TS (ATS) takes the full exploitation (myopic) rule with a certain probability, and the probability increases with the fraction of sample size to ensure that at the end of the trial, the last dose is myopic [Wang, 2021]. Simulation results show that ATS leads to higher mean clinical benefit, in some situations, close to the gold standard by the Gittins rule.

TS, including its variant ATS, may not be optimal for finally selecting the optimal dose. For this task, Russo [2016] proposed a top-two TS (TTTS) approach based on TS. Intuitively, TS may use the current best treatment too often, while to ensure the correct selection of the best treatment, it should be compared to the second best. TTTS avoids this problem of TS by forcing the use of the second best with a certain probability. It has some optimal large sample properties; its small sample properties can also be improved by acceleration. A similar approach to ATS leads to accelerated TTTS (ATTTS) [Wang and Tiwari, 2023].

9.3 Contextual bandits using dose-response models

TS and ATS approaches become inefficient when there are several dose levels to select, due to the number of parameters to be estimated. This problem can be overcome by using models to predict the response. Recall that the key step in TS is generating a posterior sample of the response for all dose levels, which can use a DR model to reduce the number of parameters to be estimated. Using models, it is also possible to select any dose at which the mean response can be predicted by a DR model. These model-based approaches are known as contextual bandits (CB) in machine learning literature, which can also be implemented by TS [Agrawal and Goyal, 2013].

As a simple example, let $g(d, \boldsymbol{\beta})$ be the mean response model, H^i be the data of the first i patients, $\hat{\boldsymbol{\beta}}$ the BB posterior sample of $\boldsymbol{\beta}$ given data H^i, then the next dose to use by TS is

$$D_{i+1} = \text{argmax}_{d \in \bar{D}} g(d, \hat{\boldsymbol{\beta}}). \tag{9.14}$$

The following algorithm shows how the TS based CB is implemented. In step 8 more than one DR model (e.g., efficacy and safety DR models)

Algorithm 1 DR modeling based contextual bandits with Thompson sampling by Bayesian bootstrap.

Require: $\bar{D}$ (a set of possible dose levels), a utility function $U(.)$, true model $g(d)$ to generate Y and model $g(d, \boldsymbol{\beta})$ to fit Y_i, empty dataset H^0.

1: Run-in:
2: **for** $i = 1$ to n_1 **do**
3: Sample D_i from $\bar{D}$ and obtain $Y_i \sim g(D_i)$.
4: $H^i \leftarrow (H^{i-1}, (D_i, Y_i))$
5: **end for**
6: **for** $i = n_1 + 1$ to n **do**
7: Generate weights $w_j, j = 1, ..., i$ from the uniform Dirichlet distribution $Dirichlet(1, ..., 1)$.
8: Fit DR-Model(s) to data H^i with weights w_js and obtain the estimated coefficients $\hat{\boldsymbol{\beta}}$.
9: Predict utilities at all dose levels

$$\hat{U}(d^k) = U(g(d^k, \hat{\boldsymbol{\beta}})), k = 1, ..., K. \tag{9.15}$$

10: Select $D_i = \text{argmax}_{d \in \bar{D}} \hat{U}(d)$.
11: Obtain $Y_i \sim g(D_i)$ and update dataset $H^i \leftarrow (H^{i-1}, (D_i, Y_i))$
12: **end for**

can be fitted. The utility may also take two or more components, e.g., $U = 0.65Eff - 0.35Tox + 0.35$ as in Lee et al. [2015].

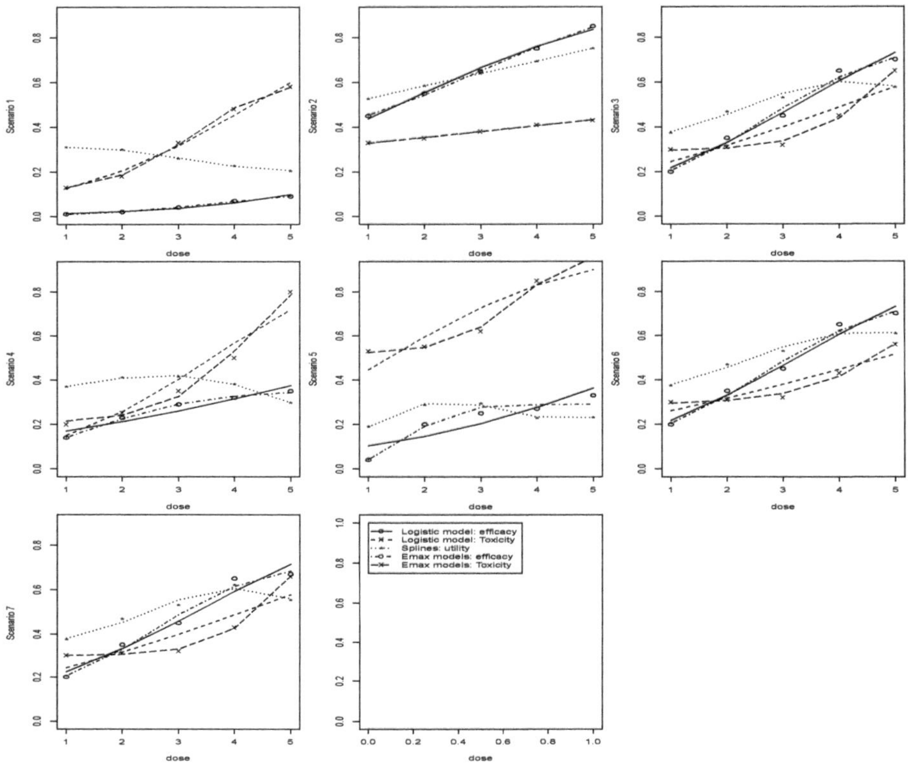

Figure 9.2
Efficacy and toxicity curves with model prediction using logistic and Emax models, and utility curves with fitted model of spline functions (df=3) in seven scenarios in Lee et al. (2015).

As an example, we take the seven hypothetical scenarios as published in Lee et al. [2015] and used in Wang and Tiwari [2025b] to examine dose-finding designs using CB. To check how commonly used DR models fit them, we fit the logistic and Emax models to the efficacy and toxicity curves and the spline functions (df=3) to the utility ($U = 0.65Eff - 0.35Tox + 0.35$) curves. The fitted models together with the data are shown in Figure 9.2. For Scenarios 1 and 2, all models fit well; while for the rest, logistic models cannot fit both toxicity and efficacy data well. The Emax models are much more flexible than the logistic models, so are the spline function models, while the logistic model cannot fit a part of a sigmoid curve with maximum effect much lower than 1 or the minimum one much higher than 0 (e.g., Scenario 5).

Then, the CB algorithm 1 is implemented with both the efficacy and toxicity models fitted in step (8). Figure 9.3 shows the mean utility for 10 interim looks with 10 patients each in the seven scenarios, with the first 10 patients

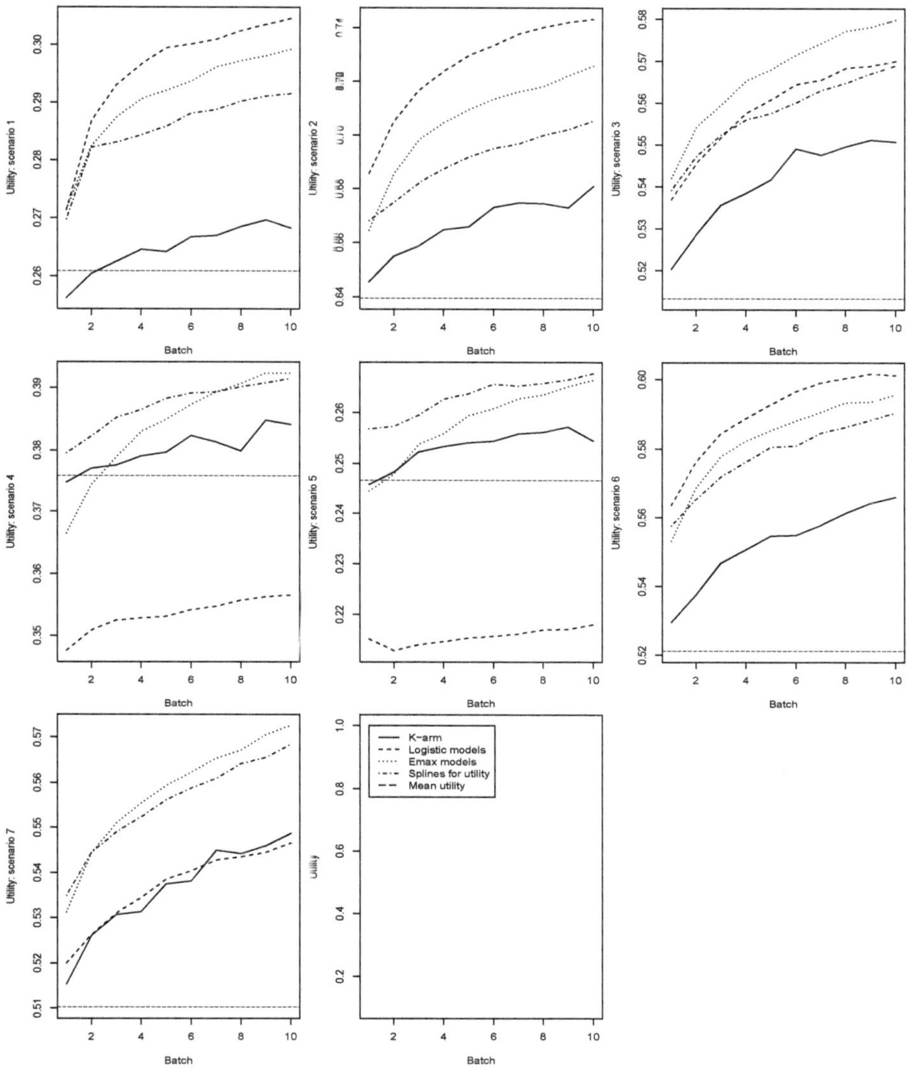

Figure 9.3
Mean trajectories of mean utility with contextual bandits (three models) and discrete armed bandits in seven scenarios of Lee et al. (2015), with up to 10 batches of 10 patients each. The first batch is randomized with equal probability.

randomly assigned to each dose with the same probability. All curves show a trend of increase with the increase of information at different rates of "learning". The logistic model-based CB shows a significant advantage over the other approaches when all models fit well (scenarios 1, 2 and 6, see Figure 9.2), showing a fast learning rate with simple models. However, this approach performs the worst in some other scenarios, e.g., Scenarios 3 and 4, and it could be even worse than the random allocation rule if the dose level selected by the model has a lower utility than the average. The Emax model-based approach generally performs among the best in all scenarios. The utility modeling approach using spline functions is another robust approach with acceptable performance over all scenarios. The K-armed bandit is robust, but with the lowest learning rate.

9.4 Contextual bandits using DER modeling

We can also combine the DE ad ER models in the CB approach. The CB approach of using DER models for dose allocation may simply follow the way of sequential prediction of responses at candidate dose levels. Taking the task of maximizing the utility as an example. The DER model-based CB algorithm is similar to that using the DR model. After having data from i patients H^i, we fit the DE and ER models and take posterior samples $\hat{\gamma}$ and $\hat{\boldsymbol{\beta}}$. Then a posterior sample of the utility of dose d is

$$\hat{U}(d) = E(g(h(d, \hat{\gamma}, \eta_i), \hat{\boldsymbol{\beta}}, \epsilon_i)), \tag{9.16}$$

and the dose for the next patient with CB is

$$D_{i+1} = \text{argmax}_{d \in \bar{D}} \hat{U}(d), k = 1, ..., K. \tag{9.17}$$

The (Algoritm 2) is similar to the DR model based.

For the DER-based CB, we cannot use the scenarios in Lee et al. [2015], since there is no exposure in them. Therefore, we use a toy example as an illustration. The following codes use three dose levels, with binary efficacy and toxicity responses, all linked to exposure with logistic models. The exposure is generated by a linear DE model. The goal is to find and use the dose with maximum utility as a linear combination of efficacy and toxicity outcomes. See the code for parameter values in these models. Since the marginal utility at each dose does not have an analytical form, we use a simulation with a very large sample size to calculate it to determine the optimal dose.

```
ddose=1:3  # Designed doses
ndose=length(ddose)
nsimu=30000  # Simulation to estimate marginal mean utility
vdose=rep(ddose,nsimu/ndose)
ci=vdose+0.5*rnorm(nsimu)
pi=1/(1+exp(4-3*ci))
qi=1/(1+exp(8-3*ci))
ui=0.65*pi-0.35*qi
lm(ui~as.factor(vdose)-1) #marginal mean utility by dose
```

Algorithm 2 DER modeling based contextual bandits with Thompson sampling by Bayesian bootstrap.

Require: $\bar{D}$ (a set of possible dose levels), a utility function $U(.)$, true model $g(c), h(d)$ to generate Y_i and C_i and model $g(d, \boldsymbol{\beta})$ and $h(d, \boldsymbol{\gamma})$ to fit Y_i and C_i, respectively, empty dataset H^0.

Run-in:
for $i = 1$ to n_1 **do**
  Sample D_i from $\bar{D}$ and obtain $C_i \sim h(D_i), Y_i \sim g(C_i)$.
  $H^i \leftarrow (H^{i-1}, (D_i, Y_i, C_i))$
end for
for $i = n_1 + 1$ to n **do**
  Generate weights $w_j, j = 1, ..., i$ from the uniform Dirichlet distribution $Dirichlet(1, ..., 1)$.
  Fit DE-Model(s) to data H^i with weights w_j and obtain the estimated coefficients $\hat{\gamma}$.
  Fit ER-Model(s) to data H^i with weights w_j and obtain the estimated coefficients $\hat{\boldsymbol{\beta}}$.
  Predict utilities at all dose levels

$$\hat{U}(d^k) = U(g(h(d^k, \hat{\gamma}), \hat{\boldsymbol{\beta}})), k = 1, ..., K. \tag{9.18}$$

  Select $D_i = \text{argmax}_{d \in \bar{D}} \hat{U}(d)$.
  Obtain $C_i \sim h(D_i), Y_i \sim g(C_i)$ and update dataset $H^i \leftarrow (H^{i-1}, (D_i, Y_i, C_i))$
end for

```
          0.2084              0.4596              0.4037  #Mean utility

simu=function(nsimu=10  # Number of simulation
   ,K=3          #Number of batches
   ,nb=15)    #sample size of each batch
   {
   Optout=NULL
   for (simu in 1:nsimu){
     Z=Y=NULL
     vopt=vuti=NULL
     Mout=NULL
     xopt=rep(ddose,nb/ndose) #init dose is design dose
     cb=db=NULL
     for (k in 1:K){           #Loop of batch
       ci=xopt+0.5*rnorm(nb) #exposure
       pi=1/(1+exp(4-3*ci))  # Pr of eff
       qi=1/(1+exp(8-3*ci))  # Pr of tox
       ui=0.65*pi-0.35*qi    #Utility
       eff=rbinom(nb,1,pi)   # binary Eff
       tox=rbinom(nb,1,qi)   # binary Tox
       Y=c(Y,eff)
       Z=c(Z,tox)
       cb=c(cb,ci)
```

```
      db=c(db,xopt)
      Mout=rbind(Mout,data.frame(db=db,cb=cb,Y=Y,Z=Z)) # Dataset appended
      len=dim(Mout)[1]       #Rows of Mout
      xopt=NULL
      util=NULL
      for(j in 1:nb){    # Thompson sampling for each subject
        bwei=rexp(len)      #Bayesian bootstrap weights
        bwei=bwei/mean(bwei)
        fitc=lm(cb~db,weights=bwei,data=Mout)$coef  #Fit DE model
        fite=glm(Y~cb,family="binomial",weights=bwei,data=Mout)$coef #ER (eff)
        fitt=glm(Z~cb,family="binomial",weights=bwei,data=Mout)$coef #ER(tox)
        vci=rep(cb,ndose)                        # exposures repeat for each in ddos
        vd0=rep(ddose,rep(len,ndose))            # same for ddose
        vdi=rep(db,ndose)                        # same for dose in data
        pd=1/(1+exp(-fite[1]-fite[2]*(cb+fitc[2]*(vd0-vdi))))  #Predicted Pr eff
        qd=1/(1+exp(-fitt[1]-fitt[2]*(cb+fitc[2]*(vd0-vdi))))  #Predicted Pr tox
        ui=65*pd-35*qd+35
        uti=lm(ui~as.factor(vd0)-1)$coef     # Mean uti for each dose over all
        d0=which(uti==max(uti))            #The optimal dose
        xopt=c(xopt,d0)                    # Add to the opt dose vectior
      }
      xopt=as.numeric(xopt)
      vopt=c(vopt,xopt)  #Keep selected dose for each simu
    }
    Optout=c(Optout,vopt)
  }
  return(Optout)     #Output simulation results
  }

#debug(simu)
UsedDose=simu(nsimu=200)
Tab3=table(UsedDose)
Tab3/sum(Tab3)
> Tab3/sum(Tab3)
UsedDose
          1           2           3
0.008888889 0.795444444 0.195666667
```

The true optimal dose is 2 and the second is 3, with mean utility 0.46 and 0.40, respectively. With the CB algorithm using DER models, we can use the optimal one in 80% time, while the worst dose was only used less than 1 %.

DR models may still be used in the CB algorithm with three doses. The next example shows that the DER modeling approach can also work for two dose levels 1 and 3, while logistic DR models do not work in this setting. For the two-dose setting, we need to change the parameters to avoid very low or high probabilities. With the following setting

```
pi=1/(1+exp(3-3*ci))
qi=1/(1+exp(6-3*ci)).
```

The codes for three doses can be easily adapted for two doses by replacing the lines for pi and qi with the two lines above. We also change the batch size from 15 to 16 so that all dose levels are used 16/2 times in the first batch. With the 2-dose setting, we have true mean utilities 0.29 and 0.33 for doses 1 and 3, respectively. With the CB algorithm using DER models, we use doses 1 and 3 31% and 69% times, respectively. This example shows the advantage of using DER models over the use of the DR model when very few dose levels are available.

9.5 Is exploration needed for allocation rules with DER modeling?

We have shown that the myopic rule can lead to convergence problems even in the ideal situation of fitting the correct logistic regression model due to lack of exploration [Iasonos et al., 2016]. Since DER modeling uses both exposure and response data, in which the ER modeling has rich exposure data, does the same problem occur? Indeed, the same problem occurs with DER modeling. The following is a simple example for when this may occur. Suppose that both the DE model $C_i = \gamma_0 + \gamma_d D_i$ and the ER model $Y_i = \beta_0 + \beta_c C_i$ are linear and are specified correctly. We even assume that the ER model is known and our goal is to find $d = \text{argmin}_{d \in \bar{D}} |E(Y_i(d)) - y^0|$. Since the ER model is known, the problem becomes $\text{argmin}_{d \in \bar{D}} |E(C_i(d) - \beta_c^{-1}(y^0 - \beta_0))|$, the same as the problem in the DR modeling. To see in which situation convergence to the right dose d^* may fail, consider $\bar{D} = (1, 2)$ and $d^* = 1$. Since the DE model is saturated, the predicted $E(C_i(d_k))$ is exactly the $\bar{c}_k$: the sample mean of C_i under d_k. Suppose that in the first 10 patients, $|E(\bar{c}_2 - \beta_c^{-1}(y^0 - \beta_0))|$ is much smaller than $|E(\bar{c}_1 - \beta_c^{-1}(y^0 - \beta_0))|$, since $\bar{c}_1$ is much higher than the target by chance, the next assigned dose is $d = 2$ with the myopic rule. However, more information on dose 2 will not solve the problem due to $\bar{c}_1$, therefore, with high probability, dose $d = 1$ will never be used, and the myopic algorithm will end with repeated use of $d = 2$. Therefore, we still need approaches such as CB with DER models.

9.6 Learning individualized dosing rules

9.6.1 Individualized dosing rules by learned DR relationship

Recall that with a simple DR model with covariates x

$$\mu(d|x) = E(Y_i(d)|x) = g(d, x, \boldsymbol{\beta}), \tag{9.19}$$

we can determine the dose d for a subject with covariates x to achieve $\mu(d|x) = y^0$ by selecting d^* so that

$$g(d^*, x, \hat{\boldsymbol{\beta}}) = y^0 \tag{9.20}$$

where $\hat{\boldsymbol{\beta}}$ are the estimated parameters. Therefore, a straightforward approach is to fit the DR or DER models to estimate the DR relationship and then determine the optimal dose based on it.

Sometimes, the optimal dose is indicated by the highest $\mu(d|x)$. In this case, it would be useful if we could write:

$$\mu(d|x) = g_0(x, \boldsymbol{\beta}_0) + g_d(d, x, \boldsymbol{\beta}_d) \tag{9.21}$$

with a separate dose-related part $g_d(d, x, \boldsymbol{\beta}_d)$ and its own parameters. Again, we do not distinguish covariates x in the two parts, but the parameters may have zero elements for those not used in each part. After fitting the model, we can find the optimal dose as

$$d^* = \text{argmax}_d g_d(d, x, \boldsymbol{\beta}_d) \tag{9.22}$$

In fact, since $g_0(x, \boldsymbol{\beta}_0)$ does not have a role in the dosing rule, it is not necessary to model it at all. Therefore, one approach is to fit $g_d(d, x, \boldsymbol{\beta}_d)$ only and let $g_0(x, \boldsymbol{\beta}_0)$ go to the residual error. This approach is useful when $g_0(x, \boldsymbol{\beta}_0)$ has many parameters to fit, while there are only a few in the $g_d(d, x, \boldsymbol{\beta}_d)$ part. However, fitting the $g_0(x, \boldsymbol{\beta}_0)$ part may be beneficial if it significantly reduces residual error (hence, making a better estimation of $g_d(d, x, \boldsymbol{\beta}_d)$) at the cost of estimating a small number of parameters. In general, the model selection rules apply here, where we treat the $g_d(d, x, \boldsymbol{\beta}_d)$ part as essential and the $g_0(x, \boldsymbol{\beta}_0)$ part as for adjustment.

9.6.2 Direct learning of individualized dose rules

The separation of parts $g_d(.)$ and $g_0(.)$ suggests that we can directly learn the dose adjustment rule without modeling the full DR relationship [Chen et al., 2016; Qian, 2016]. Suppose that the dosing rule for a subject with $\mathbf{X}_i$ can be written as $D_i = h(\mathbf{X}_i, \gamma)$ where $h(x, \gamma)$ is a known function with unknown parameters $\boldsymbol{\gamma}$. The idea is to learn the optimal dosing rule by estimating $\boldsymbol{\gamma}$ which leads to the optimal response, e.g., with the maximum mean response $g(d) = E(Y_i(d))$ as in the previous example.

The major practical difficulty is that there is often no subject with the dose given by the dosing rule $h(\mathbf{X}_i, \gamma)$, hence we cannot evaluate the response of dose $h(\mathbf{X}_i, \gamma)$ for any $\boldsymbol{\gamma}$. An approach is to borrow those with dose D_i close to it. In this way, the reward can be estimated by, e.g.,

$$\hat{V}(\gamma) = \sum_{i=1}^{n} Y_i K((D_i - h(\mathbf{X}_i, \gamma))/\sigma)/\sigma \tag{9.23}$$

where $K(.)$ is a kernel function, for example the normal density function, with SD σ. σ should sufficiently small so that the Y_is used to evaluate the $h(\mathbf{X}_i, \gamma)$ rule should have D_is close to it, but a too small one makes the estimate unstable.

The following simple example shows how the approach is used. Let $Y_i = (a_0 + \mathbf{a}_x\mathbf{X}_i)D_i - bD_i^2 + \epsilon_i$ be the response and we would like to find the dose to maximum the response. If we have fitted the model, then the optimal dose for a patient with $\mathbf{x}$ is $d^* = (a_0 + \mathbf{a}_x\mathbf{x})/2b$. Suppose we would like to find a simple dosing rule $D_i = \gamma_0 + \boldsymbol{\gamma}_x^T\mathbf{X}_i$, a simple approach is to estimate γ_0 and γ_x that maximize $\hat{V}(\boldsymbol{\gamma})$ with a proper σ. This approach seems unnecessarily complex than the direct DR model fitting one. However, it does not rely on the DR model, since, in the example above, it can find an optimal linear dosing rule for any DR model that leads to it. For example, any DR model $Y_i = (a_0 + a_x\mathbf{X}_i)D_i - bD_i^2 + g(\mathbf{X}_i) + \epsilon_i$ with bounded $g(X)$ leads to the same optimal dosing rule. We can also evaluate the reward directly for dosing rule changes, while in the DR approach we only evaluate its goodness of fit, and which may or may not have a significant impact on optimal dose, e.g., when a part of model does not fit well but this part is far from the optimal dose. This direct learning approach can take advantage of ML methods to fit a wide range of models for $\hat{V}(\boldsymbol{\gamma})$ with a penalty term to avoid overfitting.

To illustrate the implementation of the above approach, we consider a hypothetical example with a DR model $Y_i = (\beta_{d0} + \boldsymbol{\beta}_{dx}\mathbf{X}_i)D_i - \beta_d D_i^2 + \boldsymbol{\beta}_x\mathbf{X}_i + \epsilon_i$. The sample size and parameter values are given in the code below. The first scenario is that the data are generated from the optimal dosing rule adding a random error: $D_i = \gamma_0 + \gamma_x\mathbf{X}_i + V_i$, $V_i \sim N(0, 0.2^2)$. With 1000 sample size, we can find a rule that is reasonably close to the optimal one $(\gamma_0 = 0.25, \gamma_x = 0.5)$.

```
nsub=1000
sig=0.2
X1=runif(nsub)
X2=runif(nsub)
#dose=runif(nsub) # totally randomized
#Optimal dosing with random variation
dose=0.25+0.5*X1+0.2*rnorm(nsub)
yi=X2+(0.5+X1)*dose-dose^2+0.2*rnorm(nsub)

Vfun=function(beta) -mean(yi*(exp(-(dose-beta[1]-beta[2]*X1)^2/sig^2))/sig)

optim(fn=Vfun, par=c(0.1,0.3))
$par
[1] 0.2668524 0.4668580
```

The sample size needed heavily depends on the dosing rule used for the data generation. With a totally randomized dosing rule, we need a very large sample size to achieve similar precision. The reason is simple; only data with dose close to the optimal dosing line are useful. We also need to reduce σ (denoted as sig in the code).

```
nsub=500000 #500 times as above
sig=0.1 # Reduced
X1=runif(nsub)
X2=runif(nsub)
dose=runif(nsub)
```

```
#dose=0.25+0.5*X1+0.2*rnorm(nsub)
yi=X2+(0.5+X1)*dose-dose^2+0.2*rnorm(nsub)

Vfun=function(beta) -mean(yi*(exp(-(dose-beta[1]-beta[2]*X1)^2/sig^2))/sig)

optim(fn=Vfun, par=c(0.1,0.3))
$par
[1] 0.2797138 0.4749891
```

In the above, we have assumed that in the data, D_i is not confounded, i.e., its allocation does not depend on factors that may also affect Y_i. Hence, the utility of the approaches is limited to, e.g., trials with randomized doses. If the data are observed, but confounding factors are included in $\mathbf{X}_i$, the approaches detailed in Chapter 8 can be used to adjust. For example, let $e_i(d) = p(d|\mathbf{X}_i)$ be the GPS and $p(d)$ be the marginal density of D_i, using the stable weight $p(D_i)/e_i(D_i)$, the IPW adjusted reward can be written as

$$\hat{V}(\gamma) = \sum_{j=1}^{n}\sum_{i=1}^{n} \frac{Y_i p(D_i)}{e_i(D_i)} K((D_i - h(X_j, \gamma))/\sigma)/\sigma \tag{9.24}$$

In general, the direct learning approach is less efficient in terms of the sample size needed, which may not be a problem in ML using large databases. Therefore, indirect approaches that use a full DR model may still be the preferred approach in settings with small sample sizes.

9.7 Individualized dose adjustment and meta learning

Individualized dose adjustment is important for patients with narrow therapeutic windows and strong heterogeneity. A typical example is the adjustment of the dose of warfarin, an anticoagulant, which is crucial for its clinical use. Dose adjustment may be based on simple thresholds, e.g., levels of outcomes such as a biomarker that indicate the need for dose change, or a stochastic search can be used to find the dose to achieve clinical goals without the need for DR modeling. Using DR modeling allows for more efficient adjustment, especially with a few repeated measures per subject.

9.7.1 Mixed DR model-based approaches

The model-based dosing rules can be extended to using mixed models which are frequently used to fit longitudinal data. A rather general mixed DR model can be written as

$$Y_{ij} = g(D_{ij}, \boldsymbol{\beta}_i) + \epsilon_{ij} \tag{9.25}$$

where $\boldsymbol{\beta}_i = \mathbf{X}_i^T \boldsymbol{\beta} + U_i$ are random coefficients. The dose to achieve the response level y^0 for subject s with X_s is the solution to

$$g(d_s^*, X_s^T \hat{\boldsymbol{\beta}} + \hat{U}_s) = y^0 \tag{9.26}$$

where $\hat{U}_s$ is predicted based on current data from subject s. For applications, the major problem is to predict U_s when there is no or very limited data from subject s. An approach is to start from $U_s = 0$ when there are no data from subject s, then predict it with a mixed model procedure when the data are observed (Chapter 3). Along this line, Zhu and Qu [2016] used a linear mixed model

$$\log Y_{ij} = X_{ij}^T \boldsymbol{\beta}_x + Z_{ij} U_i + \beta_d \log D_{ij} + \epsilon_{ij} \tag{9.27}$$

where U_i is a random effect, but β_d is constant. This setting avoids the prediction of the random DR coefficient, hence is more stable. However, a constant β_d may not provide a good approximation if its true value has a considerable variability among subjects.

Individual dose determination using linear mixed models can be traced back to Diaz et al. [2007, 2012]. Assuming a log-linear model for the response Y_{ij} of subject i at time j with dose D_{ij} and covariates $\mathbf{X}_i$:

$$\log(Y_{ij}/D_{ij}) = a_i + \boldsymbol{\beta}_x^T \mathbf{X}_i + \varepsilon_{ij} \tag{9.28}$$

where a_i is a random intercept and ε_{ij} a random error term. The optimal dose was derived that minimizes the probability of $P(L < Y_{ij} < U)$. This approach was examined in the therapeutic drug monitoring scenario, for which the goal can be specified by controlling $P(L < Y_{ij} < U)$, and was shown to perform better than the normal approach.

9.7.2 Response-adapted individual dose adjustment

Often, patient baseline factors are not sufficient to determine the optimal dose for each individual; therefore, adjustment based on patient's response is necessary, especially for highly variable drugs and diseases in need of accurate control of symptoms or biomarkers. The INR control with warfarin is a typical example (Section 1.2.4). More accurate control may be needed for the dosing of anesthetic drugs. The idea of response-based adjustment within the patient is not new and has been used in practice. Often the adjustment is triggered by a clinical threshold; for example, we increase the warfarin dose if the patient's INR is below 2.

This type of approach is known as stochastic search, which can be written as

$$D_{ij+1} = D_{ij} + \rho_j G(\bar{H}^{ij}) \tag{9.29}$$

where $\bar{H}^{ij}$ denotes data of patient i up to jth visit and $G(.)$ is a function measuring the difference between the current response and the target, and ρ_j is a step parameter determining how fast the dose adjustment should be. This method is essentially the same as that in (9.10), but here it is within patients. A basic request for such an adjustment is that $D_{ij} \to D_i^*$ the optimal dose for subject i. However, it is also important to reach D_i^* quickly. For these purposes, a varying ρ_j which tends to 0 when $j \to \infty$ is needed.

This approach can also be viewed as an optimization approach to find d e.g., to maximize $g(d)$. Two common approaches are Gauss-Newton and gradient descent methods, for which we need at least the gradient of $g(d)$, for which the DR model should be fitted. However, many derivative-free approaches can be used as an alternative. Model-based approaches can help with the model-free ones without compromising the latter's robustness. One possibility is to use the model to calculate the gradient with a working model, yet still choose ρ_j to guarantee convergence, as we will show later.

9.7.3 Robust meta learning

The above approach adjusts D_{ij} independently, although population information can improve it. The mixed model provides this information. The risk of using this information is that some patients may be very different from others. Intuitively, we can take an adaptive approach that relies more on the model if the model prediction is similar to the empirical evidence and less if otherwise. This approach can take the form of

$$D_{ij+1} = w_j(D_{ij} + \rho_j G(\bar{H}_{ij})) + (1 - w_j)D_{ij+1}^m \tag{9.30}$$

where D_{ij+1}^m solves $g(d, \mathbf{X}_i^T\hat{\boldsymbol{\beta}} + \hat{U}_i) = y^0$, therefore it is the optimal dose based on population information, and w_j is a function of the difference in the mean response of model prediction and that of the ith patient.

9.8 Dose adjustment with dynamic DR models

In the above sections, we have assumed that the DR relationship is static and that changes due to dose adjustment quickly achieve a steady state. However, in many situations, the DR relationship is dynamic, such as in the warfarin dosing example [Henderson et al., 2010; Avery et al., 2020]. A simple model to describe the dynamic relationship for a typical patient (hence, we drop subscript i) is

$$Y_{j+1} = \beta_y Y_j + \beta_d D_j + \epsilon_{j+1} \tag{9.31}$$

with which the response at time $j + 1$ depends on the previous response and dose. This model can be expanded by including more lagged terms of both response and dose.

With dynamic DR relationships, the difficulty of dose adjustment is double. We may not be able to fit the DR model well even if we know the correct model, as data from one patient may be sparse. Even if the model is known, the optimal dose adjustment rule is often difficult to determine and implement in practice and is sensitive to model misspecification. The following are a few approaches that originate from automatic control in combination with ML.

1. Simple adjustment rule without aiming at the exact optimum, e.g., selecting next dose increment proportional to the difference between the current response and the target.
2. Fit the DR model and find (quasi) optimal dose adjustment based on it. This approach is feasible only for some simple (e.g., linear) DR models and specific loss functions as a measure of the accuracy of adjustment.
3. Model agnostic ML approaches such as Q-learning, which may take advantage of DR models
4. Meta learning that makes use of the information from both individual patients and the population as a whole.

In much of this section, we use the warfarin dataset, including simulated data based on the model fitted in Avery et al. [2020] as an example. The reason for using a simulated dataset is that the original data is **observed** with dose adjustment to achieve the target INR range. This adjustment leads to confounding bias, as we will discuss in the next section. In addition, there is a lack of data to test adjustment rules that are different from those used in clinical practice from which the data are generated. Therefore, we use simulated data to evaluate new dosing rules. Recall that the goal is to adjust the INR, which has a normal range of around 0.8 to 1.1, to the range of 2 to 3 for patients with high risk of thromboembolism.

9.8.1 Linear dose adjustment rule

We take the simulated warfarin data as an example and use the midpoint of (2, 3) $y^0 = 2.5$ as the target for adjustment for illustration. A simple dose adjustment rule

$$D_{j+1} = D_j + \rho(y^0 - Y_j) \tag{9.32}$$

is to increase the dose by ρ times of the difference between the response to dose D_j and the target: $y^0 - Y_j$. Here, ρ plays a similar role as the step size in the stochastic search for a static DR relationship. But an important difference is that here the optimal dose is not a fixed level. This simple rule only has ρ as an unknown parameter and is easy to implement. The choice of ρ is a key factor in the performance of this rule. Figure 9.4 shows the trajectories of a simulated patient with different ρs. A very small ρ leads to slow adjustment (top-left panel), while a large one may reach the target quickly but may lead to higher variability in the response later. A very large one ($\rho = 15$) resulted

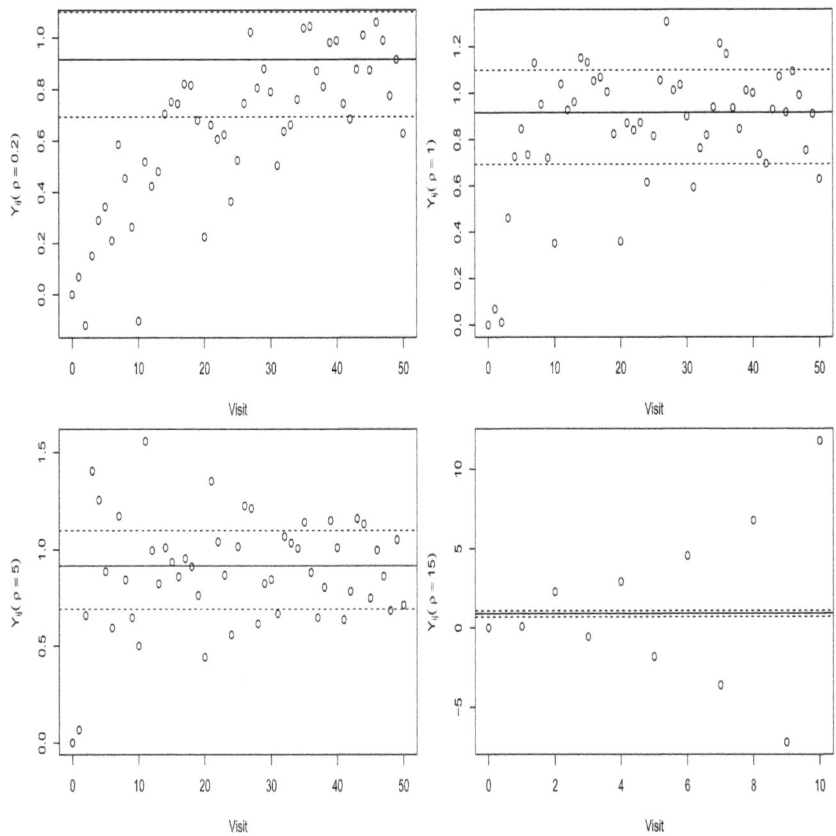

Figure 9.4
Trajectories of log-INR of a simulated patient with different ρ in the linear dose adjustment rule (9.32).

in an unstable adjustment (lower right panel), which will not happen in a real situation, as the linear model is not valid in this dose and INR range, but indicates the potential problem of over-adjustment.

To quantify the impact of the value ρ, we calculate the MSE $E((Y_j - \mu^0)^2)$ over time using 5000 simulation runs for $\rho = 0.2, 1$ and 3 (Figure 9.5). The lowest ρ has the highest MSE at most visits due to slow adjustment, although its MSE becomes the lowest at the end, while $\rho = 1$ leads to a quick initial response and MSE almost as low as that of $\rho = 0.2$. An even faster response can be achieved by $\rho = 3$, but its long-term MSE is higher than the others.

The above results suggest that 1) a constant ρ over time may not be the optimal choice in our situation, since the optimal value at the beginning and long-term maintenance seems different; 2) a varying ρ for different patients may be beneficial, since patients may reach the maintenance status at different

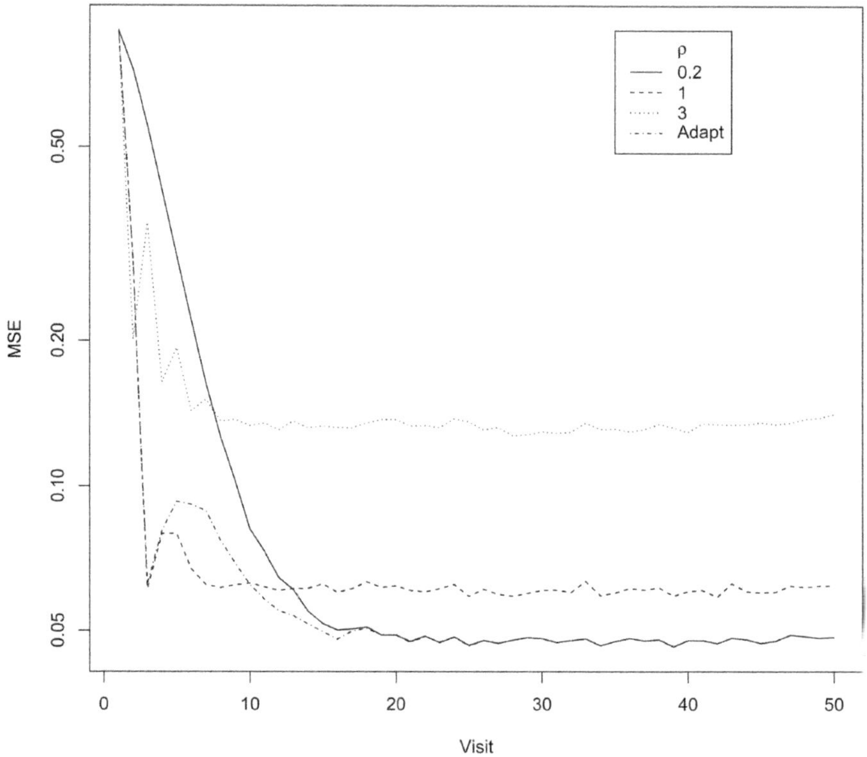

Figure 9.5
Estimated MSE: $E((Y_{ij} - \mu^0)^2)$ with different ρ and the adaptive selection that starts from $\rho = 3$ and switch to $\rho = 1$ at first reach of log(2, 3) range.

times. An adaptive approach is to use a high ρ value at the beginning and switch to a lower value when reaching the log(2, 3) range. Figure 9.5 also shows the MSE curve for adaptive selection that starts from $\rho = 3$ and switches to $\rho = 1$ at the first reach of the log(2, 3) range. We can see its advantage of being a quick responder and a good long-term maintainer. Note that these rules are not derived from the data generation model, and the adaptation is also model-independent. However, the modeling approach can improve its performance if feasible.

9.8.2 Dose adjustment as dynamic programming/automatic control problem

Here we consider dose-adjustment in view of dynamic programming and automatic control [Bertsekas, 2012]. Suppose that we adjust the dose with the dosing rule $d = h(s)$ as a function of current states s, e.g., the previous responses and doses, so that the response is as close to the target y^0 as possible in a period, and we omit randomness and consider only one patient at the moment, that is, a dose D_j in state s_j leads to a new state $s'_{j+1} = g(s_j, D_j)$ at $j + 1$. The goal is to minimize a loss function

$$Q(s_0) = \sum_{j=1}^{J} r_j + h(D_j), \tag{9.33}$$

where r_j is the risk (e.g., the difference between the actual and target states) and $h(d)$ is a cost function to penalize a high dose or a rapid dose change. Here we consider the following quadratic function in the loss function:

$$Q(s_0) = \sum_{j=1}^{J} Y_j^2 + CD_j^2, \tag{9.34}$$

where we assume the target is $y^0 = 0$, s_0 is the initial state, e.g., patients baseline and C is the cost of dose (or dose change if we replace D_j^2 with $(D_j - D_{j-1})^2$), which is often needed for reasonable dosing rules to avoid over-dose or over adjustment.

The optimal dosing rule that minimizes (9.34) generally does not have a closed form; however, the loss (9.34) in combination with a linear model is an exception. For simplicity, we consider a single patient and a simple model

$$Y_{j+1} = \beta_y Y_j + \beta_d D_j + \epsilon_j \tag{9.35}$$

where $\epsilon_j \sim N(0, \sigma_\epsilon^2)$, the target is $y^0 = 0$ and we set $D_J = 0$, since it only affects Y_{J+1} which is outside the scope of (9.34). To find the optimal dose that maximizes (9.34), we can work backwards from step $J - 1$. It is easy to find that the optimal dose is proportional to Y_{J-1}:

$$D_{J-1} = -\frac{\beta_d \beta_y}{C + \beta_d^2} Y_{J-1}. \tag{9.36}$$

Going backwards with induction, we can show that

$$D_{j-1} = -\frac{\beta_d \beta_y P_j}{C + \beta_d^2 P_j} Y_{j-1} \tag{9.37}$$

where $P_j = (\beta_y^2 C P_{j+1})/(C + \beta_d^2 P_{j+1}) + 1$. Therefore, the optimal dose is always proportional to the current response, although the coefficient changes over time.

In the above, we have assumed $D_J = 0$, since J is the stopping time. However, in many situations, there is no such fixed J. A common approach is to assume that $J \to \infty$. In this situation, backward induction does not work anymore. However, the optimal dosing rule is even simpler:

$$D_j = -\frac{\beta_d \beta_y P}{C + \beta_d^2 P} Y_j \tag{9.38}$$

where P is the solution of $P = (\beta_y^2 CP)/(C+\beta_d^2 P)+1$, a special case of a matrix equation known as Riccati Equation [Bertsekas, 2012]. It can be obtained by letting $P = P_j = P_{j+1}$ in $P_j = (\beta_y^2 CP_{j+1})/(C + \beta_d^2 P_{j+1}) + 1$, hence P can be considered P_j in steady state. However, the derivation and conditions for the system to converge, hence P_j has a steady-state, are complex and technical, hence are omitted here. The key fact is that the optimal dose is proportional to Y_j by a constant coefficient in the form of $d_j^* = KY_j$, which we will use in model-agnostic approaches.

However, the optimal d_j^*s depend on unknown parameters, which we may not know before we treat the patient. Can we estimate the coefficients during the dose adjustment (known as online identification in ML)? The optimal dosing rule leads to a model $Y_{j+1} = \beta^* Y_j + \epsilon_j$, hence β_d and β_y cannot be directly identified by the series of Y_j data. In the warfarin example, we have a population of similar patients. Hence, one approach is to use a mixed model to estimate the parameters. This approach will be explored in the meta-learning section.

9.8.3 Dose adjustment and tracking problems

Often, dose adjustment is used to force the response to track a given level y^0, which may not be zero. Suppose that this can be achieved with a steady state dose d^0, it is important for a tracking problem to find such d^0. For a dynamic systems without random term

$$Y_{j+1} = \beta_y Y_j + \beta_d D_j, \tag{9.39}$$

d^0 can be found by replacing Y_j and Y_{j+1} with y^0, and D_j by d_0, assuming d^0 yields a stable system. This leads to

$$d^0 = \frac{(1 - \beta_y)y^0}{\beta_d}. \tag{9.40}$$

We can also consider this problem in another way; since our goal is to track y^0, we can write (9.39) as

$$(Y_{j+1} - y^0) = \beta_y(Y_j - y^0) + \beta_d(D_j - d^0) + \beta_d d^0 - (1 - \beta_y)y_0 \tag{9.41}$$

The constant terms $\beta_d d^0 - (1 - \beta_y)y_0$ is often called a drift, since from time j to $j + 1$, it is added to $(Y_{j+1} - y^0)$. To avoid letting the system drift away, we need to eliminate it, which leads to the same d^0 as in (9.40). Note that the dynamic part of (9.39) is not changed by subtracting y^0 and d^0. Therefore, for tracking system (9.41), the optimal dosing rule to minimize

$$Q(s_0) = \sum_{j=1}^{J} (Y_j - y^0)^2 + C(D_{j-1} - d^0)^2 \tag{9.42}$$

is the same as that for(9.34), with Y_j and D_j replaced by $Y_j - y^0$ and $D_j - d_0$, respectively.

Although we can try to fit the model and use the rules in the previous section, this approach is not robust to model misspecification and misidentification, especially when data are sparse. Much effort has been put into making the tracking rule robust using adaptive control approaches. The next section describes a combination of adaptive control and meta-learning approaches.

9.8.4 Model agnostic meta-learning individual dose adjustment rules

The meta-learning we discuss here is different from that in Section 9.7, since we are learning the control of a dynamic system. However, the setting is similar; suppose that there are n subjects already treated with certain dosing rules and data are obtained. A typical example are the Warfarin dosing data described and used in previous chapters. But we use a simpler model for illustration:

$$Y_{ij+1} = \beta_{yi} Y_{ij} + \beta_{di} D_{ij} + \epsilon_{ij} \tag{9.43}$$

where $\beta_i \equiv (\beta_{yi}, \beta_{di}) = \beta + U_i$ are random coefficients with U_i often assumed to have normal distribution $U_i \sim N(0, \mathbf{\Sigma})$. If we trust the model, the same approach as in Section 9.7 can be used for dynamic models. That is, with a fitted mixed model, we predict $\hat{U}_i$ then $\hat{\boldsymbol{\beta}}_i = \hat{\boldsymbol{\beta}} + \hat{U}_i$. Then, the parameters in, e.g., (9.37) can be replaced by $\hat{\boldsymbol{\beta}}_i$. The prediction can be updated each time when a new pair of Y_{ij+1}, D_j is obtained. The population-level parameters $\boldsymbol{\beta}$ and $\mathbf{\Sigma}$ can also be updated by refitting the model (9.43). Although not named meta-learning, this approach is almost exactly a ML approach based on fully specified models.

Two major problems are 1) the model may be misspecified and 2) the prediction of $\hat{\boldsymbol{\beta}}_i$ may have a high variation when j is very small. An example to show the issue is the following. If patient i is an outlier, then prediction $\hat{\boldsymbol{\beta}}_i$ severely shrinks to $\boldsymbol{\beta}$, although he needs a dosing rule very different from the population-average rule. A model agnostic approach is to use the model, but with the ability to adapt for individuals.

Since dosing rules such as (9.38) depend on multiple parameters, although we can predict all parameters in the model and plug them into the dosing rule, a simper approach is to learn the dosing rule directly. Taking the tracking system as an example, let $\Delta Y_{ij} = Y_{ij} - y^0$ and $\Delta D_{ij} = D_{ij} - d_i^0$, the model (9.43) can be written as

$$\Delta Y_{ij+1} = \beta_{yi} \Delta Y_{ij} + \beta_{di} \Delta D_{ij} + \epsilon_{ij}. \tag{9.44}$$

Note that to make $\Delta Y_{ij} \rightarrow 0$, we need to find the correct d_i^0 for each subject. Although it can be estimated by inserting the individual prediction of β_{yi}, β_{di} into (9.40), this method is highly model dependent. A model-agnostic approach is to start with the population average d_0 from (9.40), and adjust according to the data of the subject i. Suppose that a population level estimate

d^0 based on the first $i-1$ subjects is available. Then we can set individual $D^0_{i1} = d^0$ and updated it each time j as

$$D^0_{ij+1} \leftarrow D^0_{ij} + \alpha_i \nabla_{D^0_{ij}} Q_i(D^0_{ij}). \tag{9.45}$$

where α_i is the learning rate and $\nabla_x Q(x)$ is the gradient of the loss function $Q(x)$. To show how this works for a specific problem, we take the loss function (9.42), but set $C = 0$ for simplicity; then we have $Q_i(D^0_{ij}) = \sum_{j=0}^{n_i} \Delta Y^2_{ij+1}$. Although we can estimate its gradient based on the individual model (9.44), the learning is not model-agnostic and potentially unstable. A preferred way is to use $\nabla_{D^0_{ij}} Q_i(D^0_{ij}) \approx -\beta_d \Delta Y_{ij}$ in which we borrow β_d from the population model; but if d^0 is approximately correct, we have $E(\beta_d \Delta Y_{ij}) \approx 0$. Therefore, with a correct learning rate α_i, we will have $D^0_{ij} \to D^0_i$ when $n_i \to \infty$.

We may also update d^0 using the same approach. With D^0_i determined, we can use the same approximate update rule

$$d^0 \leftarrow d^0 - \alpha_0 \beta_d (d_0 - D^0_i)/i \tag{9.46}$$

The following algorithm gives details on learning the draft d^0 at both individual and population levels:

Algorithm 3 Model agnostic meta learning of draft term for adaptive proportional dose adjustment.

Require: $y^0, n, n_i, K, \beta_d, \alpha$, initial value d^0
  for Subject $i = 1$ to n **do**
    Set $d^0_i = d^0$
    for Time j=0 to n_i **do**
      $D_{ij} = K\Delta Y_{ij} + d^0_{ij-1}$
      Obtain Y_{ij+1} with dose D_{ij}
      Update

$$D^0_{ij+1} \leftarrow D^0_{ij} - \alpha_i \beta_d \Delta Y_{ij+1} \tag{9.47}$$

    end for
    Update population estimate

$$d^0 \leftarrow d^0 - \alpha_0 \beta_d (d_0 - D^0_i)/i \tag{9.48}$$

  end for

A similar approach can also be applied to update K for each individual sequentially. Again, we can start from a population estimate. The update algorithm is almost the same as that for the draft; the only difference is that the gradient of with respect to K can be approximated by $\nabla_K Q_i(K) \approx \beta_d (D_{ij} - D^0_i)(Y_{ij} - y^0)$. This update can be performed in parallel with that for the draft.

The following code implements the above algorithm on a hypothetical warfarin patient with coefficients quite different from the population average in the warfarin dataset, with learning rates $\alpha = 1, 2$. The initial d_i^0 is the steady state dose based on $\hat{\boldsymbol{\beta}}$: the estimated population average coefficients of the warfarin example. Figure 9.6 shows $E(\Delta Y_{ij})$ and D_{ij}^0 over visits with model-agnostic learning for D_i^0 for a hypothetical subject with $\boldsymbol{\beta}_i = 2 \times \hat{\boldsymbol{\beta}}$.

```
 y0=log(2.5)
nrep=30
simu=function(rho=1,nsub=1000,af=1,ni=nrep,adp=0,y0=log(2.5)){
  thetai=2*theta
  d0=targ*(1-sum(theta[1:2]))/sum(thetai[3:4])
  Q=NULL
  for (sub in 1:nsub){
    #    Dj=c(y0,y0,0,0)
    y0=0
    Dj=c(y0,y0,d0,d0)
    K=rho
    d0j=d0
    yv=NULL
    for (j in 1:ni){
      yj1=sum(thetai*Dj)+rnorm(1,sd=sige)
      yv=c(yv,yj1)
      #K=K-af*(theta[3]*(yj1-targ)*yj1)#+K*yj1^2)
      dj=-K*(yj1-targ)+d0j
      d0j=d0j-af*beta[3]*(yj1-targ)
#      d0j=d0j-af*beta[3]*(mean(yv)-targ)
      Dj=c(yj1,Dj[1],dj,Dj[3])
    #  Q=rbind(Q,c(sub,j,(yj1-targ)^2))
            Q=rbind(Q,c(sub,j,(yj1-targ),d0j))
    }
  }
  Q
}

Qout=NULL
Pout=simu(af=2)
jk=lm(Pout[,3]~as.factor(Pout[,2])-1)
Qout=cbind(Qout,as.vector(jk$coefficients))
jkk=lm(Pout[,4]~as.factor(Pout[,2])-1)
Qout=cbind(Qout,as.vector(jkk$coefficients))

Pout=simu(af=1)
jk=lm(Pout[,3]~as.factor(Pout[,2])-1)
Qout=cbind(Qout,as.vector(jk$coefficients))
jkk=lm(Pout[,4]~as.factor(Pout[,2])-1)
Qout=cbind(Qout,as.vector(jkk$coefficients))

plot(1:nrep,Qout[,1],type="l", ylab="Bias/d0",ylim=range(Qout),
```

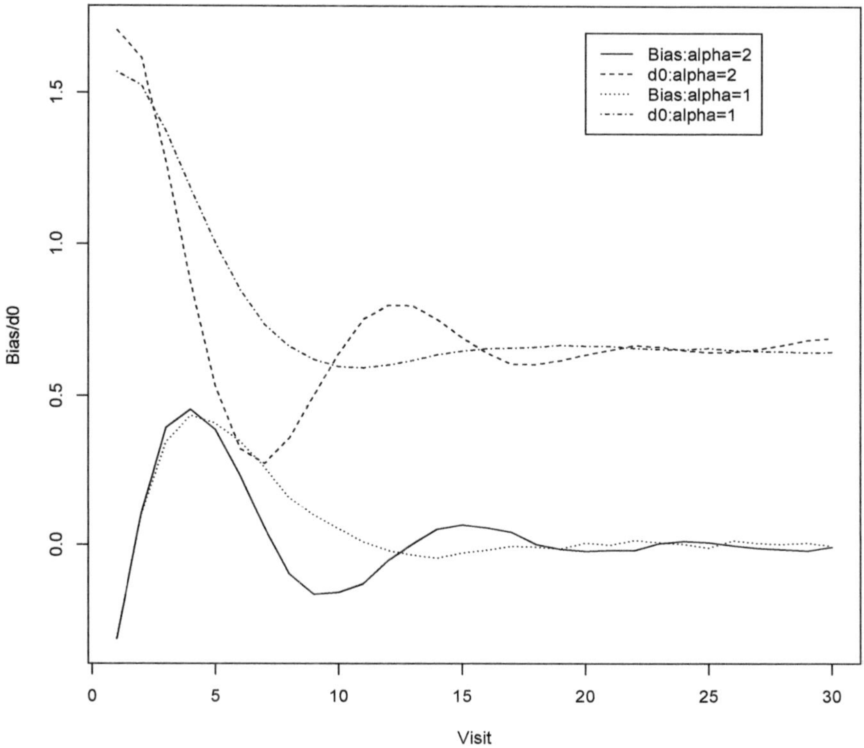

Figure 9.6
Estimated mean Bias $E(\Delta Y_{ij})$ and D_{ij}^0 by 1,000 simulated subjects over visits with model-agnostic learning for D_i^0 for a hypothetical subject with $\boldsymbol{\beta}_i = 2 \times \hat{\boldsymbol{\beta}}$: $\hat{\boldsymbol{\beta}}$ are the estimated coefficients from the Warfarin example.

```
                          xlab="Visit")
lines(1:nrep,Qout[,2],lty=2)
lines(1:nrep,Qout[,3],lty=3)
lines(1:nrep,Qout[,4],lty=4)
legend(x=20,y=1.7,legend=c("Bias:alpha=2","d0:alpha=2",
       "Bias:alpha=1", "d0:alpha=1"),lty=1:4)
```

9.8.5 The drug titration paradox

We have discussed in length dose allocation rules that aim to treat patients at the optimal dose and also to fit DER models. However, often dose changes are simply driven by the control of patient response above or below a given level or in a range. The warfarin dosing rule is one of these situations. A more extreme situation is anesthetic dose titration in which the dose level is finely adjusted to achieve the desired response level. However, analysis of these data often finds an apparent null or even negative DR relationship, known as the drug titration paradox. Some work showed with simulation that a correct DR relationship could be identified by a mixed model for repeated measures within patients [Kristensen and Agersø, 2022], while some others showed with real data that it is generally not identifiable if the paradox occurs at the patient level [Schnider et al., 2022]. In the following, we consider the paradox in the statistical aspect and show criteria for model identification. Although the criteria may not be verifiable, they can help to understand the mechanism and its connection to the causal relationship of DR.

We first consider how to identify the DR model without intercept for a single subject:

$$Y_{j+1} = \beta_d D_j + \epsilon_{j+1}, j = 1, ..., J, \tag{9.49}$$

where ϵ_js are independent error term, and we drop subscript i for simplicity. The goal is to adjust Y_j to the target level $y^0 = 0$ with an adjustment rule $D_j = h(Y_j)$, e.g., $D_j = -KY_j$ where K is a constant. Since ϵ_{j+1} is independent of D_j, we can ignore the impact on adjustment $D_j = h(Y_j)$ without creating a confounding problem and simply regress Y_{j+1} on D_j. Note that due to ϵ_j, D_j varies around dose $d = 0$. This may not be a desirable clinical property; therefore, we may stop the adjustment if $|Y_j| < \delta$, a tolerance threshold. However, unless δ is very small, there will be a portion of patients with their $|Y_j| < \delta$ and their D_j remaining unchanged. This becomes a problem, as the undesirable property of dose perturbation is necessary to identify the model. Recall that we estimate β_d by

$$\hat{\beta}_d = \frac{J^{-1}\sum_{j=1}^{J} Y_j D_j}{J^{-1}\sum_{j=1}^{J} D_j^2}. \tag{9.50}$$

For $\hat{\beta}_d$ to be consistent, we need $J^{-1}\sum_{j=1}^{J} D_j^2 \to \sigma_d^2 > 0$ when $J \to \infty$; but this fails when D_j does not maintain sufficient variability with increasing j. The problem is not only theoretical, because with a small sample size within the patient, this can happen in a large portion of patients even δ is not large.

If for all subjects, we can estimate their DR parameter $\hat{\beta}_{di}$, the marginal parameter can be estimated by

$$\hat{\beta}_d^m = n^{-1}\sum_{i=1}^{n} \hat{\beta}_{di}. \tag{9.51}$$

Without consistent estimates $\hat{\beta}_{di}$, the marginal parameter is difficult to estimate, as the use of dose and response data between subjects is subject to confounding bias due to titration and there is no reliable way to adjust for it.

We may also consider the response to dose adjustment with a dynamic model

$$Y_{j+1} = \beta_y Y_j + \beta_d D_j + \epsilon_j \tag{9.52}$$

where we do not include the intercept since it represents a shift over time, and we assume that it is eliminated by dose adjustment. With the same adjustment rule $D_j = h(Y_j)$, we cannot fit a DR model with D_j only, since D_j is no longer independent of Y_j. It is necessary to fit model (9.52) to adjust for Y_j. This is a conditional rather than a marginal DR model, but is more useful than the latter for dose adjustment purposes. Using the fit model (9.52) we can obtain consistent estimates $\hat{\beta}_y, \hat{\beta}_d$ under the same condition $J^{-1}\sum_{j=1}^{J} D_j^2 \to \sigma_d^2 > 0$ on dose adjustment rules. To justify this claim, we note that the DAG in this case is $Y_j \to D_j \to Y_{j+1}$, hence the adjustment for Y_j blocks the back door of D_j to Y_{j+1} (Chapter 8).

We may also introduce the correlation between Y_js in the model (9.49) assuming $\text{cov}(\epsilon_j, \epsilon_{j+1}) > 0$. The consequence is that ϵ_{j+1} and D_j are correlated via Y_j. However, with DAG $Y_j \to D_j \to Y_{j+1}$, conditioning on Y_j can also block the back door of D_j to Y_{j+1}, suggesting fitting a conditional model for $E(Y_{ij+1}|Y_{ij}, D_{ij})$, which results in the form of (9.52). In addition, conditional on Y_j is sufficient even when $\text{cov}(\epsilon_j, \epsilon_{j+k}) > 0$ for $k > 1$, as long as Y_{ij+1} depends only on D_{ij}. If Y_{ij+1} also depends on D_{ij-1}, we also need to condition on Y_{ij-1}.

The warfarin dose escalation data is a typical example of dose titration, since the goal is to adjust the dose to make each patient's INR within 2 and 3. Fitting a linear mixed model for log-INR

$$Y_{ij+1} = \beta_{0i} + \beta_{yi} Y_{ij} + \beta_{di} D_{ij} + \epsilon_{ij} \tag{9.53}$$

with random effects on all βs, we have

```
    Linear mixed model fit by REML ['lmerMod']
Formula: loginr ~ prey + predose + (1 + prey + predose | id)
   Data: cdata
REML criterion at convergence: 762.6149
Random effects:
 Groups   Name        Std.Dev. Corr
 id       (Intercept) 0.16151
          prey        0.12681  -0.78
          predose     0.02338  -0.47 -0.11
 Residual             0.24751
Number of obs: 9345, groups:  id, 152
Fixed Effects:
(Intercept)         prey      predose
    0.47378      0.29763      0.04372
```

showing almost no DR relationship conditional on Y_{ij}. Note that the model fitted by Avery et al. [2020] does not have an intercept and the coefficient for D_{ij} (predose in the code) is much higher. When the dose and response are in steady state, the intercept should be close to zero. But this may not be true at the population level. The following regressions of dose and log-INR on log-visit show strong trend of increase for both. Therefore, the shift over time is confounded with dose.

```
> summary(lm(dose~log(visit),data=Adata))

             Estimate Std. Error t value Pr(>|t|)
log(visit)   0.06222    0.01131    5.50 3.89e-08 ***
> summary(lm(loginr~log(visit),data=Adata))

             Estimate Std. Error t value Pr(>|t|)
log(visit)  0.030194   0.002565   11.77   <2e-16 ***
```

However, fitting models with the intercept to individual data (two subjects who did not change their dose are excluded) does not show problems. Conditional on either Y_{ij} or Y_{ij}, Y_{ij-1}, the DR coefficient β_{di} has mean 0.24, similar to that in Avery et al. [2020]. In addition, the intercepts have a mean close to zero.

```
 > Indfit=NULL
> for (id in ind){
+   sdata=warf[warf$id==id,]
+   nrep=dim(sdata)[1]
+   prey=c(NA,sdata$loginr[1:(nrep-1)])
+   predose=c(NA,sdata$dose[1:(nrep-1)])
+   prey2=c(NA,NA,sdata$loginr[1:(nrep-2)])
+   coef=lm(sdata$loginr~predose+prey)$coef
+ #  coef=lm(sdata$loginr~predose+prey+prey2)$coef
+   Indfit=rbind(Indfit,coef)
+ }
>
> apply(Indfit,2,mean,na.rm=T)
 (Intercept)      predose         prey
-0.009819386  0.238019447  0.280397127
# Using line coef=lm(sdata$loginr~predose+prey+prey2)$coef
> apply(Indfit,2,mean,na.rm=T)
(Intercept)     predose         prey       prey2
-0.03204094  0.23924335  0.25072173  0.04047869

> apply(Indfit,2,mean,na.rm=T)
 (Intercept)      predose         prey
-0.009819386  0.238019447  0.280397127
```

In summary, the identification of the warfarin DR relationship benefits from multiple repeated measures within patients and the dose adjustment occurred in most patients. In addition, linear models are easy to identify with limited repeated measures and dose adjustments. However, confounding may occur if we borrow population level information using a mixed model.

9.8.6 Off-policy learning and generalized propensity score

We start from a concrete example with a model

$$Y_{j+1} = \beta_y Y_j + \beta_d D_j + \epsilon_{j+1}, j = 1, ..., J. \tag{9.54}$$

Suppose that data Y_j, D_j are observed under a dosing rule $D_j = -KY_j + e_j$, where $e_j \sim N(0, \sigma_e^2)$, aiming to adjust Y_j close to zero. Its key feature is the random term that makes it a random dosing rule by adding e_j. Since the goal is to adjust Y_j to the target level $y^0 = 0$, we can calculate $\hat{V} = J^{-1}\sum_{j=1}^{J} Y_j^2$ as a performance measure of this dosing rule. Can we use the same data to evaluate the dosing rule of $D_j^* = -KY_j + e_j^*$, where $e_j^* \sim N(0, 0.5\sigma_e^2)$? This is a problem of off-policy learning, as is called in the ML literature, because the data are not generated by the policy (i.e., the dosing rule here) we want to evaluate.

In general settings, suppose that at each j we have a risk function $r_j(d)$ and we would like to evaluate

$$V^{\pi^*} = E_{\pi^*}(r_{j+1}(D_j)) \tag{9.55}$$

where $\pi^*(y)$ is a dosing rule depending on current state y and $r_j(d)$ is the risk when dose d is given. However, we only have data with a dosing rule $\pi(y) \neq \pi^*(y)$. Can we use the data from $\pi(y)$ to evaluate V^{π^*}? Here, we find that causal inference plays a key role in learning the DR relationship in this situation. Under some conditions, we can re-weight $r_j(\pi(Y_j))$ to estimate V^{π^*} based on generalized propensity score (GPS).

$$\hat{V}^{\pi^*} = J^{-1}\sum_{j=0}^{J-1} \frac{p^*(D_j|Y_j)}{p(D_j|Y_j)} r_{j+1} \tag{9.56}$$

where $p^*(d|y)$ and $p(d|y)$ are density functions (GPS) of dose d according to the dosing rules $\pi^*(y)$ and $\pi(y)$, respectively, and here the previous response is the confounder. To check, we write

$$\begin{aligned} E(\hat{V}^{\pi^*}) &= \int_d r_{j+1}(D_j)\frac{p^*(D_j|Y_j)}{p(D_j|Y_j)} p(D_j|Y_j)d(D_j) \\ &= \int_d r_{j+1}(D_j)p^*(D_j|Y_j)d(D_j) \\ &= E_{\pi^*}(r_{j+1}(D_j)) = V^{\pi^*} \end{aligned} \tag{9.57}$$

The following codes illustrate how to use this approach; suppose that we have data from dosing rule with $\sigma_d = 1$ and we would like to estimate V^{π^*} for $D_j^* = -KY_j + e_j$, where $e_j^* \sim N(0, 0.5^2)$.

```
nseq=30000
betay=0.5
K=0.3
```

```
sigd=1
yj=rnorm(1)
Mdata=NULL
for (j in 1:nseq){
 dj=-K*yj+sigd*rnorm(1)
 wei=dnorm(dj,-K*yj, 0.5)/dnorm(dj,-K*yj, sigd)
 yj=betay*yj+dj+rnorm(1)
 Mdata=rbind(Mdata, c(yj,dj,wei))
}
wi=Mdata[,3]/mean(Mdata[,3])
mean(Mdata[,1]^2*wi)
[1] 1.339974
```

while the true value is 1.31, therefore, the adjusted one is only slightly different from the true one. However, without adjustment, the value of $\hat{V}^{\pi}$ is 2.06, hence the adjustment is important for a valid evaluation.

It seemed that we have forgot a simple way to do this: fit the DR model (9.54), then we can evaluate any dosing rule with the prediction of the fitted model. Although the DR model approach is more efficient than the reweighting one (see the discussion in Chapter 8), it is sensitive to model misspecification. In fact, we can take advantage of both DR model and reweighing to form a doubly robust estimator. This estimator takes form

$$\hat{V}_{dr}^{\pi^*} = J^{-1}\sum_{j=0}^{J-1}\frac{p^*(D_j|Y_j)}{p(D_j|Y_j)}[r_{j+1} - m(Y_j,\pi^*(Y_j))] + m(Y_j,\pi^*(Y_j))] \tag{9.58}$$

where $m(Y_j, \pi(Y_i)) = E(r_j|Y_j, \pi(Y_j))$ is the expected reward or loss with the dosing rule $\pi(Y_j)$. $\hat{V}_{dr}^{\pi^*}$ is valid as long as $m(Y_j, D_j)$ or the GPS is correct.

We take the above example and model (9.54) to show how to estimate $m(Y_j, \pi(Y_i))$. Our goal is to estimate $E(Y_{j+1}^2|Y_j, D_j)$ with dosing rule $D_j = -KY_j + e_j$ which can be written as

$$\begin{aligned}
E(Y_{j+1}^2|Y_j, D_j) &= E[(\beta_y Y_j + \beta_d D_j + \epsilon_{j+1})^2] \\
&= E[((\beta_y - K\beta_d)Y_j + \beta_d e_j)^2] + \sigma_\epsilon^2 \\
&= (\beta_y - K\beta_d)^2 Y_j^2 + \beta_d^2\sigma_e^2 + \sigma_\epsilon^2
\end{aligned} \tag{9.59}$$

In the previous example, the dosing rule of interest only has a random component change to $e_j^* \sim N(0, 0.5\sigma_e^2)$, hence the second term changes to $0.25\beta_d^2\sigma_e^2$. After fitting the DR model, all the parameters needed in the formula (9.59) can be estimated and taken to (9.58) to estimate $\hat{V}_{dr}^{\pi^*}$.

An alternative is to use an empirical model to directly model Y_{j+1}^2 as a function of Y_j and D_j and their functions. It might be a better option if there is no established DR model, or $m(Y_j, \pi(Y_i))$ is very complex according to the DR model.

9.9 Retrospective model fitting after dose escalation

Based on a dose-finding or dose-escalation trial, although often the empirical optimal dose (i.e., the dose most frequently selected with the dose-allocation rule) is selected for further development, a retrospective model fitting provides additional information. Effort has been made for phase I dose-escalation trials. See, e.g., O'Quigley [2005].

9.9.1 Model identification issues

The conflict between treating in-trial patients with the optimal dose and determining the optimal dose for further development is also reflected in the model identification. Iasonos et al. [2016] shows such situations in the context of phase I dose-escalation trials. Without going into technical details, we recall that to identify model parameters, their information matrix should not be degenerate (that is, with rank less than p, the number of parameters in the model). However, even in the ideal situation of $\hat{d}_n^* \to d^*$, the information matrix will converge to a degenerate matrix of rank 1 for any model with the number of parameters $p > 1$.

9.9.2 Dose-allocation rules with wrong DER models

It is well known that a simple wrong DR model can be more useful in finding the optimal dose among a set of $\bar{D}$ than a correct but complex model, if it is not too wrong, as demonstrated by a comparison between a one-parameter power model and a two-parameter logistic model [Shen and O'Quigley, 1996; Iasonos et al., 2016]. Here by a not too wrong model we mean that the model does not take a suboptimal dose among $\bar{D}$ as the optimal one when it is used for prediction. However, the fitted wrong model depends not only on the model itself, but also on the distribution of the dose already allocated. Suppose that the optimal dose is to maximize $g(d)$: $d^* = \text{argmax}_{d \in \bar{D}} g(d)$. Recall that when fitting a wrong model $g(d, \boldsymbol{\beta})$ with LS, $\hat{\boldsymbol{\beta}} \to \boldsymbol{\beta}^*$:

$$\boldsymbol{\beta}^* = \text{argmin}_{\boldsymbol{\beta}} E_D(g(D_i) - g(D_i, \boldsymbol{\beta}))^2, \tag{9.60}$$

where $g(d)$ is the true DR curve, and the expectation is taking over the distribution $F_D(d)$ for D_i, which depends on the dose allocation algorithm; hence we denote it by $\boldsymbol{\beta}^*(F_D)$. A sufficient condition for not too wrong $g(d, \boldsymbol{\beta})$ is $d^* = \text{argmax}_{d \in \bar{D}} g(d, \boldsymbol{\beta}^*(F_D))$ for any F_D for which $\boldsymbol{\beta}^*$ exists. However, this seems a too strong assumption.

Due to the identification issue for any model with $p > 1$, the consistency of CRM benefits from its very simple model with $p = 1$ [Shen and O'Quigley, 1996]. However, fitting the CRM model retrospectively may also have problems if the data are not generated by CRM-guided escalation. Interestingly, a reweighting procedure can solve this problem [O'Quigley, 2005]. The weights are proportional to the dose distribution of the CRM rule, as if the trial were run by CRM. They are calculated by simulation using the CRM rule based on marginal frequencies. Their approach does not work for the cases with $p > 1$, due to the singular information matrix problem when $d^* \to d^0$.

This reweighting approach has a close connection to the off-policy evaluation in machine learning we have used above. Recall that we have used GPS for dose in (9.56) to evaluate the expected reward. The same can be used on an EE. Let $S_i(\boldsymbol{\beta}, D_i) \equiv W(D_i)(Y_i - g(D_i, \boldsymbol{\beta}))$, where $W(D_i)$ is a weight matrix and D_i is generated by the escalation rule π. As $g(D_i, \boldsymbol{\beta})$ is misspecified, when $n \to \infty$

$$S(\boldsymbol{\beta}) = n^{-1} \sum_{i=1}^{n} S_i(\boldsymbol{\beta}, D_i) \to E_{\pi}(W(D_i)(g(D_i) - g(D_i, \boldsymbol{\beta}))) \tag{9.61}$$

Suppose that for the dosing rule π^*, the solution $\boldsymbol{\beta}^*$ to $E_{\pi^*}(W(D_i)(g(D_i) - g(D_i, \boldsymbol{\beta}))) = 0$ can identify d^*, that is, $\text{argmax}_{d \in \bar{D}} g(d, \boldsymbol{\beta}^*) = \text{argmax}_{d \in \bar{D}} g(d)$. To use data from the dosing rule π to identify d^*, we weight $S_i(\boldsymbol{\beta}, D_i)$ by the ratio of GPS of π^* to that of π:

$$S_w(\boldsymbol{\beta}) = n^{-1} \sum_{i=0}^{n} \frac{p^*(D_i|H^{i-1})}{p(D_i|H^{i-1})} S_i(\boldsymbol{\beta}, D_i) \tag{9.62}$$

Then we have

$$\begin{aligned} E(S_w(\boldsymbol{\beta})) =& n^{-1} \sum_{i=0}^{n} E[\frac{p^*(D_i|H^{i-1})}{p(D_i|H^{i-1})} S_i(\boldsymbol{\beta}, D_i)] \\ &= n^{-1} \sum_{i=0}^{n} E(p^*(D_i|H^{i-1}) S_i(\boldsymbol{\beta}, D_i)|H^{i-1}) \\ &= E_{\pi^*}(W(D_i)(g(D_i) - g(D_i, \boldsymbol{\beta}))) \end{aligned} \tag{9.63}$$

Therefore, the solution to $S_w(\boldsymbol{\beta}) = 0$ can identify the optimal dose if it can be identified by π^*.

Several technical conditions are needed for the reweighting approach to work. First, we need assumptions for (9.61) to hold. These assumptions include properties of $g(d)$ and $g(d, \boldsymbol{\beta})$. Second, and more important, the dosing rule π should cover the dose range of π^*. This is satisfied if π is ergodic, that is, all dose levels are used when $n \to \infty$. In practice, it is too restricting, for example, in a phase I dose-escalation trial, since the high end of dose levels are often never reached. In fact, we only need $p(d|H^{i-1}) > 0$ if $p^*(d|H^{i-1}) > 0$ for any d. Also, π^* need not be a sequential rule, and $p^*(D_i|H^{i-1})$ can be a constant.

Relevant to this topic is the work on regression models as a functional of the independent variable (here the dose) [Buja et al., 2019], in which a model is called well-specified if it is identified when the distribution of dependent variables has acceptable changes. Reweighting was proposed as a diagnosis of well-specification. Reweighting may also be considered as a way to emphasize the key part of the DR curve. For example, if the best and second best doses are in one neighborhood region, placing heavy weights in this region may distinguish the two doses when the model is severely misspecified globally but well behaved locally.

9.10 Dosing for normal range control and Quantile DR relationship

Often, chronic use of a drug is to keep the measure of biomarkers within the normal range. Such situations are plentiful, but we will take Warfarin dosing [Henderson et al., 2010; Avery et al., 2020] as an example to show how quantile DR relationship can be used to evaluate dosing rules at the population level.

9.10.1 Modeling probability of outside of normal range

Until now, we have mostly focused on the DER relationships of the means. Suppose that the model is

$$Y_{ij} = \gamma D_i + \boldsymbol{\beta}^T \mathbf{X}_i + \epsilon_{ij} \tag{9.64}$$

where ϵ_{ij} is random error. Our goal is for a given $\mathbf{X}$ to determine d to maximum $P(d, \mathbf{X}) \equiv P(L < \gamma d + \boldsymbol{\beta}^T \mathbf{X} + \epsilon_{ij} < U)$. If ϵ_{ij} are not symmetrically distributed, the optimal dose d^* is to make $\gamma d^* + \boldsymbol{\beta}^T \mathbf{X}$ at the midpoint of (L, U) However, to deal with arbitrary ϵ_{ij}, a better solution is to model directly $P(L < Y_{ij} < U)$. For this purpose, it is better to use two separate models

$$\begin{aligned} P(L < Y_{ij} | D_i, \mathbf{X}_i) &= g^{-1}(\gamma_L D_i + \boldsymbol{\beta}_L^T \mathbf{X}_i) \\ P(U < Y_{ij} | D_i, \mathbf{X}_i) &= g^{-1}(\gamma_U D_i + \boldsymbol{\beta}_U^T \mathbf{X}_i) \end{aligned}$$

where $g(.)$ is a link function, e.g., $g^{-1}(l) = \text{expit}(l)$ and the two probabilities have their own coefficients. The models can be fitted to indicators for $L < Y_{ij}$ and $U < Y_{ij}$. Then, one can calculate $P(d, \mathbf{X}) = P(L < Y_{ij} | d, \mathbf{X}) - P(U < Y_{ij} | d, \mathbf{X})$. This approach is less efficient, in particular, when the occurrence of outside (L, U) is rare and the sample size is small. However, it provides the flexibility to allow different DR relationships for the lower and upper bounds. The optimal dose does not have an explicit form, but is easy to find with a numerical optimizer such as R-function optim. Although the optimal dose depends on $\mathbf{X}$, the relationship is simply linear. Suppose that d_1 is the dose with control of $P(L < Y_{ij} | d_1, \mathbf{X}_1)$, then the dose d_2 for a subject with $\mathbf{X}_2$

satisfies, e.g.,

$$\gamma_l d_1 + \boldsymbol{\beta}_L \mathbf{X}_1 = \gamma_l d_2 + \boldsymbol{\beta}_L \mathbf{X}_2 \tag{9.65}$$

The same equation also holds for the upper bound.

When there is a subject effect in a mixed effect model with $\boldsymbol{\beta}_i = \boldsymbol{\beta} + \mathbf{u}_i$

$$Y_{ij} = \gamma D_i + \boldsymbol{\beta}_i^T \mathbf{X}_i + \epsilon_{ij} \tag{9.66}$$

although $P(d, \mathbf{X})$ can still be estimated, we need to estimate the distribution of $\mathbf{u}_i + \epsilon_{ij}$. In popPK approach, often normal distributions are assumed for the two components, hence the estimation depends on both distributions. The two-model approach can also be extended to include random coefficients, although it may suffer further when Y_{ij} outside of the range rarely occurs.

9.10.2 Quantile dose-response relationship

Quantile dose-response (QDR) relationship shows how quantiles change with dose. This relationship may be marginal for a population or conditional on certain baselines or covariates. This type of relationship is often estimated in popPKPD modeling approaches using model prediction based on specific distributions of random components in it. Here we use the warfarin example to show the quantile DR model approach as an alternative.

The standard approach to assess the distribution of response given dose d is quantile regression (QR). First we ignore repeated measures and consider the quantile $Q_Y(\tau|D, X) \equiv \min(y : P(Y \leq y|D, X) = \tau)$ we may use a similar linear model

$$Q_Y(\tau|D_i, \mathbf{X}_i) = \beta_d(\tau) D_i + \boldsymbol{\beta}_x(\tau)^T \mathbf{X}_i \tag{9.67}$$

for a $0 \leq \tau \leq 1$. The coefficients also depend on τ. Although this model has some similarity to the model fitting the $L < Y_i$ indicator, here the fixed is τ, rather than the normal range. Fitting the model with a number of τ values covering (0,1), particularly at the two ends, one can have a good understanding of the distribution of Y for given dose and $\mathbf{X}$. Estimating quantiles is not new. In popPK analysis, often the 10/90% quantiles of exposure for the whole population together with the DE curve based on a mixed model are presented. However, the difference is that the QR approach directly models the quantiles-dose relationship, while the mixed model models the mean dose relationship. The QR approach allows different models for different values of τ, therefore, it is more flexible.

The QR models can be extended to include fixed and/or random effects in a similar way as how we construct mixed-effect models. However, fitting such a QR model is much more difficult. For example, even a QR model with only a fixed subject-level intercept and dose cannot be fitted to the warfarin dataset for $\tau = 0.1, 0.9$. In this case, a common remedy is to fit them as random effects. However, for warfarin data, using random effects means borrowing between subjects leading to substantial loss of DR effects, just as happened when fitting the mixed model to the same data.

However, we can explore other approaches to estimate the quantile DR relationship. Recall the model for log-INR can be written as

$$Y_{ij+1} = \beta_{yi} Y_{ij} + \beta_{di} D_{ij} + \epsilon_{ij} \tag{9.68}$$

with random coefficients β_{yi} and β_{di}. The popPKPD approach commonly predicts β_{yi} and β_{di} using a mixed model with the assumption of a normal distribution for them. For the warfarin dataset, they can be estimated by fitting the individual model for all patients, except two who had no dose change. Given estimates $\hat{\beta}_{yi}$ and $\hat{\beta}_{di}$, if we ignore ϵ_{ij} at the moment, we can estimate

$$P(Y_{ij+1}|Y_{ij} = y, D_{ij} = d) \tag{9.69}$$

by the quantile of $\hat{\beta}_{yi} y + \hat{\beta}_{di} d$. To take ϵ_{ij} into account, we can add pooled residuals $\hat{\epsilon}_{ij}$ and estimate the quantiles of $\hat{\beta}_{yi} y + \hat{\beta}_{di} d + \hat{\epsilon}_{ij}$. Figure 9.7 shows the two types of quantiles for $Y_{ij} = 0.5$. For comparison, we also include raw data with $0.25 < Y_{ij} < 0.75$. The quantile curves show reasonable coverage of the raw data, although we cannot check their correctness due to the lack of data with exactly $Y_{ij} = 0.5$. Although the above approach estimates QDR relationships, it depends on fitted mean models at subject level. However, the approach does not need the specification of distributions for random effects and ϵ_{ij}.

9.11 Comments and bibliographic notes

This chapter covers a wide range of topics related to dose allocation, adjustment in clinical trials, and clinical practice. We take the view of learning the DR relationship in parallel with dose allocation, which may be considered as a ML approach. We follow the idea of ML, especially reinforcement learning [Sutton et al., 1998], but avoid technical details in ML, in particular, the asymptotic properties such as the asymptotic learning rate. They are less relevant in the context of clinical trials due to the small sample size. Contextual bandits are a powerful tool for dose-finding. We focus on practical aspects such as model selection, robustness, and implementation. The use of DER modeling for this purpose is rather new, but it seems a promising approach to be developed.

A special topic is dose adjustment with dynamic models, in particular model-agnostic approaches. This area overlaps with reinforcement learning and automatic control [Bertsekas, 2012]. The approach presented has a root in adaptive control, with technical complexity far beyond the scope of the book. We take a rather intuitive approach, e.g., for deriving the adaptive rule of tracking the target response level without relying on control theory.

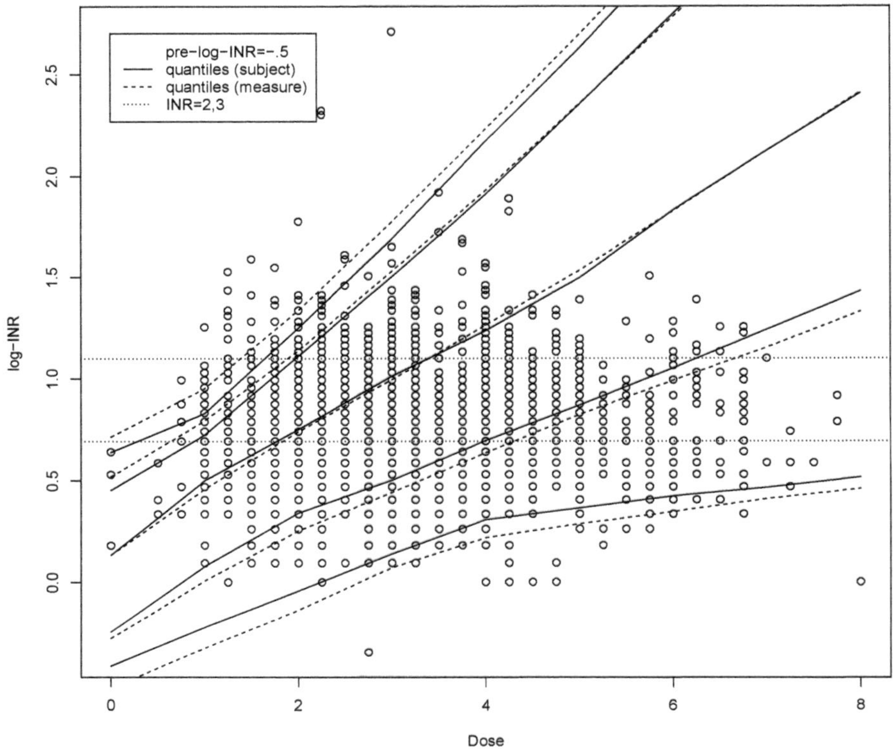

Figure 9.7
Predicted (0.1,0.2,0.5,0.8,0.9) quantiles of warfarin by dose when $Y_{ij} = 0.5$. The dots are observed data with $0.25 < Y_{ij} < 0.75$.

Another new topic covered here has a close connection to causal inference is the off-policy learning in ML when the data are from a dosing rule in practice, and we would like to use the data to evaluate another dosing rule. We avoid the technical difficulty of the ML part, but make use of the causal inference methods in Chapter 8.

The paradox of dose titration is important in both practical and theoretical aspects. We show its connection to model identification and causal inference of mixed models, with the warfarin example.

10

Appendices

The appendices include two types of materials: some basic statistical concepts, methods and theoretical results that are well known, but listed here for convenience. The others are rather non-standard and not covered in common textbooks, in particular, model fitting and inference with misspecified models in both frequentist and Bayesian aspects.

10.1 Basic statistical concepts

This section describes some basic statistical concepts, starting in the frequentist framework and extending to the Bayesian framework later. A statistical analysis starts with data and the model from which the data are generated. In a parametric model, there are unknown but fixed parameters to be estimated. Often not all parameters are of our interest, as some are nuisance parameters. We use the data to estimate the parameters, hence parameter estimates are functions of the data. A function of data independent of any unknown parameter is called a *statistic*. A parameter estimate $\hat{\theta}$ that on average equals the true value, i.e., $E(\hat{\theta}) = \theta$ is an *unbiased* estimate.

We often consider the asymptotic properties of parameter estimates when the sample size is large. An important property called consistency refers to that the estimate based on n samples $\hat{\boldsymbol{\theta}}_n$ tends to the true $\boldsymbol{\theta}$ when $n \to \infty$, namely the difference between them can be made as small as we like by increasing the sample size n, and this is denoted by $\hat{\boldsymbol{\theta}}_n \to \boldsymbol{\theta}$. Note that a consistent estimate may not be unbiased with a finite sample size. An estimate is called asymptotic unbiased if the bias diminishes to zero with increasing sample sizes. An unbiased estimate may not be consistent since its variation may not necessarily diminish with n, but counterexamples are rare in common situations in this book.

Even when two random series a_n and b_n all converge to 0, one may converge faster than the other. The rate is often measured by a power function n^r. We denote $a_n = O(n^{-1})$ if $a_n/n \to C$: a constant and $a_n = o(n^{-1})$ if $a_n/n \to 0$. There are also different types of convergence, although differences between them are often not a practical concern and we do not always distinguish

DOI: 10.1201/9781003457008-10

them. The common ones we use here are convergence in probability, denoted as $a_n \to_p a$, if

$$\lim_{n\to\infty} P(|a_n - a| > \epsilon) = 0 \tag{10.1}$$

for any $\epsilon > 0$, and convergency in distribution (also known as weakly convergency), denoted by $a_n \to_d a$, if the distribution function of a_n converges to that of a: $F_{a_n}(.) \to F_a(.)$. Formally, it is called a cumulative distribution function, but we drop "cumulative" in the whole book for simplicity. A shorthand for a_n asymptotically following, e.g., a normal distribution is $a_n \sim_d N(\mu, \sigma^2)$. Convergence in probability implies convergence in distribution, while the reverse is not true. However, a weak convergence to a constant is equivalent to the convergence in probability to the same constant.

An important aspect of statistical inference is hypothesis testing. For example, in a model

$$Y_i = \beta_0 + \beta_c C_i + \varepsilon_i \tag{10.2}$$

one key question to answer is if $\beta_c = 0$, i.e., C_i has no effect on Y_i. The question can be answered by testing a hypothesis $H_0 : \beta_c = 0$ based on the observed data. Put in another way, we examine whether there is sufficient evidence in the observed data against H_0, if so we reject H_0. When testing a hypothesis, we may commit two types of mistakes; one is to reject a H_0 that is true, while the other is not to reject a H_0 which is not true. The two types of mistakes are called type I and type II errors, respectively. The amount of evidence against H_0 is measured by the probability of making a Type I error, a common level in practice is 5%. Therefore, hypothesis testing is a task to control the type I error at a given level and to maximize the probability of not committing a type II error. The probability is known as the power of the test. However, the power depends on the true value of the parameter. Obviously, the power of a test is higher when $\beta_c = 1$ than when $\beta_c = 0.5$. A test controlling its type I error at α (referred to as a test of level α) is a uniformly most powerful test (UMP) if its power is not less than other tests of the same level α for any β. As an example, suppose that $Y_1, ..., Y_n$ follows normal distribution with $Y_i \sim N(\mu, \sigma^2)$ and we would like to test $H_0 : \mu \leq 0$, then test statistic

$$t = \bar{y}./\sqrt{S^2/n}, \tag{10.3}$$

where S^2 is the sample variance, follows the t-distribution with $n-1$ degree of freedom. Therefore, if we would like to test $H_0 : \mu \leq 0$ at 5% level, we reject it when $t > t_{n-1,0.95}$, where $t_{n-1,0.95}$ is the 95% percentile of the t distribution. However, to test $H_0 : \beta = 0$ we need a two-sided 5% test which reject H_0 when $t > t_{n-1,0.975}$ or $t < t_{n-1,0.025}$. A common test we use based on $\hat{\theta}_n \sim N(0, se^2)$, where se is the standard error of $\hat{\theta}$. Then $\hat{\theta}/se \sim N(0, 1)$.

Relevant to both parameter estimation and hypothesis testing is the confidence interval (CI) of a parameter. A $1-\alpha$ CI is a function of the data, which covers the true β value with probability $1-\alpha$, if the experiment and the test are repeated infinitely. $1-\alpha$ CI is not unique, but often the one with the shortest length is unique. Under some situations, the CI may consist of more than one intervals. But we will not consider these situations here.

10.2 Model fitting and parameter estimation

Given a DER model, the key step is to fit the model to the data by estimating the parameters. There are many methods in the frequentist toolbox.

10.2.1 Maximum likelihood estimation

The maximum likelihood estimate (MLE) approach is the most commonly used approach in statistics to fit statistical model, estimate model parameter and test hypotheses regarding model parameters. Suppose we observe response and dose data $Y_1, ..., Y_n, D_1, ..., D_n$ but the dose data are considered as fixed. The likelihood function for $Y_1, ..., Y_n$ is defined as the product of individual density functions:

$$L(\boldsymbol{\theta}) = \prod_{i=1}^{n} f(Y_i, \boldsymbol{\theta}) \tag{10.4}$$

where $\boldsymbol{\theta}$ contains all parameters. For example, when $Y_i \sim N(\mu, \sigma^2)$ with mean μ and variance σ^2, the likelihood function is

$$L(\mu, \sigma^2) = \prod_{i=1}^{n} \frac{1}{\sqrt{2\pi\sigma^2}} \exp(-\frac{(Y_i - \beta^T D_i)^2}{2\sigma^2}). \tag{10.5}$$

The MLE for μ and σ^2 are the values that maximize $L(\mu, \sigma^2)$. To this end, it is often to use the log-likelihood function

$$l(\mu, \sigma^2) = logL(\mu, \sigma^2) = -n\log(\sigma^2)/2 - \sum_{i=1}^{n} \frac{(Y_i - \beta^T D_i)^2}{2\sigma^2} + C \tag{10.6}$$

Taking derivatives with respect to β we obtain the score functions

$$\begin{aligned} \frac{\partial l(\beta, \sigma^2)}{\partial \beta} &\propto \sum_{i=1}^{n} D_i^T (Y_i - \beta^T D_i) \\ \frac{\partial l(\beta, \sigma^2)}{\partial \sigma^2} &= -n\sigma^{-2}/2 + \sum_{i=1}^{n} (Y_i - \beta^T D_i)^2 \sigma^{-4}/2. \end{aligned} \tag{10.7}$$

The MLE of β and σ^2 can be obtained by solving the score equations formed by setting the score functions equal to zero leading to $\hat{\beta} = (\sum_{i=1}^{n} D_i^T D_i)^{-1} \sum_{i=1}^{n} Y_i D_i$ and $\hat{\sigma}^2 = n^{-1} \sum_{i=1}^{n} (Y_i - \hat{\beta}^T D_i)^2$.

In general, write the log-likelihood function for $\mathbf{Y}$ as $l(\boldsymbol{\theta})$, its derivatives with respect to $\boldsymbol{\theta}$:

$$S(\boldsymbol{\theta}) \equiv \frac{\partial l(\boldsymbol{\theta})}{\partial \boldsymbol{\theta}} \tag{10.8}$$

is called score function and the MLE $\hat{\boldsymbol{\theta}}$ is the solution to score equations $S(\boldsymbol{\theta}) = 0$.

Under some technical conditions that we skip here, MLE $\hat{\boldsymbol{\theta}}$ is consistent, that is, $\hat{\boldsymbol{\theta}} \to \boldsymbol{\theta}$. A key condition for the consistency of $\hat{\boldsymbol{\theta}}$ is $E(S(\boldsymbol{\theta})) = 0$, which is satisfied by the score function. This condition plays a central role in generalized estimating equation (GEE) in the next section. Also, under some technical conditions the MLE follows asymptotic normal distributions

$$\sqrt{n}(\hat{\boldsymbol{\theta}} - \boldsymbol{\theta}) \sim N(0, nI^{-1}(\boldsymbol{\theta})) \tag{10.9}$$

where

$$I(\boldsymbol{\theta}) = E(\frac{\partial^2 l(\mathbf{Y}, \boldsymbol{\theta})}{\partial \boldsymbol{\theta} \partial \boldsymbol{\theta}^\top}) \tag{10.10}$$

is the Fisher's information matrix. We can also write $\hat{\boldsymbol{\theta}} \sim N(\boldsymbol{\theta}, I^{-1}(\boldsymbol{\theta}))$. However, (10.9) contains more information, as it shows that $\hat{\boldsymbol{\theta}}$ has a convergence rate $\sqrt{n}$.

For several models, the score function has a simple form

$$S(\boldsymbol{\theta}) = \sum_{i=1}^{n} \mathbf{X}_i^T W_i (Y_i - \mu_i(\eta_i)) \tag{10.11}$$

with $E(Y_i) = \mu_i(\eta_i)$, $\eta_i = \mathbf{X}_i^T \boldsymbol{\theta}$ and W_i are weights. The models include $Y_i = \mathbf{X}_i^T \boldsymbol{\theta} + \varepsilon_i$ assuming normality for Y_i. Less obviously, they also include the Poisson model $Y_i \sim Poisson(\mu_i(\eta_i))$ with log link $\eta_i = \log(E(Y_i))$ and logistic model $Y_i \sim Bin(\mu_i(\eta_i))$ with logit link $\eta_i = \text{logit}(E(Y_i))$. For these two models the score function has a general form

$$S(\boldsymbol{\theta}) = \sum_{i=1}^{n} \mathbf{X}_i^T \frac{\partial \mu_i(\eta_i)}{\partial \eta_i} \text{var}(Y_i)^{-1} (Y_i - \mu_i(\eta_i)) \tag{10.12}$$

but with the link functions above $\partial \mu_i(\eta_i)/\partial \eta_i = \text{var}(Y_i)$. Even in the general form 10.12, a weighted LS algorithm can be used to estimate $\boldsymbol{\theta}$, which is more stable than a general-purpose maximization algorithm.

10.2.2 Profile likelihood

The profile likelihood approach [Murphy and Van der Vaart, 2000] is a useful tool in exposure-response modeling, since it may provide an easy alternative to deal with technical difficulties when an additional parameter is added to a model and convergence cannot be achieved.

Suppose a model contains parameters $\boldsymbol{\beta}$ and λ and one is interested in inference for λ. The profile likelihood method fits the model fixing λ at different values. Specifically, suppose that $L(\boldsymbol{\beta}, \lambda)$ is the likelihood function, for each given λ value, the profile likelihood finds the MLE for $\boldsymbol{\beta}$ and calculates

$$L^*(\lambda) = \max_{\boldsymbol{\beta}} L(\boldsymbol{\beta}, \lambda) \tag{10.13}$$

Profile likelihood is useful when fixing λ, $\boldsymbol{\beta}$ is easy to estimate. In the case of the QT model, for fixed $\Delta(=\lambda)$, it is a linear mixed model and can be easily fitted. $L^*(\lambda)$ may be treated as an approximation to the marginal likelihood function for λ. Again, since the profile likelihood is derived from the full likelihood function, REML should not be used when fitting the model for profile likelihood approach. Plotting $L^*(\lambda)$ around its peak is a good way to assess the impact of λ in the model. We can also calculate an approximate CI by finding the intercepts of the curve and a horizontal line of corresponding significance level. Note that the approximation may be poor if λ and $\boldsymbol{\beta}$ have a strong association (in terms of orthogonality between them measured by the relative size of $\partial^2 \log(L(\boldsymbol{\beta}, \lambda))/\partial\boldsymbol{\beta}\partial\lambda$). Adjustment can be applied to improve this approach [Murphy and Van der Vaart, 2000].

10.2.3 Generalized estimating equation

Recall that the score function for several models has the general form (10.12). This leads to the ideal of quasi-likelihood that first specifies the score function as (10.12) assuming that it comes from a "qausi" likelihood function, hence the MLE of the quasi-likelihood is the solution to the score equation (10.12). For example, in Chapter 2 we have introduced over-dispersion models with negative- and beta-binomial distributions. It is in principle less efficient than the MLE, but often the efficiency loss is very small.

In fact, (10.12) does not need to have a distribution model behind it. For a wide range of situations, equations not derived from likelihood functions may also be used in the same way as the score equations. The quasi-likelihood approach was further developed into generalized estimation equations (GEE). A set of GEEs are equations

$$\mathbf{S}(\boldsymbol{\theta}) = 0 \tag{10.14}$$

based on the model and observed data, e.g., as (10.12). A GEE estimate $\hat{\boldsymbol{\theta}}_{GEE}$ is the solution to the equations. For common GEEs $\hat{\boldsymbol{\theta}}_{GEE}$ can be obtained from software such as SAS proc GENMOD and R function glm(.), both allow the user to specify the mean, link and variance functions. Some software for Poisson or logistic regressions in fact allows Y_i to be non-integer. Although a warning may be given, e.g., by R function glm(.), the estimate and SE are correct.

Under some technical conditions, $\hat{\boldsymbol{\theta}}_{GEE}$ is consistent. A key condition for this is that, let $\boldsymbol{\theta}_0$ be the true values,

$$E(S(\boldsymbol{\theta})) = 0 \tag{10.15}$$

for $\boldsymbol{\theta} = \theta_0$ and $E(S(\boldsymbol{\theta})) \neq 0$ for any $\boldsymbol{\theta} \neq \boldsymbol{\theta}_0$. Therefore, this equation identifies the model parameters. Furthermore, expanding the GEE around its estimate $\hat{\boldsymbol{\theta}}$

$$0 = \mathbf{S}(\hat{\boldsymbol{\theta}}) + \frac{\partial \mathbf{S}(\hat{\boldsymbol{\theta}})}{\partial \boldsymbol{\theta}}(\boldsymbol{\theta} - \hat{\boldsymbol{\theta}}) + o(\boldsymbol{\theta} - \hat{\boldsymbol{\theta}}), \tag{10.16}$$

where $o(a)$ is a higher order term of a, we can derive

$$\sqrt{n}(\hat{\boldsymbol{\theta}} - \boldsymbol{\theta}) \sim N(0, n\mathbf{F}^{-1}\text{var}(\mathbf{S}(\boldsymbol{\theta}))\mathbf{F}^{-1}) \tag{10.17}$$

with $\mathbf{F} = E(\partial \mathbf{S}(\hat{\boldsymbol{\theta}})/\partial \boldsymbol{\theta})$. $\mathbf{F}^{-1}\text{var}(\mathbf{S}(\boldsymbol{\theta}))\mathbf{F}^{-1}$ is known as the sandwich variance estimate. When $\mathbf{S}(\boldsymbol{\theta})$ has the form

$$S(\boldsymbol{\theta}) = \sum_{i=1}^{n} \frac{\partial \mu_i(\boldsymbol{\theta})}{\partial \boldsymbol{\theta}} \mathbf{W}_i(\mathbf{Y}_i - \boldsymbol{\mu}_i(\boldsymbol{\theta}))/n \tag{10.18}$$

we can derive

$$\mathbf{F} = \sum_{i=1}^{n} \frac{\partial \mu_i(\boldsymbol{\theta})}{\partial \boldsymbol{\theta}} \mathbf{W} \frac{\partial \mu_i(\boldsymbol{\theta})}{\partial \boldsymbol{\theta}}^T \tag{10.19}$$

and

$$\text{var}(\mathbf{S}(\boldsymbol{\theta})) = \frac{\partial \mu_i(\boldsymbol{\theta})}{\partial \boldsymbol{\theta}} \mathbf{W}\text{var}(\mathbf{R}_i)\mathbf{W} \frac{\partial \mu_i(\boldsymbol{\theta})}{\partial \boldsymbol{\theta}}^T . \tag{10.20}$$

where $\mathbf{R}_i = \mathbf{Y}_i - \boldsymbol{\mu}_i(\boldsymbol{\theta})$. In practice, we can replace $\text{var}(\mathbf{R}_i)$ by its empirical estimate. The sandwich estimate is valid as long as the mean model for $\mathbf{Y}_i$ is correctly specified. In summary, although the GEE estimator may be less efficient, it is more robust than MLE.

10.3 Model misspecification

Here we consider how a model behaves when it is misspecified (i.e., different from the true model that generates the data). As a simple example, suppose that the data are generated from a quadratic curve $Y_i = a + bX_i^2 + \varepsilon_i$ but a linear model $Y_i = a + bX_i + \varepsilon_i$ is fitted to the data. Intuitively, the linear model would act as the best linear approximation to the quadratic curve. In fact, if the data are generated from model $Y_i = g_0(X_i) + \varepsilon_i$ but are fitted by a (misspecified) model $Y_i = g(X_i, \boldsymbol{\beta}) + \varepsilon_i$ with X_i taking finite values $X_1, ..., X_K$ with sampling proportions $w_1, ..., w_K$, then the LS estimate $\hat{\boldsymbol{\beta}}_{LS} \to \boldsymbol{\beta}^*$ and

$$\boldsymbol{\beta}^* = \text{argmin}_\theta \sum_{k=1}^{K} w_k (g_0(X_i) - g(X_i, \boldsymbol{\beta}))^2 \tag{10.21}$$

[White, 1981]. Furthermore, asymptotically, $\sqrt{n}(\hat{\boldsymbol{\beta}}_{LS} - \boldsymbol{\beta}^*) \sim_d N(\boldsymbol{\beta}^*, \mathbf{V}^*)$, where $\mathbf{V}^*$ has a sandwich form such as (10.20), as the variance of the GEE estimate. In practice, we can replace unknown parameters in $\mathbf{V}^*$ with their estimate to obtain $\hat{\mathbf{V}}^*$, since $\hat{\mathbf{V}}^* \to \mathbf{V}^*$ almost surely, under some conditions [White, 1981, 1982] This property shows a very important fact that the limit of the parameter estimate for a misspecified model depends not only on the two models but also on the distribution of X_i.

For MLE with a misspecified likelihood function, a classical work is White [1982], who showed that MLE makes the misspecified likelihood function the best approximation to the true one. Let $f_0(Y_i|\mathbf{X}_i)$ be the true density of Y_i and $f(Y_i|\mathbf{X}_i, \boldsymbol{\beta})$ be the misspecified density, all conditional on $\mathbf{X}_i$ and $\mathbf{X}_i \sim F_x(x)$. Then $\hat{\boldsymbol{\beta}}_{MLE} \to \boldsymbol{\beta}^*$ and

$$\boldsymbol{\beta}^* = \text{argmin}_\beta \int_{\mathbf{X}_i} E_Y(log(f_0(Y_i|\mathbf{X}_i)) - f(Y_i|\mathbf{X}_i, \boldsymbol{\beta}))dF_x(\mathbf{X}_i) \qquad (10.22)$$

where $E_Y(log(f_0(Y_i|\mathbf{X}_i)) - f(Y_i|\mathbf{X}_i, \boldsymbol{\beta}))$ is the Kullback-Leibler divergence and the expectation is taken over $f_0(Y_i|\mathbf{X}_i)$. Under some technical conditions, the asymptotic normality of $\hat{\boldsymbol{\beta}}_{MLE}$ also holds, hence $\sqrt{n}(\hat{\boldsymbol{\beta}}_{MLE} - \boldsymbol{\beta}^*) \sim_d N(0^*, \mathbf{V}^*)$. The results apply to a wide range of estimators that maximizes/minimizes a function such as the squared loss function, known as M-estimators. Since often maximizing a function is equivalent to solving the equations by setting its derivatives to zero, the M-estimators are equivalent to some EE/GEE estimators, which is also known as Z-estimators.

Some "less harmful" misspecifications are those on the variability of the response. For example, fitting a Poisson model to a beta-binomial model can be considered as using a wrong model, although the key coefficients β are estimated correctly. However, its SEs are underestimated without adjustment, as $\text{var}(Y_i|\mathbf{X}_i)$ is misspecified. In fact, the sandwich variance estimate adjusts it implicitly as it uses an empirical variance estimate rather than that based on the Poisson distribution. The overdispersion models, which have an overdispersion parameter, can be considered as an explicit adjustment. Estimation of this parameter can be considered as a *calibration* for variance. But the GEE approach together with the sandwich variance estimate automatically takes it into account.

10.4 Approximate and generalized Bayesian analyses and model misspecification

Here we give a very brief review of recent developments in this very active research area. We have shown that $\sqrt{n}(\hat{\theta} - \theta^*) \sim_d N(0, \boldsymbol{\Sigma})$ for frequentist approaches ranging from MLE to GEE with correct and misspecified models (in which case θ^* is not the true value θ, but the values that make the misspecified model the best approximation to the true one). The goal is to develop similar theoretical results and methods in the Bayesian framework. In fact, with properly specified priors and the correct model, we have the posterior distribution of θ that satisfies $\sqrt{n}(\theta - \hat{\theta}) \sim_d N(0, \mathbf{\Sigma}_b)$, where $\hat{\theta}$ is the MLE. The result looks like a mirror image of $\sqrt{n}(\hat{\theta} - \theta) \sim_d N(0, \mathbf{\Sigma})$, since here $\hat{\theta}$ is observed and θ is a random variable in Bayesian framework. Similar results hold when a wrong model (no θ value makes it the true data generation model) is used in Bayesian analysis [Kleijn and Van der Vaart, 2012]. In this case, we have $\sqrt{n}(\theta - \hat{\theta}^*) \sim_d N(0, \mathbf{\Sigma}_b)$, where θ^* is the value θ that minimizes the Kullback-Leibler divergence of the misspecified model from the true model.

Let $l(Z_i|\theta)$ be the log-density of Z_i, an approach to take misspecified models into account is to add a parameter η in the (generalized) Bayes posterior distribution

$$\pi(\theta|Z^n) \propto \exp(-\eta \sum_{i=1}^{n} l(Z_i|\theta))\pi_0(\theta) \tag{10.23}$$

to control the contribution of the data $Z^n = (Z_1, ..., Z_i)$. To see how η is determined, consider a toy example with $Z_i \sim N(\mu, \sigma^2)$, but we use a misspecified model with fixed $\sigma^2 = 1$. Therefore, the variance of the generalized Bayesian posterior for μ would be $(\eta n)^{-1}$, while the sandwich variance estimate is $\hat{\sigma}^2/n$, where $\hat{\sigma}^2$ is the sample variance of Z_i. An approach to determine η is to match the variances, so we have $\hat{\eta} = \hat{\sigma}^{-2}$, which makes (10.23) approximately the same as the Bayesian posterior with a correct model. When there are multiple parameters, this approach can be adapted by matching the Fisher information number [Lyddon et al., 2019], but in this general situation, calibration with η may not be able to fully correct model misspecification.

For some problems such as constructing a credible interval $C_\alpha^\eta(Z^n)$ based on (10.23) conditional on the data Z^n, η can be determined by matching it with the frequentist coverage

$$c_\alpha(\eta) = P(\theta \in C_\alpha^\eta(Z^n)). \tag{10.24}$$

Although it is unknown, we can estimate it by bootstrapping the data:

$$\hat{c}_\alpha(\eta) = B^{-1} \sum_{b=1}^{B} I(\hat{\theta}_n \in C_\alpha^\eta(Z_b^n)). \tag{10.25}$$

where Z_b^n is the bth set of bootstrapped data. With this estimate, we can search for $\hat{\eta}$ so that $\hat{c}_\alpha(\hat{\eta}) \approx 1 - \alpha$.

The asymptotic properties in the scenarios of the misspecified model suggest that we may replace the log-likelihood function $l(Z_i|\theta)$ with a quasi-likelihood or even a general loss function [Lyddon et al., 2019] that has no connection to a likelihood but captures the difference between the observed and model-predicted responses. With a general loss function, (10.23) is known as the Gibbs posterior, and its calibration by η is the key in its use [Martin and Syring, 2022]. Its asymptotic properties can be borrowed directly since we can consider the general loss function as a misspecified log-likelihood function. Therefore, we also have $\sqrt{n}(\theta - \hat{\theta}^*) \sim_d N(0, \Sigma_b)$, and the θ^* value minimizes the Kullback-Leibler divergence of $\exp(-\eta \sum_{i=1}^{n} l(Z_i|\theta))$ from the true likelihood function.

10.5 Bootstrap and Bayesian bootstrap

Bootstrap is a procedure to reconstruct the distribution of data using a set of observations. The idea behind bootstrap is to take samples from the observations so that the samples behave like they were sampled from the population the observation come from. Suppose that we observe c_i and $Y_i, i = 1, ..., n$ and would like to fit a model

$$Y_i = \beta_0 + \beta c_i + \varepsilon_i \tag{10.26}$$

to make statistical inference for β. To use bootstrap, we sample from c_is and Y_is in pairs, with or without replacement to form c_i^b and $Y_i^b, i = 1, ..., n$, then fit them to the model and obtain estimates β^b. After repeating these steps for B times, we can either using samples $\beta^1, ..., \beta^B$ construct confidence intervals or calculating variance for $\hat{\beta}$, the LS estimate for β by fitting the model to the original dataset.

There are other resampling methods in this case. One way is to fit the model to the original data and obtain the residuals $\hat{\varepsilon}_i = Y_i - \hat{\beta}_0 - \hat{\beta} c_i$. The residuals are then sampled with replacement to obtain $\hat{\varepsilon}_i^b, i = 1, ..., n$. Then, bootstrap samples for Y_i can be constructed as $Y_i^b = \hat{\beta}_0 - \hat{\beta} c_i + \hat{\varepsilon}_i^b$. When the model is correct, this approach is more accurate than the direct sampling scheme.

Bayesian bootstrap (BB) is a Bayesian counterpart of bootstrap proposed in Rubin [1981]. Its implementation is very simple and does not require specification of prior and likelihood. Taking the model (10.26) as an example, for Bayesian bootstrap, instead of taking samples from c_i and Y_i, we weight them by a Dirichlet distribution $D(1, 1, ..., 1)$. In practice, the weight can be easily generated from exponentially distributed samples $-\log(U_i)$, where U_i is sampled from the uniform distribution. Then, bootstrap samples $\hat{\beta}^b$ are obtained using weighted LS fitting the original data, but the weights change for each b. There are a number of interpretations for Bayesian bootstrap. It can be considered as weighted likelihood approach [Newton and Raftery, 1994], or an empirical likelihood approach. Since the ordinary bootstrap is equivalent to weighting the pairs with integer (rather than exponential) weights, BB can also be considered as a smoothed version of the ordinary bootstrap. In practice, it may also be easier to implement than ordinary bootstrap.

BB has some interesting asymptotic properties, which make it a powerful tool for approximate Bayesian analysis. We know that the posterior distribution of θ satisfies $\sqrt{n}(\theta - \hat{\theta}) \sim_d N(0, \mathbf{\Sigma}_b)$. Let $\hat{\theta}_b, b = 1, ..., B$ be the BB sample of θ, then we have the posterior distribution of θ that satisfies $\sqrt{n}(\hat{\theta}^b - \hat{\theta}) \sim_d N(0, \mathbf{\Sigma}_b)$, that is, the BB posterior sample has the same asymptotic distribution of the posterior sample. This property holds when the log-likelihood is replaced with a general loss function; in this case, we have $\sqrt{n}(\hat{\theta}^b - \hat{\theta}^*) \sim_d N(0, \mathbf{\Sigma}_b^*)$ and $\mathbf{\Sigma}_b^*$ is the frequentist sandwich variance. Therefore, the BB sample is automatically calibrated for model misspecification. However, as we have seen in the example in Chapter 7, the calibration may need a larger sample size than the direct calibration by matching variances.

10.6 Connection with power prior and borrowing external data for DR modeling

The use of loss function and its general or Gibbs posterior distribution is closely connected to power priors, an approach widely used to borrow external data [Ibrahim et al., 2015] and its application on DR modeling in bridging trials [Ollier et al., 2020]. The power prior has exactly the same for as (10.23), but is proposed in different context. Suppose that $Z^t \equiv (Y_i, ..., Y_n, D_1, ..., D_n)$ are observed data from a trial and $Z^e \equiv (Y_{n+1}, ..., Y_{n+m}, D_{n+1}, ..., D_{n+m})$ are external data. External data may be "wrong" in the sense that they present a different DR relationship from the trial data. The goal is to estimate the DR relationship in the trial as accurately as possible, potentially using external data as well, but also to mitigate the risk of pooling wrong data. Let β be the DR parameters to be estimated, the power prior is defined as

$$\pi(\beta|Z^e) = p(Z^e|\beta)^\eta \pi(\beta). \tag{10.27}$$

The goal is to find the posterior distribution given both datasets:

$$\pi(\beta|Z^t, Z^e) = p(Z^t|\beta)p(Z^e|\beta)^\eta \pi(\beta) \tag{10.28}$$

The power prior (10.27) has the same form as (10.23) and is defined with full distributional specification. However, the log-likelihood can be replaced by a loss function. With some technical conditions, we can show that the asymptotic properties of Gibbs posteriors are valid for $\pi(\beta|Z^t, Z^e)$, given that η is properly calibrated [Wang et al., 2025a].

Intuitively, we would like to calibrate the power prior so that $\eta \approx 1$ if Z^t and Z^e are similar, and $\eta \approx 0$ otherwise. The remaining question is how to measure the difference between Z^t and Z^e. Although the similarity between the distributions of Z^e and Z^t, e.g., measured by the KL divergence, is the ultimate criterion, it is not necessary for an approximate Bayesian approach to DR modeling. Recall that the loss function can be specified as

$$l(\beta) = (Y_i - g(D_i, \beta))^2 \tag{10.29}$$

and the divergency of $g(d, \beta)$ from the true model $g^*(d)$ can be measured by $min_\beta E_D(g^*(D) - g(D,\beta))^2$, but if we consider D_is as fixed, then its empirical version is

$$D(g^*(d), g(d,\beta)) = \min_\beta n^{-1} \sum_{i=1}^{n} (g^*(D_i) - g(D_i, \beta))^2 \tag{10.30}$$

and which is independent of the distribution of Y_i given D_i. Hence, for DR modeling, the similarity should be measured by the difference in the shape of the DR curves.

Sometimes, we may take a more practical approach and focus on β, assuming that the DR model in the trial data is correct. Data Z^e are different from Z^t in two situations: 1) the model is also correct for Z^e but the value of β is different; 2) the model is wrong for Z^e. To focus on the essence, we consider a very simple situation with 1) $n = m$, $\text{var}(Y_i) = \sigma^2$ and assume that the DR model is linear and the data are centered so that we have $Y_i = \beta D_i + \epsilon_i$ in which only β is to be estimated. Using the loss function (10.29) in the Z^e and Z^t parts in (10.28), we have the

$$l(\beta) = \sum_{i=1}^{n} (Y_i - \beta D_i)^2 + \eta \sum_{i=n+1}^{n+m} (Y_i - \beta D_i)^2 \tag{10.31}$$

For fixed η and assuming $\sum_{i=1}^{n} D_i^2 = \sum_{i=n+1}^{n+m} D_i^2$, minimizing it leads to

$$\hat{\beta} = \frac{\hat{\beta}_t + \eta\hat{\beta}_e}{1+\eta} \tag{10.32}$$

where $\hat{\beta}_t$ and $\hat{\beta}_e$ are the estimates of β based on Z^t and Z^e, respectively. We can also calculate its bias as

$$\hat{\delta} = \eta(\hat{\beta}_e - \hat{\beta}_t)/(1+\eta). \tag{10.33}$$

We can also find η that minimizes the MSE of $\hat{\beta}$

$$\hat{\eta} = \frac{\text{var}\hat{\beta}_t}{\hat{\delta}^2 + \text{var}\hat{\beta}_e} \tag{10.34}$$

To make statistical inference, we can take the BB approach that includes the estimation of $\hat{\beta}_e, \hat{\beta}_t$ and $\hat{\eta}$ (and more steps such as adjustment for covariates if needed). Let $\hat{\beta}^b$ be the BB sample of (10.32), we have

$$\sqrt{n}(\hat{\beta}^b - \beta_t) \sim_d N(0, \sigma_b^2) \tag{10.35}$$

where β_t is the true value of β for Z^t. To see why $\hat{\eta}$ can mitigate the impact of bias, we note that the variances in (10.34) converge to zero, but the bias does not. Hence, $\hat{\eta} \to 0$ in probability. Details can be find in, e.g., Wang et al. [2025a].

The above obviously holds when the model is correct for both Z^e and Z^t. It also holds when the model is wrong for Z^e, e.g., the true DR model is nonlinear for Z^e. In general, $\hat{\delta}$ will not be zero when $n \to \infty$, hence we still have $\hat{\eta} \to 0$. Although not easy to happen, it may also be possible that the linear approximation to the nonlinear DR model for Z^e results in a $\hat{\beta}_e$ very similar to $\hat{\beta}_t$. In this case, we still have (10.35) approximately. Interestingly, if we use a BB to fit the model to Z^e data, the variance of $\hat{\beta}_e$ consists of two parts, one part represents the variation we would obtain when a correct model was fitted, and another part represents the variability due to the variability of distribution of D_i. Therefore, σ_b^2 also represents the uncertainty due to model misspecification. However, how to interpret and use it in the context of model misspecification is unclear.

10.7 Dynamic and causal inference models

The dynamic nature of DER relationships for time-varying dose changes can be captured by dynamic models such as (9.39). Here we explore the relationship between dynamic models and causal models developed for dynamic treatments, in particular, marginal structural models (MSM) and nested structure models (NSM) [Robins, 2000; Vansteelandt and Joffe, 2014], but our scope is limited to simple models only.

Consider the simple dynamic model

$$Y_{t+1} = \beta_y Y_t + \beta_d D_t + \epsilon_t \tag{10.36}$$

We can write Y_t in terms of Y_0 and dosing history $\bar{D}_{t-1} = (D_0, ..., D_{t-1})$:

$$Y_t = \beta_y^t Y_0 + \beta_d \sum_{j=1}^{t} \beta_y^{t-j-1} D_j + \epsilon_t^* \tag{10.37}$$

where $\epsilon_t^* = \sum_{j=1}^t \beta_y^{t-j-1}\epsilon_t$. An easy way to introduce subject-level random effect is to assume that Y_0 is a random variable, e.g., $Y_0 \sim N(0, \sigma^2)$.

A DR MSM models the marginal relationship between mean response at time t and dosing history $\bar{D}_{t-1}$, e.g., the mean HbA1c at week 12 in a type II diabetes trial. It can be written as

$$E(Y_t(\bar{D}_{t-1})) = \beta_0^* + \beta_d^* Cum(\bar{D}_{t-1}) \tag{10.38}$$

where $Cum(\bar{D}_{t-1})$ is a function of $\bar{D}_{t-1}$. For the dynamic model, we have $\beta_0^* = \beta_y^t Y_0, \beta_d^* = \beta_d$ and $Cum(\bar{D}_{t-1}) = \sum_{j=1}^t \beta_y^{t-j-1} D_j$, hence the cumulative effect of dose change depends on the model dynamic. The MSM can be fitted without knowing the dynamic model behind it, since β_0^* is a single parameter and $\beta_d^* Cum(\bar{D}_{t-1})$ can be approximated by lagged D_ts or spline functions of them.

The above approach works for prefixed dosing strategy, e.g., loading dose 2mg on day 1 and daily dose 1mg afterward. However, an adjustment is required if the dose depends on confounding factors, e.g., for patients older than 65 years, the loading dose will be 1mg then 0.5mg afterward, if the response is also age dependent. A direct adjustment with confounders included in MSM can be used, alternatively, an IPW with GPS may be more appropriate if many potential confounders should be adjusted for.

NSMs are alternatives to MSM for modeling dynamic treatments. A simple NSM in our context can be written as a contrast of the mean response with dose D_t and that with a reference dose (which is set to 0 for simplicity) while fixing the future dose at 0 [Vansteelandt and Joffe, 2014]:

$$E(Y_T(D_t|\bar{D}_{t-1}, \bar{L}_t)) - E(Y_T(0|\bar{D}_{t-1}, \bar{L}_t)) = g(D_t, \bar{D}_{t-1}, \bar{L}_t) \qquad (10.39)$$

where $\bar{L}_t$ is a collection of covariates up to time t, including previous responses $Y_t, ..., Y_0$. Taking the dynamic model (10.36) as an example, we can derive the mean response at T as

$$g(D_t, \bar{D}_{t-1}, \bar{L}_t) = g(D_t, Y_t) = \beta_y^{T-t}(Y_t + \beta_d D_t) \qquad (10.40)$$

which can be considered as a decay in the rate of β_y from the state $(Y_t + \beta_d D_t)$ at t to time T, which corresponds to the response of a dynamic system to a pulse input and reflects the dynamic nature of the system. However, the simplicity of this case is due to the Markov property of model (10.36). In the NSM, β_d represents the direct DR relationship. For a marginal DR relationship, we need to use (10.37), in which we also need β_y. Although for binary or categorical treatments, the NSM can be fitted directly, in most cases, we need to fit the entire dynamic model; the process of estimating the MSM from the NSM is the g-computation, the common approach to make population level inference after fitting an NSM [Robins, 2000; Vansteelandt and Joffe, 2014].

Bibliography

Aalen, O., Borgan, O., and Gjessing, H. (2008). *Survival and event history analysis: a process point of view.* Springer Science & Business Media.

Abrahamowicz, M., Bartlett, G., Tamblyn, R., and Du Berger, R. (2006). Modeling cumulative dose and exposure duration provided insights regarding the associations between benzodiazepines and injuries. *Journal of Clinical Epidemiology*, 59(4):393–403.

Agrawal, S. and Goyal, N. (2013). Thompson sampling for contextual bandits with linear payoffs. In *International conference on machine learning*, pages 127–135. PMLR.

Akaike, H. (2003). A new look at the statistical model identification. *IEEE Transactions on Automatic Control*, 19(6):716–723.

An, H., Justin, T. L., Aubrey, G. B., Marron, J. S., and Dittmer, D. P. (2019). dr4pl: A stable convergence algorithm for the 4 parameter logistic model. *R J.*, 11(2):171.

Andersen, P. K. and Keiding, N. (2002). Multi-state models for event history analysis. *Statistical Methods in Medical Research*, 11(2):91–115.

Atkinson, A., Donev, A., and Tobias, R. (2007). *Optimum experimental designs, with SAS*, volume 34. OUP Oxford.

Austin, P. C. (2012). Generating survival times to simulate cox proportional hazards models with time-varying covariates. *Statistics in Medicine*, 31(29):3946–3958.

Avery, P., Clairon, Q., Henderson, R., James Taylor, C., and Wilson, E. (2020). Robust and adaptive anticoagulant control. *Journal of the Royal Statistical Society Series C: Applied Statistics*, 69(3):503–524.

Bates, D., Mächler, M., Bolker, B., and Walker, S. (2015). Fitting linear mixed-effects models using lme4. *Journal of Statistical Software*, 67(1): 1–48.

Bates, D. M. and Watts, D. G. (1988). *Nonlinear regression analysis and its applications*, volume 2. Wiley New York.

Bauer, R. J. (2010). Nonmem users guide: introduction to nonmem 7. *Ellicott City: ICON Development Solutions*, pages 1–61.

Beal, S. L. and Sheiner, L. B. (1982). Estimating population kinetics. *Critical Reviews in Biomedical Engineering*, 8(3):195–222.

Bender, R., Augustin, T., and Blettner, M. (2005). Generating survival times to simulate cox proportional hazards models. *Statistics in Medicine*, 24(11):1713–1723.

Bennett, J. and Wakefield, J. (2001). Errors-in-variables in joint population pharmacokinetic/pharmacodynamic modeling. *Biometrics*, 57(3):803–812.

Bernardo, J. M. and Smith, A. F. (2009). *Bayesian theory*, volume 405. John Wiley & Sons.

Bertsekas, D. (2012). *Dynamic programming and optimal control: Volume I*, volume 4. Athena scientific.

Bissiri, P. G., Holmes, C. C., and Walker, S. G. (2016). A general framework for updating belief distributions. *Journal of the Royal Statistical Society: Series B (Statistical Methodology)*, 78(5):1103–1130.

Bonate, P. L. (2006). *Pharmacokinetic-pharmacodynamic modeling and simulation.* Springer.

Bonate, P. L. (2011). Modeling tumor growth in oncology. *Pharmacokinetics in Drug Development: Advances and Applications, Volume 3*, pages 1–19.

Bonate, P. L. (2013). Effect of assay measurement error on parameter estimation in concentration–qtc interval modeling. *Pharmaceutical Statistics*, 12(3):156–164.

Breidt, F. J. and Opsomer, J. D. (2017). Model-assisted survey estimation with modern prediction techniques.

Bretz, F., Pinheiro, J. C., and Branson, M. (2005). Combining multiple comparisons and modeling techniques in dose-response studies. *Biometrics*, 61(3):738–748.

Brown, D. W., Greene, T. J., Swartz, M. D., Wilkinson, A. V., and DeSantis, S. M. (2021). Propensity score stratification methods for continuous treatments. *Statistics in Medicine*, 40(5):1189–1203.

Buckley, J. and James, I. (1979). Linear regression with censored data. *Biometrika*, 66(3):429–436.

Buja, A., Brown, L., Berk, R., George, E., Pitkin, E., Traskin, M., Zhang, K., and Zhao, L. (2019). Models as approximations i. *Statistical Science*, 34(4):523–544.

Cameron, A. C. and Trivedi, P. K. (2005). *Microeconometrics: methods and applications*. Cambridge University Press.

Cameron, A. C. and Trivedi, P. K. (2013). *Regression analysis of count data*. Number 53. Cambridge University Press.

Carroll, R. J. and Ruppert, D. (2017). *Transformation and weighting in regression*. Chapman and Hall/CRC.

Carroll, R. J., Ruppert, D., Stefanski, L. A., and Crainiceanu, C. M. (2006). *Measurement error in nonlinear models: a modern perspective*. Chapman and Hall/CRC.

Chen, G., Zeng, D., and Kosorok, M. R. (2016). Personalized dose finding using outcome weighted learning. *Journal of the American Statistical Association*, 111(516):1509–1521.

Claret, L., Girard, P., Hoff, P. M., Van Cutsem, E., Zuideveld, K. P., Jorga, K., Fagerberg, J., and Bruno, R. (2009). Model-based prediction of phase iii overall survival in colorectal cancer on the basis of phase ii tumor dynamics. *Journal of Clinical Oncology*, 27(25):4103–4108.

Clayton, D. et al. (1992). Models for the analysis of cohort and case-control studies with inaccurately measured exposures. *Statistical Models for Longitudinal Studies of Health*, pages 301–331.

Cook, R. J., Lawless, J. F., et al. (2007). *The statistical analysis of recurrent events*. Springer.

Cox, D. R. (1972). Regression models and life-tables. *Journal of the Royal Statistical Society: Series B (Methodological)*, 34(2):187–202.

Crippa, A. and Orsini, N. (2016). Dose-response meta-analysis of differences in means. *BMC Medical Research Methodology*, 16:1–10.

Crowther, M. J. and Lambert, P. C. (2013). Simulating biologically plausible complex survival data. *Statistics in Medicine*, 32(23):4118–4134.

Csajka, C. and Verotta, D. (2006). Pharmacokinetic–pharmacodynamic modelling: history and perspectives. *Journal of Pharmacokinetics and Pharmacodynamics*, 33:227–279.

Daimon, T., Hirakawa, A., and Matsui, S. (2019). *Dose-finding designs for early-phase cancer clinical trials: A brief guidebook to theory and practice*. Springer.

Davidian, M. and Giltinan, D. M. (2017). *Nonlinear models for repeated measurement data*. Routledge.

De Boor, C. (1978). *A practical guide to splines*, volume 27. Springer New York.

Diaz, F. J., Cogollo, M. R., Spina, E., Santoro, V., Rendon, D. M., and de Leon, J. (2012). Drug dosage individualization based on a random-effects linear model. *Journal of Biopharmaceutical Statistics*, 22(3):463–484.

Diaz, F. J., Rivera, T. E., Josiassen, R. C., and de Leon, J. (2007). Individualizing drug dosage by using a random intercept linear model. *Statistics in Medicine*, 26(9):2052–2073.

Diggle, P. (2002). *Analysis of longitudinal data.* Oxford University Press.

Efron, B. (1988). Logistic regression, survival analysis, and the Kaplan-Meier curve. *Journal of the American statistical Association*, 83(402):414–425.

Ette, E. I. and Williams, P. J. (2007). *Pharmacometrics: the science of quantitative pharmacology.* John Wiley & Sons.

Fitzmaurice, G., Davidian, M., Verbeke, G., and Molenberghs, G. (2008). *Longitudinal data analysis.* CRC Press.

Fleming, T. R. and Harrington, D. P. (2013). *Counting processes and survival analysis.* John Wiley & Sons.

Florian, J. A., Tornøe, C. W., Brundage, R., Parekh, A., and Garnett, C. E. (2011). Population pharmacokinetic and concentration—qtc models for moxifloxacin: pooled analysis of 20 thorough qt studies. *The Journal of Clinical Pharmacology*, 51(8):1152–1162.

Fong, C., Hazlett, C., and Imai, K. (2018). Covariate balancing propensity score for a continuous treatment: Application to the efficacy of political advertisements. *The Annals of Applied Statistics*, 12(1):156–177.

Food and Drug Administration (2023). Optimizing the dosage of human prescription drugs and biological products for the treatment of oncologic diseases guidance for industry.

Gajewski, B. J., Meinzer, C., Berry, S. M., Rockswold, G. L., Barsan, W. G., Korley, F. K., and Martin, R. (2019). Bayesian hierarchical emax model for dose-response in early phase efficacy clinical trials. *Statistics in Medicine*, 38(17):3123–3138.

Gelman, A., Carlin, J. B., Stern, H. S., and Rubin, D. B. (1995). *Bayesian data analysis.* Chapman and Hall/CRC.

Gelman, A., Jakulin, A., Pittau, M. G., and Su, Y.-S. (2008). A weakly informative default prior distribution for logistic and other regression models. *Bayesian Analysis.*

Gibaldi, M. and Perrier, B. (1982). *Pharmacokinetics.* Dekker.

Gittins, J. C. (1979). Bandit processes and dynamic allocation indices. *Journal of the Royal Statistical Society Series B: Statistical Methodology*, 41(2):148–164.

Graham, D. J., McCoy, E. J., and Stephens, D. A. (2015). Doubly robust dose-response estimation for continuous treatments via generalized propensity score augmented outcome regression. *arXiv preprint arXiv:1506.04991*.

Graham, D. J., McCoy, E. J., and Stephens, D. A. (2016). Approximate Bayesian inference for doubly robust estimation. *Bayesian Analysis*, 11: 47–69.

Henderson, R., Ansell, P., and Alshibani, D. (2010). Regret-regression for optimal dynamic treatment regimes. *Biometrics*, 66(4):1192–1201.

Hendry, D. J. (2014). Data generation for the cox proportional hazards model with time-dependent covariates: a method for medical researchers. *Statistics in Medicine*, 33(3):436–454.

Hernan, M. A. and Robins, J. M. (2023). *Causal inference: what if.* CRC Press.

Hindmarsh, A. C. (1982). RS Stepleman et al. (eds.), North-Holland, Amsterdam, 1983 (vol. 1 of imacs transactions on scientific computation), pp. 55–64.

Hirano, K. and Imbens, G. W. (2004). The propensity score with continuous treatments. *Applied Bayesian Modeling and Causal Inference from Incomplete-data Perspectives*, 226164:73–84.

Hoeting, J. A., Madigan, D., Raftery, A. E., and Volinsky, C. T. (1999). Bayesian model averaging: a tutorial (with comments by M. Clyde, David Draper and EI George, and a rejoinder by the authors. *Statistical Science*, 14(4):382–417.

Holford, N., Black, P., Couch, R., Kennedy, J., and Briant, R. (1993a). Theophylline target concentration in severe airways obstruction—10 or 20 mg/l? a randomised concentration-controlled trial. *Clinical Pharmacokinetics*, 25:495–505.

Holford, N., Hashimoto, Y., and Sheiner, L. B. (1993b). Time and theophylline concentration help explain the recovery of peak flow following acute airways obstruction: population analysis of a randomised concentration controlled trial. *Clinical Pharmacokinetics*, 25(6):506–515.

Houede, N., Thall, P. F., Nguyen, H., Paoletti, X., and Kramar, A. (2010). Utility-based optimization of combination therapy using ordinal toxicity and efficacy in phase I/II trials. *Biometrics*, 66(2):532–540.

Houk, B. E., Bello, C. L., Poland, B., Rosen, L. S., Demetri, G. D., and Motzer, R. J. (2010). Relationship between exposure to sunitinib and efficacy and tolerability endpoints in patients with cancer: results of a pharmacokinetic/pharmacodynamic meta-analysis. *Cancer Chemotherapy and Pharmacology*, 66:357–371.

Hsiao, C. (2022). *Analysis of panel data.* Cambridge University Press.

Iasonos, A., Wages, N. A., Conaway, M. R., Cheung, K., Yuan, Y., and O'Quigley, J. (2016). Dimension of model parameter space and operating characteristics in adaptive dose-finding studies. *Statistics in Medicine*, 35(21):3760–3775.

Ibrahim, J. G., Chen, M.-H., Gwon, Y., and Chen, F. (2015). The power prior: theory and applications. *Statistics in Medicine*, 34(28):3724–3749.

Imai, K. and Van Dyk, D. A. (2004). Causal inference with general treatment regimes: Generalizing the propensity score. *Journal of the American Statistical Association*, 99(467):854–866.

Imbens, G. W. (2000). The role of the propensity score in estimating dose-response functions. *Biometrika*, 87(3):706–710.

Imbens, G. W. and Newey, W. K. (2009). Identification and estimation of triangular simultaneous equations models without additivity. *Econometrica*, 77(5):1481–1512.

International Council for Harmonisation (2023). Ich m15: Guideline on general principles for model-informed drug development.

Kalbfleisch, J. D. and Prentice, R. L. (2002). *The statistical analysis of failure time data.* John Wiley & Sons.

Kawakatsu, S., Bruno, R., Kågedal, M., Li, C., Girish, S., Joshi, A., and Wu, B. (2021). Confounding factors in exposure–response analyses and mitigation strategies for monoclonal antibodies in oncology. *British Journal of Clinical Pharmacology*, 87(6):2493–2501.

Kleijn, B. J. and Van der Vaart, A. W. (2012). The Bernstein-von-mises theorem under misspecification. *Electron. J. Statist.*, 6:354–381.

Klein, J. P. (1992). Semiparametric estimation of random effects using the cox model based on the em algorithm. *Biometrics*, pages 795–806.

Ko, H. and Davidian, M. (2000). Correcting for measurement error in individual-level covariates in nonlinear mixed effects models. *Biometrics*, 56(2):368–375.

Kristensen, N. R. and Agersø, H. (2022). Dose/exposure–response modeling in dose titration trials: overcoming the titration paradox. *CPT: Pharmacometrics & Systems Pharmacology*, 11(12):1592–1603.

Lacroix, B. D., Friberg, L. E., and Karlsson, M. O. (2012). Evaluation of ippse, an alternative method for sequential population pkpd analysis. *Journal of Pharmacokinetics and Pharmacodynamics*, 39:177–193.

Lai, T. L. and Robbins, H. (1985). Asymptotically efficient adaptive allocation rules. *Advances in Applied Mathematics*, 6(1):4–22.

Langford, O., Aronson, J. K., van Valkenhoef, G., and Stevens, R. J. (2018). Methods for meta-analysis of pharmacodynamic dose–response data with application to multi-arm studies of alogliptin. *Statistical Methods in Medical Research*, 27(2):564–578.

Lawless, J. F. and Nadeau, C. (1995). Some simple robust methods for the analysis of recurrent events. *Technometrics*, 37(2):158–168.

Lee, J., Thall, P. F., Ji, Y., and Müller, P. (2015). Bayesian dose-finding in two treatment cycles based on the joint utility of efficacy and toxicity. *Journal of the American Statistical Association*, 110(510):711–722.

Li, F., Ding, P., and Mealli, F. (2023). Bayesian causal inference: a critical review. *Philosophical Transactions of the Royal Society A*, 381(2247):20220153.

Lin, D. Y. and Wei, L.-J. (1989). The robust inference for the cox proportional hazards model. *Journal of the American Statistical Association*, 84(408):1074–1078.

Lin, W. (2013). Agnostic notes on regression adjustments to experimental data: Reexamining freedman's critique. *The Annals of Applied Statistics*, 7(1).

Lindsey, J. K. (2000). *Applying generalized linear models.* Springer Science & Business Media.

Lindstrom, M. J. and Bates, D. M. (1990). Nonlinear mixed effects models for repeated measures data. *Biometrics*, pages 673–687.

Longford, N. T. (1995). Random coefficient models. In *Handbook of statistical modeling for the social and behavioral sciences*, pages 519–570. Springer.

Lyddon, S. P., Holmes, C., and Walker, S. (2019). General Bayesian updating and the loss-likelihood bootstrap. *Biometrika*, 106(2):465–478.

Margossian, C. C., Zhang, Y., and Gillespie, W. R. (2022). Flexible and efficient Bayesian pharmacometrics modeling using stan and torsten, part i. *CPT: Pharmacometrics & Systems Pharmacology*, 11(9):1151–1169.

Martin, R. and Syring, N. (2022). Direct gibbs posterior inference on risk minimizers: Construction, concentration, and calibration. In *Handbook of statistics*, volume 47, pages 1–41. Elsevier.

Martinussen, T. and Scheike, T. H. (2006). *Dynamic regression models for survival data*, volume 1. Springer.

McCandless, L. C., Douglas, I. J., Evans, S. J., and Smeeth, L. (2010). Cutting feedback in Bayesian regression adjustment for the propensity score. *The International Journal of Biostatistics*, 6(2).

McCullagh, P. (2019). *Generalized linear models*. Routledge.

McCulloch, C. E. and Searle, S. R. (2004). *Generalized, linear, and mixed models*. John Wiley & Sons.

Minematsu, T., Ohtani, H., Yamada, Y., Sawada, Y., Sato, H., and Iga, T. (2001). Quantitative relationship between myocardial concentration of tacrolimus and qt prolongation in guinea pigs: pharmacokinetic/pharmacodynamic model incorporating a site of adverse effect. *Journal of Pharmacokinetics and Pharmacodynamics*, 28:533–554.

Morita, S., Thall, P. F., and Müller, P. (2008). Determining the effective sample size of a parametric prior. *Biometrics*, 64(2):595–602.

Murphy, S. A. and Van der Vaart, A. W. (2000). On profile likelihood. *Journal of the American Statistical Association*, 95(450):449–465.

Nedelman, J. R., Rubin, D. B., and Sheiner, L. B. (2007). Diagnostics for confounding in pk/pd models for oxcarbazepine. *Statistics in Medicine*, 26(2):290–308.

Nelsen, R. B. (2006). *An introduction to copulas*. Springer.

Neuenschwander, B., Branson, M., and Gsponer, T. (2008). Critical aspects of the Bayesian approach to phase i cancer trials. *Statistics in Medicine*, 27(13):2420–2439.

Newton, M. A. and Raftery, A. E. (1994). Approximate Bayesian inference with the weighted likelihood bootstrap. *Journal of the Royal Statistical Society Series B: Statistical Methodology*, 56(1):3–26.

Niu, J., Straubinger, R. M., and Mager, D. E. (2019). Pharmacodynamic drug–drug interactions. *Clinical Pharmacology & Therapeutics*, 105(6):1395–1406.

Oksendal, B. (2013). *Stochastic differential equations: an introduction with applications*. Springer Science & Business Media.

Ollier, A., Morita, S., Ursino, M., and Zohar, S. (2020). An adaptive power prior for sequential clinical trials–application to bridging studies. *Statistical Methods in Medical Research*, 29(8):2282–2294.

O'malley, R. E. et al. (1991). *Singular perturbation methods for ordinary differential equations*, volume 89. Springer.

O'Quigley, J. (2005). Retrospective analysis of sequential dose-finding designs. *Biometrics*, 61(3):749–756.

Ouellet, D., Patel, N., Werth, J., Feltner, D., McCarthy, B., Stone, R., Mitchell, D., and Lalonde, R. (2006). Oii-a-2: The use of a clinical utility index in decision making to select an insomnia compound. *Clinical Pharmacology & Therapeutics*, 79(2):P3–P3.

Overgaard, R. V., Jonsson, N., Tornøe, C. W., and Madsen, H. (2005). Non-linear mixed-effects models with stochastic differential equations: implementation of an estimation algorithm. *Journal of Pharmacokinetics and Pharmacodynamics*, 32:85–107.

Parmigiani, G. and Inoue, L. (2009). *Decision theory: Principles and approaches.* John Wiley & Sons.

Pearl, J. (2022). Causal diagrams for empirical research (with discussions). In *Probabilistic and causal inference: The works of Judea Pearl*, pages 255–316.

Pinheiro, J. and Bates, D. (2000). *Mixed-effects models in S and S-PLUS.* Springer Science & Business Media.

Pintilie, M. (2006). *Competing risks: a practical perspective.* John Wiley & Sons.

Pompe, E. (2021). Introducing prior information in weighted likelihood bootstrap with applications to model misspecification. *arXiv preprint arXiv:2103.14445.*

Pompe, E. and Jacob, P. E. (2021). Asymptotics of cut distributions and robust modular inference using posterior bootstrap. *arXiv preprint arXiv:2110.11149.*

Prentice, R. L. (1982). Covariate measurement errors and parameter estimation in a failure time regression model. *Biometrika*, 69(2):331–342.

Putter, H., Fiocco, M., and Geskus, R. B. (2007). Tutorial in biostatistics: competing risks and multi-state models. *Statistics in Medicine*, 26(11):2389–2430.

Qian, M. (2016). Personalized dose finding using outcome weighted learning comment.

R Core Team (2013). R: A language and environment for statistical computing.

Ray, K. and van der Vaart, A. (2020). Semiparametric Bayesian causal inference. *The Annals of Statistics*, (48):2999–3020.

Reddy, V. P., Kozielska, M., Suleiman, A. A., Johnson, M., Vermeulen, A., Liu, J., de Greef, R., Groothuis, G. M., Danhof, M., and Proost, J. H. (2013). Pharmacokinetic–pharmacodynamic modeling of antipsychotic drugs in patients with schizophrenia part i: The use of panss total score and clinical utility. *Schizophrenia Research*, 146(1-3):144–152.

Rizopoulos, D. (2012). *Joint models for longitudinal and time-to-event data: With applications in R*. CRC Press.

Rizopoulos, D., Verbeke, G., and Lesaffre, E. (2009). Fully exponential Laplace approximations for the joint modelling of survival and longitudinal data. *Journal of the Royal Statistical Society Series B: Statistical Methodology*, 71(3):637–654.

Robert, C. P. et al. (2007). *The Bayesian choice: from decision-theoretic foundations to computational implementation*, volume 2. Springer.

Robins, J. M. (2000). Marginal structural models versus structural nested models as tools for causal inference. In *Statistical models in epidemiology, the environment, and clinical trials*, pages 95–133. Springer.

Rogers, J. A., Maas, H., and Pitarch, A. P. (2023). An introduction to causal inference for pharmacometricians. *CPT: Pharmacometrics & Systems Pharmacology*, 12(1):27–40.

Rosenbaum, P. R. and Rubin, D. B. (1983). The central role of the propensity score in observational studies for causal effects. *Biometrika*, 70(1):41–55.

Rubin, D. B. (1978). Bayesian inference for causal effects: The role of randomization. *The Annals of Statistics*, pages 34–58.

Rubin, D. B. (1981). The Bayesian bootstrap. *The Annals of Statistics*, pages 130–134.

Rubin, D. B. (2005). Causal inference using potential outcomes: Design, modeling, decisions. *Journal of the American Statistical Association*, 100(469):322–331.

Ruppert, D., Wand, M. P., and Carroll, R. J. (2003). *Semiparametric regression*. Number 12. Cambridge University Press.

Russo, D. (2016). Simple Bayesian algorithms for best arm identification. In *conference on learning theory*, pages 1417–1418. PMLR.

Russo, D. J., Van Roy, B., Kazerouni, A., Osband, I., Wen, Z., et al. (2018). A tutorial on Thompson sampling. *Foundations and Trends® in Machine Learning*, 11(1):1–96.

SAS Institute Inc. (2011). Base sas® 9.3 procedures guide: Statistical procedures.

Schnider, T. W., Minto, C. F., Luginbühl, M., and Egan, T. D. (2022). The drug titration paradox: more drug does not correlate with more effect in individual clinical data. *British Journal of Anaesthesia*, 129(6):861–867.

Schoenfeld, D. A. (1983). Sample-size formula for the proportional-hazards regression model. *Biometrics*, pages 499–503.

Schwarz, G. (1978). Estimating the dimension of a model. *The Annals of Statistics*, pages 461–464.

Senn, S. S. (2008). *Statistical issues in drug development*, volume 69. John Wiley & Sons.

Sheiner, L. B. (1997). Learning versus confirming in clinical drug development. *Clinical Pharmacology & Therapeutics*, 61(3):275–291.

Sheiner, L. B. (2002). Is intent-to-treat analysis always (ever) enough? *British Journal of Clinical Pharmacology*, 54(2):203.

Shen, L. Z. and O'Quigley, J. (1996). Consistency of continual reassessment method under model misspecification. *Biometrika*, 83(2):395–405.

Stan Development Team (2023). Stan modeling language users guide and reference manual, version 2.32.

Stephens, D. A., Nobre, W. S., Moodie, E. E., and Schmidt, A. M. (2023). Causal inference under mis-specification: adjustment based on the propensity score (with discussion). *Bayesian Analysis*, 18(2):639–694.

Stram, D. O. and Lee, J. W. (1994). Variance components testing in the longitudinal mixed effects model. *Biometrics*, pages 1171–1177.

Sun, J. (2006). *The statistical analysis of interval-censored failure time data*, volume 3. Springer.

Sun, L., Mi, K., Hou, Y., Hui, T., Zhang, L., Tao, Y., Liu, Z., and Huang, L. (2023). Pharmacokinetic and pharmacodynamic drug–drug interactions: research methods and applications. *Metabolites*, 13(8):897.

Sutton, R. S., Barto, A. G., et al. (1998). *Reinforcement learning: An introduction*, volume 1. MIT Press Cambridge.

Sylvestre, M.-P. and Abrahamowicz, M. (2008). Comparison of algorithms to generate event times conditional on time-dependent covariates. *Statistics in Medicine*, 27(14):2618–2634.

Sylvestre, M.-P. and Abrahamowicz, M. (2009). Flexible modeling of the cumulative effects of time-dependent exposures on the hazard. *Statistics in Medicine*, 28(27):3437–3453.

Terza, J. V., Basu, A., and Rathouz, P. J. (2008). Two-stage residual inclusion estimation: addressing endogeneity in health econometric modeling. *Journal of Health Economics*, 27(3):531–543.

Therneau, T. and Grambsch, P. (2000). *Modeling survival data: Extending the Cox model.* Springer.

Tosteson, T. D., Buonaccorsi, J. P., and Demidenko, E. (1998). Covariate measurement error and the estimation of random effect parameters in a mixed model for longitudinal data. *Statistics in Medicine*, 17(17): 1959–1971.

Van der Vaart, A. W. (2000). *Asymptotic statistics*, volume 3. Cambridge University Press.

VanderWeele, T. (2015). *Explanation in causal inference: methods for mediation and interaction.* Oxford University Press.

Vansteelandt, S. and Joffe, M. (2014). Structural nested models and g-estimation: the partially realized promise. *Statistical Science*, 29:707–731.

Vegetabile, B. G., Griffin, B. A., Coffman, D. L., Cefalu, M., Robbins, M. W., and McCaffrey, D. F. (2021). Nonparametric estimation of population average dose-response curves using entropy balancing weights for continuous exposures. *Health Services and Outcomes Research Methodology*, 21:69–110.

Verbeke, G. and Lesaffre, E. (1997). The effect of misspecifying the random-effects distribution in linear mixed models for longitudinal data. *Computational Statistics & Data Analysis*, 23(4):541–556.

Villar, S. S., Bowden, J., and Wason, J. (2015). Multi-armed bandit models for the optimal design of clinical trials: benefits and challenges. *Statistical Science: A Review Journal of the Institute of Mathematical Statistics*, 30(2):199.

Wadsworth, I., Hampson, L. V., Bornkamp, B., and Jaki, T. (2020). Exposure–response modelling approaches for determining optimal dosing rules in children. *Statistical Methods in Medical Research*, 29(9):2583–2602.

Wadsworth, I., Hampson, L. V., and Jaki, T. (2018). Extrapolation of efficacy and other data to support the development of new medicines for children: a systematic review of methods. *Statistical Methods in Medical Research*, 27(2):398–413.

Wang, J. (2001). Optimal design for linear interpolation of curves. *Statistics in Medicine*, 20(16):2467–2477.

Wang, J. (2005). A semi-parametric approach to fitting a nonlinear mixed pk/pd model with an effect compartment using sas. *Pharmaceutical Statistics*, 4(1):59–69.

Wang, J. (2012a). Dose as instrumental variable in exposure–safety analysis using count models. *Journal of Biopharmaceutical Statistics*, 22(3):565–581.

Wang, J. (2012b). Semiparametric hazard function estimation in meta-analysis for time to event data. *Research Synthesis Methods*, 3(3):240–249.

Wang, J. (2014). Determining causal exposure-response relationships with randomized concentration-controlled trials. *Journal of Biopharmaceutical Statistics*, 24(4):874–892.

Wang, J. (2021). Response-adaptive trial designs with accelerated Thompson sampling. *Pharmaceutical Statistics*, 20(3):645–656.

Wang, J., Donnan, P. T., Steinke, D., and MacDonald, T. M. (2001). The multiple propensity score for analysis of dose–response relationships in drug safety studies. *Pharmacoepidemiology and Drug Safety*, 10(2):105–111.

Wang, J. and Li, W. (2014). Test hysteresis in pharmacokinetic/pharmacodynamic relationship with mixed-effect models: an instrumental model approach. *Journal of Biopharmaceutical Statistics*, 24(2): 326–343.

Wang, J. and Quartey, G. (2012). Nonparametric estimation for cumulative duration of adverse events. *Biometrical Journal*, 54(1):61–74.

Wang, J. and Tiwari, R. (2023). Adaptive designs for best treatment identification with top-two Thompson sampling and acceleration. *Pharmaceutical Statistics*, 22(6):1089–1103.

Wang, J. and Tiwari, R. (2025a). Approximate Bayesian analysis for borrowing external controls for randomized controlled trials with dynamic borrowing and covariate balancing adjustment. *Pharmaceutical Statistics*, 24 (https://doi.org/10.1002/pst.2474).

Wang, J. and Tiwari, R. (2025b). Optimal dose selection in phase i/ii dose finding trial with contextual bandits: a case study and practical recommendations. *Journal of Biopharmaceutical Statistics*, pages 1–27.

Wang, J., Zhang, H., and Tiwari, R. (2025a). Robust Bayesian approaches for leveraging external controls in drug development: recent advances, statistical and regulatory challenges. In *Handbook of statistics*, volume 53. Elsevier.

Wang, J., Zhang, Z., and Tiwari, R. (2025b). The benefit of dose-exposure-response modeling in the estimation of dose-response relationship and dose optimization: some theoretical and simulation evidence. arXiv:2508.04186

Wang, J., Zhang, Z., and Tiwari, R. (2025c). Robust estimation of causal dose-response relationship using exposure data with dose as an instrumental variable. arXiv:2508.04215.

Wang, N. and Davidian, M. (1996). A note on covariate measurement error in nonlinear mixed effects models. *Biometrika*, 83(4):801–812.

Wang, Y., Sung, C., Dartois, C., Ramchandani, R., Booth, B., Rock, E., and Gobburu, J. (2009). Elucidation of relationship between tumor size and survival in non-small-cell lung cancer patients can aid early decision making in clinical drug development. *Clinical Pharmacology & Therapeutics*, 86(2):167–174.

Wei, L.-J., Lin, D. Y., and Weissfeld, L. (1989). Regression analysis of multivariate incomplete failure time data by modeling marginal distributions. *Journal of the American Statistical Association*, 84(408):1065–1073.

White, H. (1981). Consequences and detection of misspecified nonlinear regression models. *Journal of the American Statistical Association*, 76(374):419–433.

White, H. (1982). Maximum likelihood estimation of misspecified models. *Econometrica: Journal of the Econometric Society*, pages 1–25.

Whitehead, A. (2002). *Meta-analysis of controlled clinical trials*. John Wiley & Sons.

Whitehead, J. and Williamson, D. (1998). Bayesian decision procedures based on logistic regression models for dose-finding studies. *Journal of Biopharmaceutical Statistics*, 8(3):445–467.

Wu, L., Hu, X. J., and Wu, H. (2008). Joint inference for nonlinear mixed-effects models and time to event at the presence of missing data. *Biostatistics*, 9(2):308–320.

Wu, L., Liu, W., and Hu, X. (2010). Joint inference on HIV viral dynamics and immune suppression in presence of measurement errors. *Biometrics*, 66(2):327–335.

Yin, A., Moes, D. J. A., van Hasselt, J. G., Swen, J. J., and Guchelaar, H.-J. (2019). A review of mathematical models for tumor dynamics and treatment resistance evolution of solid tumors. *CPT: Pharmacometrics & Systems Pharmacology*, 8(10):720–737.

Zellner, A. (1986). On assessing prior distributions and Bayesian regression analysis with g-prior distributions. *Bayesian Inference and Decision Techniques*.

Zhang, L., Beal, S. L., and Sheiner, L. B. (2003). Simultaneous vs. sequential analysis for population pk/pd data i: best-case performance. *Journal of Pharmacokinetics and Pharmacodynamics*, 30:387–404.

Zhang, Z., Wang, J., and Xi, D. (2024). An instrumental variable approach to learning the causal exposure–response relationship in a randomized dose comparison trial. *Statistics in Biopharmaceutical Research*, pages 1–11.

Zhang, Z., Zhou, J., Cao, W., and Zhang, J. (2016). Causal inference with a quantitative exposure. *Statistical Methods in Medical Research*, 25(1):315–335.

Zhao, S., van Dyk, D. A., and Imai, K. (2020). Propensity score-based methods for causal inference in observational studies with non-binary treatments. *Statistical Methods in Medical Research*, 29(3):709–727.

Zhou, M. (2001). Understanding the cox regression models with time-change covariates. *The American Statistician*, 55(2):153–155.

Zhu, X. and Qu, A. (2016). Individualizing drug dosage with longitudinal data. *Statistics in Medicine*, 35(24):4474–4488.

Zohar, S., Katsahian, S., and O'Quigley, J. (2011). An approach to meta-analysis of dose-finding studies. *Statistics in Medicine*, 30(17):2109–2116.

Index

For Product Safety Concerns and Information please contact our EU representative GPSR@taylorandfrancis.com
Taylor & Francis Verlag GmbH, Kaufingerstraße 24, 80331 München, Germany

www.ingramcontent.com/pod-product-compliance
Ingram Content Group UK Ltd.
Pitfield, Milton Keynes, MK11 3LW, UK
UKHW020354280226
468510UK00008B/115

* 9 7 8 1 0 3 2 5 9 6 2 5 9 *